Angela Brown
12-7-89

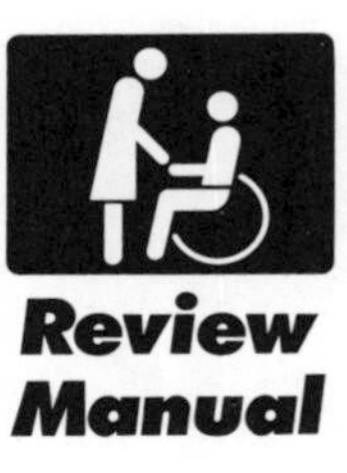

American Red Cross Nurse Assistant Training Preparation for Competency Evaluation

Developed by the American Red Cross
with financial support from Beverly Enterprises, Inc.

Acknowledgements

The American Red Cross Preparation for Competency Evaluation is based on the Nurse Assistant Training course developed at American Red Cross national headquarters during 1988-89. Financial support for course development and the field test of course materials and training was provided by Beverly Enterprises, Inc.

Chapters participating in the development of the Preparation for Competency Evaluation include:

Massachusetts Bay Chapter, Boston, MA
Hawkeye Chapter, Waterloo, IA

The American Red Cross Nurse Assistant Training course was developed under the guidelines established by the 1987 Omnibus Budget Reconciliation Act of the 100th Congress of the United States, Subtitle C, Nursing Home Reform, and on information provided by the Health Care Financing Administration of the U.S. Department of Health and Human Services, the National Citizens' Coalition for Nursing Home Reform, and, where applicable, state regulations regarding nurse assistant training.

Chapters supporting the Nurse Assistant Training project throughout development of the training course and participating in the 1989 field test include:

Dallas County Chapter, Dallas, TX
Greater Kansas City Chapter, Kansas City, MO
Massachusetts Bay Chapter, Boston, MA
Metropolitan Atlanta Chapter, Atlanta, GA
Pasadena Chapter, Pasadena, CA
Pittsburgh-Allegheny Chapter, Pittsburgh, PA
Seattle-King County Chapter, Seattle, WA

Advisory Committee Members

Bobbie Primus, Ed.D., M.P.H., R.N. (Chair)
Coordinator of Special Projects
University of Central Florida

Carolyn Branson, R.N.
Health Services Specialist
American Red Cross
Eastern Operations Headquarters

Julieann Crevatin, M.P.A.
Administrator of Nursing Services
American Red Cross
Seattle-King County Chapter

David M. Eisenberg, Ph.D.
Director, Long Term Care
Philadelphia Corporation for Aging

Pat Fenton, R.N.
Director of Nursing
American Red Cross
Pittsburgh-Allegheny Chapter

Faye Flowers, R.N.
American Red Cross
Southeastern Michigan Chapter

Sue Freeman, R.N.
American Red Cross
Greater Kansas City Chapter

Katherine Graves, R.N.
Health Services Specialist
American Red Cross
Midwestern Operations Headquarters

Kathy Holmes, R.N.
Nursing Coordinator
American Red Cross
Greater Kansas City Chapter

Theresa Lang, R.N.
Board Member
American Red Cross
Greater Minneapolis Area Chapter

Sharon Oswald, R.N.
Director, Quality Assurance
Beverly Enterprises

Dean Owens, R.N.
American Red Cross
Mobile County Chapter

Richard Perry
International Vice President/Director,
Professional Division
United Food & Commercial Workers
International Union
AFL-CIO/CLC

Virginia Powell
Nurse Assistant
Beverly Enterprises

Ann Robbins, R.N.
Nursing Director
American Red Cross
Dallas County Chapter

David Schulke
Staff
Senate Special Committee on Aging

Beth Schulman
International Vice President/Director,
Professional Division
United Food & Commercial Workers
International Union
AFL-CIO/CLC

Amanda Sefton, R.N.
American Red Cross
Indianapolis Area Chapter

Marilyn Self, R.N.
Director of Nursing Services
American Red Cross
Metropolitan Atlanta Chapter

Gerald M. Shea
Director, Health Care Division
Service Employees International
AFL-CIO/CLC

Sally Sohner, R.N.
American Red Cross
Los Angeles Chapter

Ruth Stryker-Gordon, R.N., M.A.
Professor Emeritus
University of Minnesota

Rosemary Sullivan, R.N.
Coordinator of Occupational Training
American Red Cross of Massachusetts Bay

Henrietta Villaescusa, R.N.
President
National Association of Hispanic Nurses

Audrey S. Weiner, M.P.H.
Assistant Administrator
Hebrew Home for the Aged at Riverdale, N.Y.

Ruth A. Wong, R.N., M.P.H.
Director, Nursing and Health Services
American Red Cross
Pasadena Chapter

Panel of Expert Reviewers

Susan Alford
Director of Quality Assurance
Beverly Enterprises—Central Division

Frank Baskin, M.S.W.
Independent Consultant
Lowell, Massachusetts

Eileen Blaustein, M.S.N., R.N.
Director of Nursing
Carroll Manor Nursing Home
Hyattsville, Maryland

Martha Bohn, M.S.W., A.C.S.W.
Beverly Enterprises

Sarah Burger, M.S.N.
National Coalition for Nursing Home Reform

Rose Cebulka, R.N.
American Red Cross
Pittsburgh-Allegheny Chapter

Margaret Cohn, B.S.N., M.P.H., Ph.D.
Nursing Home Intervention Project
College of Health and Human Development
Pennsylvania State University

Martha D'Erasmo, R.N., M.P.H.
Manager, Health Care Services
Coopers and Lybrand

Shirley Ellis
Director of Ombudsman Program
Board of Aging, Long Term Care
Wisconsin Ombudsman

Lois Evans, D.N.Sc.
University of Pennsylvania
School of Nursing

Thomas Fairchild, Ph.D.
Center for Studies in Aging
North Texas State University

Donald Gelfand, Ph.D.
Associate Professor
University of Maryland
School of Social Work

Ann Gotshall, R.N., M.S.
Volunteer
American Red Cross
Seattle-King County Chapter

Ann Grant, R.N., C.N.P.
Nurse Practitioner
Dallas, Texas

Anita Heygster
Health Care Financing Administration
U.S. Department of Health and Human Services

Elma Holder
Executive Director
National Citizen Coalition for Nursing Home Reform

Bette Hortsman, R.P.T.
Allied Health Limited
Morton Grove, Illinois

Thomas E. Hoyer, Jr.
Health Care Financing Administration
U.S. Department of Health and Human Services

Judy Johnson
Director of Quality Assurance
Beverly Enterprises—Central Division

Joan M. Kiernat, M.S., O.T.R.
Institute of Gerontology
Phoenix, Arizona

Mary T. Knapp, M.S.N., C.R.N.P.
Member-at-large, Executive Committee Council on Gerontological Nursing
John Whitman and Associates

Sheryl Leudeke, M.A., C.T.R.S.
Director of Social Services
Beverly Enterprises-Eastern Division

Lois Liggett, R.P.T
Wilson Health Care Center
Gaithersburg, Maryland

Nancy Mace, R.N.
Member, National Board of Directors
ADRDA

Pam Maraldo, Ph.D., R.N., F.A.A.N.
Executive Director
National League for Nursing

John McConnell, M.S.N., R.N.
Director of Nursing
Stoddard Baptist Nursing Home
Washington, D.C.

Mary Ousley, R.N.
Kenwood House
Richmond, Kentucky

Leonard Peterson, C.S.P.
Assistant Director, Risk Management
Beverly Enterprises

Nina Phillips, R.N., O.N.C.
Director of Staff Development
Wisconsin Avenue Nursing Home
Beverly Enterprises

Michael Salamon, Ph.D.
Psychologist
Woodmere, New York

Lucy Theilheimer
Senior Program Specialist
Health Advocacy Services Section
American Association of Retired Persons

Justine Thompson, R.N.
Director of Nursing
Golden Acres
Dallas, Texas

Richard Thorp, M.D.
Executive Vice President
American College of Health Care Administrators

Toby A. Turner, M.N., R.N., C.
Senior Staff Specialist
Center for Nursing Practice
American Nurses' Association

Susan Noble Walker, Ed.D., R.N.
Chairperson, Executive Committee Council on
Gerontological Nursing
Northern Illinois University School of Nursing

Mary Walsh, R.N., F.A.A.N., D.S.
Retired Associate Professor of Nursing
Catholic University

Jean Wesley, M.N., R.N.
Director, Geriatric Education and Consulting
Hutchinson, Kansas

Carter Williams, M.S.W.
Private Practice

Bruce K. Wilson, R.N., Ph.D.
Pan-American University

Nurse Assistant Training Program Development Team

Bruce Spitz
Project Director

Carol Hunter-Geboy, Ph.D.
Manager, Development Team

Margaret Casey, R.N.
Associate Project Director

Debbi Accame
Photographer

Judy Armbrister
Editor

Cindy Apodaca
Project Assistant

Jean Canale, M.P.H.
Project Associate

David Fado
Desk Top Publisher

Earl Harbert
Operations Specialist

Barbara Hunt
Photographer

Rima Kamal
Production Manager

Ann Martin, R.N.
Writer/Consultant

Kathleen Masucci, R.N.
Writer/Consultant

Jack Pardue
Illustrator

Lynda Ramsey
Project Secretary

Sina Samad
Desk Top Publisher

Jeanne Shields, R.N.
Technical Consultant

Rosemary Sullivan, R.N.
Writer/Consultant

Ellen Tishman, R.N.
Project Assistant

Karen Tracy
Project Assistant

Angie Turner-Elliot, R.N.
Writer/Consultant

Elsa Williams
Editor

Instructions for Facilitators

Below are guidelines for staff developers or registered nurses preparing to facilitate the review process detailed in the American Red Cross Preparation for Competency Evaluation.

The Preparation for Competency Evaluation was designed as a self-paced instructional workbook so experienced nurse assistants can review for state competency evaluation with minimal assistance. Beginning nurse assistants should be referred to their local American Red Cross chapter/station for the Nurse Assistant Training course.

Review Options

This workbook can be used in either of two ways:

- Self-directed review, or
- Facilitated review

Self-directed review

This option allows nurse assistants to review information and skills on their own. However, it does not provide the encouragement or feedback necessary if a learner has not had success in an academic setting, nor does it provide the verbal instruction necessary for the low-literacy learner.

Facilitated review

This option allows nurse assistants to review information and skills under the supervision and reinforcement of a facilitator (either American Red Cross personnel or long-term care facility staff) when one is available.

Facilitated review can be provided using a classroom model or consultation model:

- *Classroom Model*—The facilitator monitors the review process in a formal classroom setting. Classroom hours are identified and a schedule is established for nurse assistants to complete the workbook. The facilitator allows learners to work individually at their own pace, but is available on site to answer questions as they arise and to assist with review of skills.

- *Consultation Model*—The facilitator is only available to meet with learners at designated locations and during specified hours. Nurse assistants must review material independently; they may meet with the facilitator as needed.

Your Role as a Facilitator

As a facilitator, it is your responsibility to ensure that nurse assistants understand how to use the Preparation for Competency Evaluation workbook correctly.

The workbook consists of two parts, *Review Information* and *Core Skills*. You should give this workbook to nurse assistants individually if the consultation model is being used or during the first classroom session if the classroom model is being used. Clear instructions should also be given regarding the format and usage of the two parts of the workbook.

Part 1

Using clear, simple language you should outline the following steps for using Part 1, *Review Information*:

- Carefully read all information in a section before you try to answer the review questions.

- Try to answer each review question on your own. Re-read the written information in the text to find the answers if you need to. Do not look at the answers to any questions until you have completed all three questions in one section.

- Check your answers by turning the workbook upside down and reading the correct answers.

- If you have answered a question incorrectly or if you could not answer a question, you should re-read the material and try to answer that question again before going on to the next section.

- Circle any question that you missed more than once or could not find the answer to.

- Ask your facilitator about questions that are still unclear after you review all of the materials.

Remind nurse assistants to review *Hints to Improve Your Test-Taking Ability* and the *Practice Test* in Unit 5. Highlight important concepts and review the sample test questions and answers.

Part 2

There are 23 core skills in this workbook that must be mastered before a nurse assistant attempts to take a state competency evaluation. These skills are fundamental and nurse assistants should already be familiar with them. However, nurse assistants should be encouraged to review core skills and to practice any skill which has not been previously mastered.

Give clear, simple instructions for using Part 2, *Core Skills*.

- Review each skill sheet, including precautions and procedures, in the correct sequence as illustrated.

- Practice skills that you need to review. Work at your own pace using the skill sheets.

- Ask your facilitator to demonstrate a skill if you are unsure how to do it.

Facilitating Skills Practice

Facilitation of skills practice is an important component of this review process and another of your responsibilities as a facilitator. You should be prepared to demonstrate all of the core skills found in Preparation for Competency Evaluation. As you facilitate skills practice, you will need to:

- Answer questions related to skills execution.
- Help nurse assistants practice correctly by providing explanations, prompting and encouragement.
- Observe nurse assistants practicing skills for competency. Skill sheets may be checked off as they master steps in a skill.
- Demonstrate core skills if nurse assistants have questions about precautions or procedures.

Emphasis during review and practice of core skills should be on the following:

- *Sequence*—The specific components that are part of a skill must be completed in the correct sequence.
- *Accuracy*—Nurse assistants must pay attention to important details, such as universal precautions, proper body mechanics, and respecting residents' rights.
- *Attitude*—Nurse assistants must always respect the resident's feelings, needs, and rights at all times, remembering the principles of privacy, dignity, communication, and independence.
- *Consistency*—Skills must always be performed the same way in accordance with established nursing procedures.
- *Safety*—Nurse assistants must ensure their own safety and the safety of the resident.
- *Economy of time and effort*—Skills must be organized and performed efficiently.

As a facilitator you should provide nurse assistants with continual feedback on their progress during all skills practice sessions.

Equipment You Will Need

The ideal setting for skills practice is a laboratory with the necessary equipment. The list below includes all equipment, arranged by skill, you will need to help nurse assistants practice the skills in this workbook.

Skill 1: Handwashing

Sink with running water
Liquid soap or soap dispenser
Paper towels
Wastebasket

Skills 2 and 3: Putting on and Taking Off Disposable Gloves, Mask, and Gown

Isolation gown
Disposable mask
Disposable gloves
Linen or trash hamper

Skill 4: Making an Occupied Bed

Complete resident unit
Laundry hamper
Top and bottom sheet
Blanket
Bedspread
Pillow and pillowcase

Skill 5: Positioning

Bed
Pillow
Sheets, including a draw sheet
Blanket or towel
Foot support
Hand roll

Skill 6: Moving the Resident From Bed to Chair

Bed
Safety belt
Wheelchair
Chair
Blanket

Skill 7: Passive Range of Motion

None

Skill 8: Complete Bed Bath

Basin
Bath blanket
Bed
Bedspread
Blanket
Bedpan
Chair
Disposable bed protector
Disposable gloves
Lotion
Soap
Soap dish
Towels
Washcloths
Plastic trash bag

Skill 9: Brushing and Flossing Teeth

Toothbrush
Toothpaste
Mouthwash
Glass
Emesis basin
Dental floss
Disposable gloves
Plastic trash bag

Skill 10: Denture Care

Towels
Disposable gloves (optional)
Plastic trash bag
Tissues

(continued on next page)

Washcloths
Toothettes or lemon glycerine swabs
Emesis basin
Glass
Denture cup
Toothbrush
Toothpaste
Mouthwash

Skill 11: Mouth Care for the Unconscious Resident

Towels
Toothettes or lemon glycerine swabs
Disposable gloves
Plastic trash bag
Emesis basin
Mouthwash
Glass

Skill 12: Brushing and Combing Hair

Brush
Comb
Hand mirror (optional)

Skill 13: Shaving

After-shave lotion
Basin
Disposable razor
Towel
Washcloth
Disposable gloves
Plastic trash bag
Shaving cream
Soap
Hand mirror
Styptic pencil (optional)

Skill 14: Cleaning and Trimming Fingernails

Towel
Washcloth
Nail clippers
Emery board or file
Orange stick
Basin
Soap
Lotion

Skill 15: Giving Footcare and Cleaning Toenails

Towel
Washcloth
Orange stick
Basin
Soap
Lotion

Skills 16 and 17: Dressing/ Undressing

Clothing

Skill 18: Assisting With a Bedpan or Urinal

Bedpan
Bedpan cover
Disposable gloves
Plastic trash bag
Urinal
Toilet tissue
Basin
Washcloth
Soap
Powder

Skill 19: Taking an Oral Temperature With a Glass Thermometer

Cotton balls or tissues
Thermometer sheath (optional)
Watch with second hand
Pencil and paper
Oral thermometer
Thermometer holder

Skill 20: Taking a Rectal Temperature With a Glass Thermometer

Lubricating jelly
Watch with second hand
Thermometer sheath (optional)
Disposable gloves (optional)
Plastic trash bag
Cotton balls or tissues
Pencil and paper
Rectal thermometer
Thermometer holder

Skill 21: Counting a Pulse

Watch with second hand
Pencil and paper

Skill 22: Counting Respiration

Watch with second hand
Pencil and paper

Skill 23: Taking Blood Pressure

Sphygmomanometer and correct size cuff
Alcohol wipes
Pencil and paper
Stethoscope

Table of Contents

Acknowledgements iii

Instructions for Facilitators xi

Table of Contents xix

Introduction 1

PART 1: REVIEW INFORMATION 5

Unit 1: Working in Long-Term Care 7

Module 1: Introduction to Long-Term Care 9

Module 2: Role of the Nurse Assistant 13

Unit 2: Foundation for Caring 17

Module 1: Understanding Residents in Long-Term Care 19

Module 2: The Human Body and the Process of Aging 27

Module 3: Understanding the Rights of Residents in Long-Term Care 47

Module 4: Communication 51

Module 5: Principles of Care 61

Unit 3: Core Skills for Caring 63

Module 1: Infection Control 67

Module 2: Taking Care of a Resident's Environment 75

Module 3: Maintaining Mobility 85

Module 4: Personal Care 91

Module 5: Nutrition 105

Module 6: Elimination 115

Module 7: Vital Signs 127

Unit 4: Special Skills for Caring 137

Module 1: Modifying Care 139

Module 2: Death and Dying 157

Module 3: Restorative Nursing 161

Unit 5: Getting Ready for Your Competency Evaluation 165

Hints to Improve Your Test-Taking Ability 167

Practice Test 171

PART 2: CORE SKILLS 177

Skill 1: Hand Washing 179

Skill 2: Putting On a Gown, Mask, and Disposable Gloves 183

Skill 3: Taking Off Soiled Disposable Gloves, Mask, and Gown 185

Skill 4: Making an Occupied Bed 189

Skill 5: Positioning 201

Skill 6: Moving the Resident From Bed to Chair 219

Skill 7: Performing Passive Range of Motion 233

Skill 8: Giving a Complete Bed Bath 247

Skill 9: Brushing and Flossing 265

Skill 10: Denture Care 269

Skill 11: Mouth Care for the Unconscious Resident 273

Skill 12: Brushing and Combing Hair 277

Skill 13: Shaving 279

Skill 14: Cleaning and Trimming Fingernails 283

Skill 15: Giving Foot Care and Cleaning Toenails 287

Skill 16: Dressing the Resident 291

Skill 17: Undressing the Resident 295

Skill 18: Assisting With a Bedpan or Urinal 297

Skill 19: Taking an Oral Temperature With a Glass Thermometer 303

Skill 20: Taking a Rectal Temperature With a Glass Thermometer 307

Skill 21: Counting a Radial Pulse 313

Skill 22: Counting Respiration 315

Skill 23: Taking Blood Pressure 317

Glossaries 321

Common Abbreviations 323

General Glossary 327

Introduction

Each morning thousands of people wake up in long-term care facilities. Many will stay only long enough for recovery and/or rehabilitation; others will live out their lives there. As a nurse assistant, you give residents most of their care. A resident's quality of life is based on the quality of care you give.

Since you have been working in long-term care, you know that to give quality care you need both information and skills. All states have started a testing procedure to measure the knowledge and skills of nurse assistants working in long-term care facilities. States are calling their test a competency evaluation for nurse assistants; the competency evaluation will test how well you know both information and skills.

The American Red Cross Preparation for Competency Evaluation is designed to help you review information and skills for your state's competency evaluation. This workbook has two parts. Part 1 reviews the information, and Part 2 reviews core skills you need to know for your competency evaluation. The workbook is self-paced. That means you can go through this material as fast or as slow as you want. Take as much time as you need.

How to Review the Text Material

Follow these steps when you review the text material in Part 1:

- Carefully read all information in a section before you try to answer the review questions.

- Try to answer each review question on your own. Re-read the information in the text to find the information you need to answer a question. Do not look at the answers to any questions until you have completed all three questions in one section.

- Check your answers by turning the workbook upside down and reading the correct answers.
- If you have answered a question incorrectly or if you could not answer a question, you should re-read the material and try to answer that question again before going on to the next section.
- Circle any question that you missed a second time or could not find the answer to.
- Ask your facilitator or your supervisor about questions that are still unclear after you review all of the materials.

Remember to take all the time that you need. Only you can decide when you know this material well enough to take your state's competency evaluation.

How to Use the Skill Material

Part 2 of the Preparation for Competency Evaluation includes 23 core skills that you need to know. You will be asked to demonstrate several of these skills when you take your state competency evaluation. These skills are things you do every day, and you probably already know how to do them. But it is still important that you review these core skills and practice any skill you do not know well.

Each skill is reviewed on one skill sheet. A skill sheet lists the precautions and procedures for a core skill. Precautions are things you need to remember to do or not to do. The procedure for a skill is all of the steps you must take, in the right order. To help you remember how you do a skill, each skill sheet is illustrated.

Review or practice skills at your own pace using these skill sheets. You may want to review a skill when it is mentioned in the text material (Part 1) or you may want to finish the text material before reviewing any of the skills.

When you review and practice the core skills, remember these important points:

- Order—The specific steps of a skill must be done in the correct order.
- Accuracy—Pay attention to important details, such as universal precautions and proper body mechanics.
- Attitude—Respect the resident's feelings, needs, and rights at all times, remembering the principles of privacy, dignity, communication, and independence.
- Consistency—Skills must always be performed the same way in accordance with established nursing procedures.
- Safety—You must ensure your own safety and the safety of the resident.
- Economy of time and effort—Skills must be organized and performed efficiently.

Test-Taking Review

Included in the Preparation for Competency Evaluation (Unit 5) is both Test-Taking Tips and a sample written evaluation of 25 multiple choice questions. Review this unit carefully before you take your state competency evaluation.

Take your time with this workbook. It is yours to keep and use. You can write in it or make notes if it will help you review and prepare. Reviewing for the state competency evaluation is a hard job but once you pass the test you will feel great! Good luck and thank you for all your work as a nurse assistant.

PART 1: REVIEW INFORMATION

Unit 1: Working in Long-Term Care

In this unit, you will review some general information about working in long-term care. First, you will go over what is meant by a long-term care facility and its purpose. Then, your role as a nurse assistant in a long-term care facility will be discussed as well as some of the personal qualities you need to be a good nurse assistant.

Unit 1, Working in Long-Term Care

Module 1: Introduction to Long-Term Care

Do you know what most people call a nursing home today?

A "long-term care facility" is another name for a nursing home. It means basically the same thing, but more health care workers say long-term care facility today. A long-term care facility is for people who need care for longer than a hospital stay.

The purpose of a long-term care facility is to help residents stay as independent—or able to take care of themselves—as possible by meeting their physical and psychosocial needs. Physical needs have to do with the residents' bodies. Psychosocial needs have to do with their hearts, minds, and souls.

Review Questions

1. A long-term care facility is another name for a

   Nursing home.

2. Psychosocial needs have to do with hearts,

   Hearts minds, and souls.

3. Physical needs have to do with the residents'

   Bodies.

Answers: 1. nursing, 2. minds, 3. bodies

Do you know who is "captain" of the health care team?

Many employees with different skills are needed to make sure that residents' needs are met. This group of employees who work together in long-term care is called the health care team. As a nurse assistant, you are one of the most important members of the health care team. Members of the health care team assist the resident in different ways, but the resident is the one in charge.

Some members of the health care team are:

1. Resident—The "captain" of the team. The resident is in charge of and decides about the kind of care they need, with help from other team members. If the resident cannot decide, the resident's family can.

2. Registered nurse (RN)—Supervises other members of the nursing care team as they plan and provide resident care and activities.

3. Licensed practical nurse (LPN) or licensed vocational nurse (LVN)—Helps plan and supervise some types of care under direction of a registered nurse.

4. Nurse assistant (NA)—Helps plan care and assists the resident with care under supervision of a licensed nurse.

5. Physician—Writes medical orders and prescriptions for medication when needed.

6. Administrator—Directs the overall operation of the entire facility.

7. Dietitian—Supervises the food services.

8. Social worker—Helps admit and discharge residents. Works with residents and their families if they need someone to talk to about their problems.

Review Questions

1. Many employees with different ____________ are needed to make sure residents' needs are met.

2. The ____________ is the captain of the team.

3. A nurse assistant helps plan care and assists the resident with care under the supervision of a ____________ nurse.

Answers: 1. skills, **2.** resident, **3.** licensed

Do you know the many ways a family can help in the care of a resident?

The family is another important member of the health care team, and like residents, families are very different. Some families play a big role in the care of the resident. Other families do not want to play a big role. But all families should be invited and encouraged to help with decision making and care.

Families can help in many ways:

- Give you information about the resident

  Likes and dislikes (activities, foods, colors)
  Cultural and religious practices
  Habits (sleeping, bathing, elimination)
  Feelings and fears
  Past history (career, children, hobbies)

- Play a role in the resident's care

  Feeding
  Ambulation (moving from place to place)
  Hair care and nail care
  Bathing and back rub

- Give the resident emotional support

  Visiting or phoning
  Sending cards, letters, and photos
  Listening to and talking with the resident
  Showing affection (hugging and touching)
  Helping the resident take part in social activities

- Play a role in decision making

  Care planning and levels of care
  Medication
  Restrictions on movement (restraining)
  Discharge planning
  Needed support services

- Give financial support

Review Questions

1. The ____________ is another important member of the health care team.
2. The family can help by giving information, assisting in care, providing ____________ support, helping in decision making, and giving financial support.
3. All families should be invited and encouraged to help with ____________ ____________ and care.

Answers: 1. family, 2. emotional, 3. decision making

Unit 1, Working in Long-Term Care

Module 2: Role of a Nurse Assistant

Do you know who spends more time with residents than anyone else?

Nurse assistants probably spend more time with residents than anyone else in a long-term care facility. You can influence the "quality of life" of a resident more than any other staff member; it is your job to see that each resident has a good "quality of life."

As a nurse assistant, you are an important member of the health care team. A nurse assistant helps residents in long-term care do anything they cannot do by themselves.

As a nurse assistant, some of your duties are to:

- Assist residents with personal care.
- Take and record vital signs.
- Record food intake and output.
- Assist residents with eating, elimination, exercise, walking, and movement.
- Respect residents' rights at all times.
- Notice and report any changes in a resident's condition.
- Communicate positively with residents.

Review Questions

1. The ____________ ____________ probably spends more time with residents than anyone else in a long-term care facility.

2. A nurse assistant can influence the ____________ ____________ ____________ of a resident.

3. A nurse assistant takes and records ____________ signs.

Answers: 1. nurse assistant, **2.** quality of life, **3.** vital

Do you know some of the personal qualities you must have to be a good nurse assistant?

To be a good nurse assistant, certain personal qualities are necessary. Some of the qualities you need to be a good nurse assistant are listed below. As you read this list, can you think of some other qualities?

- Health/hygiene

  Eat a well-balanced diet.
  Get plenty of rest.
  Practice good body mechanics.
  Never take alcoholic beverages before or during work and never take illegal drugs.
  Prevent spread of disease by washing your hands the right way.

Show that you care about your appearance by bathing daily, shampooing often, using deodorant, and wearing clean clothing.
Wear comfortable shoes that provide support.

- Social

Be able to get along with other people.
Be a good listener.
Be able to talk with residents, families, and other staff members.
Be able to tell someone when you have a problem or need something.

- Character

Keep private information to yourself.
Be truthful.
Be polite to residents, families, and staff.
Treat others with respect.
Be dependable.
Be reliable.
Never accept money from residents or families.
Be energetic.

Review Questions

1. To be a good nurse assistant, certain personal ______________ are necessary.

2. To be a good nurse assistant, you must have certain personal qualities, such as preventing spread of disease by ______________ ______________ ______________ the right way.

3. To be a good nurse assistant, one characteristic you must have is to be polite to ______________, ______________, and ______________.

Answers: 1. qualities, **2.** washing your hands, **3.** residents, families, staff

Unit 2: Foundation for Caring

Now that you have reviewed some general information on long-term care, this unit focuses on building a foundation for caring. To build this foundation for caring, first you need to understand the residents: who are they, what are their needs, how does the aging process affect their bodies, and what are their rights. Second, you will review the importance of good communication both to you and the resident. Third, you will review the Principles of Care. These six principles, or responsibilities, are very important and should be a routine part of everything you do for the residents.

Unit 2, Foundation for Caring

Module 1: Understanding Residents in Long-Term Care

In this module, you will review some very important concepts about working in a long-term care facility. First, who are the residents? You know them best, but do you know why most of them are in a long-term care facility? Then, you will look at the basic human needs we all have and how you can help residents satisfy those needs. Finally, you will examine your own feelings about aging. As a nurse assistant in a long-term care facility, it's very important for you to understand the aging process and know the "truth" about getting older.

Did you know that there are more female than male residents in long-term care facilities?

Who are the residents in long-term care? Think about residents you have worked with. Here is some basic information about residents in long-term care:

- The average resident is 85 years old.
- Most of the residents are women.
- All the residents have suffered some kind of loss.
- All the residents have special needs that can best be met in the nursing home.
- Most elderly residents have a disability caused by one of five chronic diseases: heart disease, arthritis, cancer, stroke, or Alzheimer's disease.
- Residents who are not elderly most likely have a disability caused by a spinal cord injury.

Review Questions

1. The average resident is __85__ years old.

2. __Most__ of the residents are women.

3. Most elderly residents have a disability caused by one of five chronic __diseases__.

Answers: 1. 85, 2. most, 3. diseases

Understanding Basic Human Needs

Did you know that the residents have the same needs that you do?

We all need five basic things to live and be happy:

- Independence
- Respect
- Love
- Safety
- Comfort

Residents in nursing homes have the same needs you do, but it may be harder for them to make sure those needs are met. Because you spend more time than anyone else with a resident and know the resident best, you may be the one person who can tell when a resident has an unmet need and offer help.

It is your responsibility to help residents try to meet their social and emotional needs as well as physical needs. Residents whose needs are being met will be happier, live longer, and have a better "quality of life" than residents whose needs are not being met. You can help residents have "quality" in their life. See the chart below for some tips. As you think of other ways you can help residents, make notes in the margins.

Need	**What You Can Do**
Independence	Help residents take part in their care Teach residents to do things for themselves Use prosthetic or assistive devices to help residents be more independent
Respect	Show respect at all times Keep residents informed Recognize improvements the resident has made Listen to what residents have to say Help residents get together with other residents they like
Love	Give smiles and hugs to residents Be friendly to residents Be kind and considerate Arrange for the resident to have privacy with a partner Use a gentle touch to communicate that you care

Need	What You Can Do
Safety	Have side rails up when needed
	Lock wheelchair wheels
	Answer call lights as quickly as possible
	Check on residents often to see if they need anything
	Check food temperature
Comfort	Make sure residents can sleep comfortably
	Make sure resident is warm
	Make sure resident is positioned properly
	Make sure resident is dressed warmly
	Assist residents to exercise

Review Questions

1. The five basic things we need to live and be happy are independence, respect, ______, safety, and comfort.
2. ______ in nursing homes have the same needs you do.
3. Residents whose needs are being met will be ______, live longer, and experience a better quality of life.

Answers: 1. love, **2.** Residents, **3.** happier

Examining Your Feelings About Aging

How do you feel about growing older?

The residents in your care may have fears about growing older and being in a nursing home. If the residents have fears or bad feelings about aging, they may have bad feelings about themselves.

One of the most important things you can do is to keep in mind the good things about being older and help residents share their good experiences. What are some good things about being an older adult? Work is done; there is time now to do things they have wanted to do;

they have wisdom to share with younger people; they can watch children achieve, grandchildren grow; they can pass on their memories of things that have happened.

Aging is not a disease or a punishment. It is just another stage of life. If we are lucky enough to live that long, each of us will be an older person one day. We can learn from older adults how to grow old successfully.

Now for some facts about aging. As you review these facts, think about the residents you are caring for and how you can help them.

- Right now, about 1 out of 10 people in the United States is over 65 and the number is growing.

- Only 1 out of every 20 people over age 65 lives in a nursing home or other long-term care facility. Most of these people are 75 years old or older.

- Physical strength lessens with age. Studies have shown that many older people have less muscle strength than younger people. However, regular exercise can stop or help slow down the loss of strength as we age.

- The ability to see generally gets poorer as we get older. But some people have good vision well into their 80s. Older people are more likely to be farsighted, have cataracts, have trouble telling the difference between certain colors (especially blues), and have trouble adjusting to a fast change in the amount of light when, for example, they are going into a dim building from a sunny, outdoor area.

- Only about one-third of people age 65 and older have some hearing loss, but the number grows as people reach their 70s and 80s. Older people who have trouble hearing may not respond when spoken to or may say the wrong thing because they did not hear correctly. Others could think older people are confused or antisocial if they do not know about the hearing problem.

- Loss of teeth is not a normal part of getting older; however, a large number of people 65 years and older have lost many or all of their teeth.

- People usually get shorter as they get older, starting around age 55. The discs that are between each vertebra in our spine (backbone) shrink, and the spine, which keeps us standing up straight, gets shorter.

- Sexual interest and sexual desire are present in older people. In one large study of healthy men between the ages of 60 and 94, over half of the men reported that they were still sexually active (having intercourse). Many older people do not show an interest in sex because they are widowed or are not romantically involved with anyone. This is especially true in long-term care facilities where the residents are mostly women.

- Most old people are healthy enough to keep up their normal activities. When questioned, only about one out of five old people says that health is a big problem.

When caring for residents, you may be aware of any negative attitudes or feelings you have about older people and residents in nursing homes. To feel more comfortable, spend time talking with older people so you can get to know them. Remember that residents are not all alike. Respect the feelings and attitudes of residents even if you do not feel the same way. Let the residents know in every way that you care—show them and tell them.

Remember how much residents give up when they come to live in the nursing home. Talking about their former lives or careers will make them feel better about themselves. Try to help a new resident make friends in the facility.

Review Questions

1. Physical ____________ decreases with age.
2. Sexual ____________ and sexual ____________ are present in older people.
3. When caring for residents, you should be aware of any negative ____________ feelings you may have about older people and residents in nursing homes.

Answers: **1.** strength, **2.** interest, desire, **3.** attitudes

Unit 2, Foundation for Caring

Module 2: The Human Body and the Process of Aging

Did you know that aging is a normal process, not an illness?

This module reviews the physical changes that occur to the body systems as we age. You can assist the residents and give them the best possible care if you understand the process of aging. By assisting residents to do as much for themselves as possible, you can help the residents stay independent and improve their self-esteem.

This is a long but very important module. All 10 of the body's systems are reviewed. Take your time. For each of the body's systems, you will review the changes that may occur with aging and how you can help residents.

Before discussing the body's systems, let's review some general information about aging. The three aspects of aging are:

- Chronological: how many years old you are
- Physical: how well your body works
- Psychological: how old you act or how old you feel

Some basic things about the aging process are:

- Aging begins when we are born and continues all our life.
- Aging is a normal process, not an illness.
- Our body cells wear out but are continually replaced while a person is growing. As we age, our body's ability to replace worn out cells slows down, and as a result, some body parts don't work as well.

- No one ages just like anyone else. Each person's body is unique and individual. For example, you may develop a problem seeing, but your hearing may be as good as ever, or vice versa.
- Aging may be affected by health habits and heredity as well as by environmental and psychological factors.

Review Questions

1. The three aspects of aging are chronological, ___Phical___, and psychological.
2. Aging begins when we are ___born___ and continues all our life.
3. Aging is a ___Normal___ process, not an illness.

Answers: 1. physical, 2. born, 3. normal

Sensory System

Did you know that as people age, they may have a harder time adjusting to changes in lighting?

The sensory system is made up of our five senses—sense of hearing, sight, touch, taste, and smell. Our senses take information from the environment, or what is going on around the body. That information is then sent by nerves to the brain, where it is used to help the body react to the environment.

As we age, the following changes can occur:

Sight	Less ability to focus on close objects; things are not as clear.
	Difficulty adjusting to changes in lighting
	Less ability to distinguish colors
Hearing	As people age, they may lose their hearing, especially for high frequency sounds.
Taste and Smell	Both taste and smell lessen.
Touch	As people age, they may have less sensation when they feel temperature, pain, pressure, etc.

Here are some ways you can help the resident's sensory system work as well as possible.

If a resident does not see well:

1. Stand where the resident can see you.
2. Say who you are when you go into the resident's room.
3. Keep the resident's room well lighted.
4. Do not move the resident's furniture and belongings; the resident needs to know where to find them.

If a resident cannot hear well:

1. Touch the resident or be sure you are seen when going into the resident's room.
2. Face the resident at eye level and speak directly to them.

3. Speak slowly in a low pitched tone.

4. Reduce background noises (such as television, radio, or other people talking) as much as possible.

5. If necessary, write the message to ensure communication.

If a resident has a poor sense of touch:

1. Check bath water temperature to make sure it is not too hot.

2. Never allow a resident to sit outdoors in the heat or cold long enough to become overheated or chilled.

3. Check the resident's skin daily for signs of pressure or for other injuries they may not realize they have.

If a resident's sense of taste and smell are not good:

1. Food may need more seasoning. Encourage use of lemon, spices, and herbs but discourage adding salt.

2. Smell can be improved by bringing material closer to the resident's nose.

Review Questions

1. The sensory system is made up of our __5__ senses.

2. As people age, they may lose their hearing, especially for __high__ frequency sounds.

3. Both __taste__ and smell decrease with age.

Answers: 1. five, 2. high, 3. taste

Integumentary System (Skin, Hair, and Nails)

Did you know that as we age, our skin loses some of the protective layer of fatty tissue?

The integumentary system is made up of our skin, hair, and nails. The skin is the largest organ in the body. It covers and protects the body against infection.

As the skin ages, the following changes occur:

- Hair loses color.
- Some of the skin loses protective layer of fatty tissue.
- The oil glands produce less oil.
- Skin bruises more easily because aging blood vessels under the skin break more easily. Bedsores occur more easily.

- Nails become thick and lose their shape because they grow out unevenly.

Some of the ways you can help the resident keep this system working as well as possible include:

- Keep the skin clean, dry, and well-lubricated so skin will not tear.

- Provide padding to bony areas and change the resident's position often.

- Use little soap. Soap is very drying to skin.

- Handle resident very gently to avoid hurting thin, fragile skin.

- Keep resident's nails clean and filed smoothly so the resident will not scratch and hurt their skin.

- Keep your own nails cut and filed smoothly, too, so you won't scratch or bruise the resident.

- Shampoo the resident's hair regularly and brush daily to stimulate scalp to produce oil.

- Keep elderly residents warmly dressed. They often feel cold because they have less fatty tissue.

- Report to charge nurse right away any:

  Blue-gray skin color (cyanosis)

  Breaks, swelling, redness, or complaint of pain in the skin

  Redness, swelling, or complaint of pain around nails

Review Questions

1. As the skin ages, the oil glands produce ______ oil.

2. Use little soap because soap is very ______ to the skin.

3. Keep elderly residents warmly dressed. They often feel ______ because they have less fatty tissue.

Answers: 1. less, 2. drying, 3. cold

Musculoskeletal System (Muscles and Bones)

Did you know that exercise may slow the aging process?

The musculoskeletal system is made up of muscles and bones, and allows the body to move. Movement is necessary to keep joints flexible. This system also protects internal organs.

As our musculoskeletal system ages, the following changes may occur:

- Bones are not as strong because of mineral loss.
- Joints may stiffen and be harder to move.
- Tissue in the backbone shrinks; height is reduced.
- Muscles become weaker, causing a lessening of strength.

- Muscles become less elastic.

Many factors influence the aging process in this system, especially exercise and diet. The more you exercise and keep muscles and bones flexible, the more slowly aging occurs. Remember, changes vary from person to person.

Some ways you can help a resident keep this system working as well as possible are:

- Encourage self-care.
- Position the resident carefully and change their position often.
- Do range of motion exercises (exercises that move joints) as ordered.
- Use safety measures to protect residents from falls that can result in fractures and other injuries, e.g., properly fitting shoes, walking cane, safe walking area with no rugs, and well-lighted rooms.

Review Questions

1. The musculoskeletal system is made up of muscles and ___bones___.

2. As the system ages, bones are not as strong because of ___Mineral___ loss.

3. To keep this system working as well as possible, do range of motion ___exercises___ as ordered.

Answers: 1. bones, **2.** mineral, **3.** exercises

Nervous System

Did you know that the nervous system is like a communications center?

The nervous system controls and organizes all body activities. The nervous system is like a communications center. Messages are sent to the brain from all parts of the body and from the five senses. The brain organizes the information it gets and tells the body what to do.

The following changes may occur as this system ages:

- After age 25, there is a slow but steady loss of nerve cells. That loss causes no changes in behavior or performance unless a person has an injury, disease, or poor nutrition.
- The sending of messages from the body to the brain slows down, causing the body to react more slowly. For example, it may take longer for the hand to get the message that it is touching something hot.
- Learning may be slower.

You can help the resident keep this system working as well as possible by:

- Giving more time for activities
- Giving more time for learning
- Reporting to the charge nurse right away if any change in the resident's behavior, such as depression or confusion, occurs

Review Questions

1. ________________ are sent to the brain from all parts of the body and from the five senses.
2. After age ________ there is a slow but steady loss of nerve cells.
3. Report to the charge nurse right away if there is any change in the resident's ________________.

Answers: 1. Messages, **2.** 25, **3.** behavior

Respiratory System (Breathing)

Did you know that breathing puts oxygen into the body and takes carbon dioxide out?

The respiratory system allows the body to breathe. Breathing is one of our most important body functions. Breathing air in and out puts oxygen into the body and takes carbon dioxide out of the body.

The following changes may occur as the respiratory system ages:

- Lungs become less elastic; less air can be inhaled and exhaled.
- The rib cage changes and chest muscles become weaker.
- The number of air sacs in the lungs decreases, making breathing more difficult. The resident must breathe faster to get enough oxygen in and carbon dioxide out.

- Oxygen exchange is decreased.

To keep this system working as well as possible, you can:

- Remind the resident to take deep breaths often during the day. Deep breathing fills the lungs with air and helps the lungs stay more flexible.
- Give the resident time to rest between daily activities.
- Encourage the resident to stop smoking.
- Report right away any of the following problems to the charge nurse:

  Shortness of breath
  Difficulty breathing
  Blue-gray color (cyanosis) of skin
  Unusual confusion (confusion is often the first sign of pneumonia)

Review Questions

1. The respiratory system allows the body to

_______________.

2. Breathing air in and out puts oxygen into the body and takes __________ __________ out of the body.

3. To keep the respiratory system working as well as possible, you should encourage the resident to stop _______________.

Answers: 1. breathe, **2.** carbon dioxide, **3.** smoking

You have reviewed 5 of the 10 systems—you're halfway there. Remember, as you go over the material, especially the ways you can help a resident, see if you can think of other ways you can help.

Cardiovascular System (Circulation)

Did you know that the cardiovascular system pumps blood carrying food and oxygen to the body cells through the blood vessels?

The cardiovascular system pumps blood carrying food and oxygen to the body cells through the blood vessels. It also takes away waste products from the cells. The whole cardiovascular system depends on the heart pumping the blood through the blood vessels.

The following changes occur as the cardiovascular system ages:

- Heart loses elasticity.

- Blood vessels become narrower and less elastic. The heart must work harder to supply blood to internal organs and to hands and feet.

- The amount of blood pumped out with each heart beat (contraction) is less, resulting in less oxygen in the system and less reserve energy for the person.

Here are some ways you can help this system work as well as possible:

- Give resident more time to complete tasks and more time to rest.
- Encourage regular exercise.
- Check skin often.
- Encourage healthy eating.
- Avoid smoking.
- Monitor vital signs.

- Report to the charge nurse right away any of the following problems:

  Shortness of breath
  Change in vital signs
  Skin discoloration on injury

Review Questions

1. The whole cardiovascular system depends on the ______________ pumping the blood through the blood vessels.

2. As the cardiovascular system ages, blood vessels become ________________ and less elastic.

3. To help the cardiovascular system work as well as possible, encourage regular _______________.

Answers: 1. heart, 2. narrower, 3. exercise

Digestive System

Did you know that as we age, we digest food more slowly?

The digestive system breaks down food into nutrients that are used by the body. The system also gets rid of the materials that are not used by the body.

As our body continues aging, the changes that occur in the digestive system are:

- Less salivation
- Loss of muscle tone results in food being digested more slowly
- Less digestive juices
- Nutrients are not absorbed as efficiently, resulting in some vitamin and iron loss as well as possible weight loss.

Here are some ways you can help make sure this system works as well as possible:

- Encourage resident to drink liquids.
- Give good oral hygiene.
- Provide privacy and time for going to the bathroom.
- Encourage exercise to help stimulate bowel activity.
- Encourage residents to eat high fiber foods, such as cereal, whole wheat bread, fruits, and vegetables.
- Make sure resident has regular bowel movements.
- Allow the resident enough time for eating and completely chewing food before swallowing.
- Be sensitive to the eating patterns of residents. Many older residents do better with frequent small meals than a few larger ones.
- Report to the charge nurse right away any:

  Change in the resident's appetite
  Change in bowel habits
  Signs of nausea and vomiting

Review Questions

1. The digestive system gets rid of the materials that are not used by the ______________.
2. As we age, ________________ are not absorbed as efficiently, resulting in some vitamin and iron loss as well as possible weight loss.
3. To help the digestive system work as well as possible, encourage residents to drink ______________.

Answers: 1. body, **2.** nutrients, **3.** liquids

Urinary System

Did you know that an older person may need to pass urine more often?

The urinary system:

- Removes wastes from the bloodstream
- Makes urine
- Keeps the fluid balanced in the body

The following changes may occur as the urinary system changes:

- The kidneys may get smaller in size and weight so they don't work as well to filter wastes from the blood. Kidneys can become less efficient in removing drugs from the bloodstream.

- The bladder, ureters, and urethra are less elastic. The bladder can hold less urine.

- The older person may need to pass urine more often, especially at night.

- The bladder loses muscle tone, which causes a person to be unable to empty the bladder completely. An older person may feel the urge to urinate again right away.

You can help this system work as well as possible by:

- Answering call lights right away, and taking residents to the bathroom when asked

- Encouraging the resident to sit on toilet for a few minutes after voiding to make sure bladder is empty

- Providing privacy when assisting the resident in toileting needs

- Encouraging resident to drink liquids by offering fresh water and other liquids often

- Reporting to charge nurse right away if:

  Urine is cloudy
  Urine is bloody
  Urine has a foul odor

Review Questions

1. The urinary system produces ________________.

2. As the urinary system ages, the bladder, ureters, and urethra are less ________________.

3. To keep the urinary system working as well as possible, encourage the resident to sit on the toilet for a few minutes after voiding to make sure the bladder is ________________.

Answers: 1. urine, **2.** elastic, **3.** empty

Endocrine System

Did you know that the endocrine system is made up of many glands located in different parts of the body?

The endocrine system is made up of many glands. These glands are located in different parts of the body and make substances called hormones that regulate the activity of organs and cell groups throughout the body.

The following changes may occur as the endocrine system ages:

- In females, production of hormones in the ovaries slows down over a period of years. This is called menopause or "change of life" and causes the monthly menstrual cycle to become irregular and finally to stop, ending a woman's ability to have children.

- In males, production of the hormone testosterone slows down but does not stop.

- The most important age-related change in the pancreas is the decrease in insulin and the possibility of adult onset of diabetes mellitus.

You can help make this system work as well as possible by observing and reporting any of these symptoms to the charge nurse:

- Decreased activity or sluggish response
- Abnormal feeling of being cold
- Excessive thirst
- Frequent urination of large quantities of urine
- Itching of skin and genital area
- Blurred vision
- Tingling and numbness of the hands and feet

Review Questions

1. The endocrine system is made up of many ____________________.

2. The most important age-related change in the pancreas is the decrease in ____________________.

3. To help make the endocrine system work as well as possible, observing and reporting any change to the ____________ ____________ is important.

Answers: 1. glands, 2. insulin, 3. charge nurse

Reproductive System

Did you know that the most important change in the female reproductive system is menopause?

The reproductive system allows humans to reproduce and to have sexual intercourse.

The following changes may occur as the reproductive system ages:

- The most important change in males is that the prostate gland gets bigger, which squeezes the urethra and interferes with the passage of urine.
- Older men may have a slower sexual response—it takes them longer to get an erection and may take longer to have an orgasm during intercourse.
- The most important change in the female is the ending of menstruation or menopause. Menopause usually occurs between the ages of 45 to 55 and ends the female ability to reproduce. This results in a decrease in production of hormones, causing dryness and sensitivity in the vagina and vulva area.
- Because vaginal secretions decrease, there may be discomfort during sexual intercourse.
- Older men and women may not lose their desire for sexual stimulation or their ability to achieve sexual satisfaction. Elderly residents who have lost their partners may masterbate for sexual pleasure. And privacy needs to be given at appropriate times.

Some ways you can help this system work as well as possible are:

- Keep male genital area clean.

- Report to the charge nurse any of these problems with urination:

  Voiding frequently in small amounts
  Painful urination

- Keep female genital area clean.

- Report any of these problems:

  Odor
  Redness
  Irritation
  Discharge
  Bleeding
  Pain

Review Questions

1. The reproductive system allows humans to ____________________ and to have sexual intercourse.

2. The most important change in males is enlargement of the ____________ __________.

3. To help the reproductive system work as well as possible, keep the ____________ area clean.

Answers: 1. reproduce, 2. prostate gland, 3. genital

Unit 2, Foundation for Caring

Module 3: Understanding the Rights of Residents in Long-Term Care

Did you know that residents must be informed in words and in writing at the time of admission of their legal rights?

What do we mean by a person's rights? Can you think of a right that you know you have? Sometimes people have to work hard to be sure they get certain rights. Examples from history, the media, or community experience show this: women and the right to vote; blacks and the right to equal opportunities for education jobs and housing; children and the right to protection from abuse, etc. Rights that are guaranteed by law have often been won because people demanded them and marched or demonstrated to get laws written or changed. Residents in long-
term care have won legal rights because their friends, families, and even nurse assistants who cared have fought for them. Today, all long-term care facilities must have a list of residents' rights, and they must be given to each resident at admission.

Here is a list of rights that all residents have and some ways you can help protect those rights. You should also review your state's Bill of Rights for nursing home residents.

Right	What You Can Do
1. Know about all their rights	Remind the resident and family to meet with the social worker. Tell the resident and family about the state ombudsman program.

Right	What You Can Do
2. Know what care will cost.	Refer the resident to the social worker. Give the resident any literature the nursing home has about costs.
3. Know about their own medical condition.	Encourage the resident to talk with the charge nurse or physician and ask specific questions about their condition.
4. Choose the people who will take care of them.	Make sure the charge nurse knows which caregivers the resident likes. Provide consistency in care (same staff).
5. Help plan their care and treatment.	Be sure to involve the resident and their family in writing the care plan. (Remember the resident is the head of the team.)
6. Have their needs taken care of.	Do everything possible to take care of a resident's needs. Communicate the resident's needs to other team members.
7. Make a complaint.	Tell other team members about the complaint. Change care to meet the resident's needs.
8. Be free from abuse.	Never abuse a resident. Report incidence(s) of abuse.

Right	What You Can Do
9. Be free from restraints.	Never use restraints without a doctor's order.
10. Be treated with dignity and respect.	Ask for permission to provide care. Involve the resident in their care.
11. Have privacy.	Ask for permission to provide care. Keep the resident covered when providing care. Pull the curtain when providing care.
12. Manage their own money matters.	Never take money for care. Never discuss a resident's finances.
13. Send and receive mail that has not been opened.	Deliver mail to residents. Offer assistance to open or read mail.
14. Practice their religion.	Help the resident get to religious services. Call in clergy if requested.
15. Use their own clothing and possessions.	Make sure the resident gets dressed every day. Make sure the resident's possessions are marked.
16. Be alone with their partner or spouse.	Provide privacy Help the resident plan visiting time.
17. Refuse care or treatment.	Offer to come back at a better time (in a few minutes). Work with the charge nurse to change the care plan if necessary.

Review Questions

1. Today, all long-term care facilities must have a list of residents' ______________, and they must be given to each resident at ____________________.

2. Never use a restraint without a ________________ order.

3. To protect a resident's right to receive mail that has not been opened, you might offer ______________________ to open or read mail.

Answers: 1. rights, admission **2.** doctor's, **3.** assistance

Unit 2, Foundation for Caring

Module 4: Communication

Did you know that you communicate every day both verbally and nonverbally?

Communication is one of your primary responsibilities as a nurse assistant. One of the most important parts of being with other people is how we communicate, or exchange messages, with them. For residents in a nursing home who are away from the people they know and love, seeing and talking with other people are especially important.

Nonverbal Communication

A lot of what we communicate to other people is nonverbal. Nonverbal means "without words." Instead of talking or writing our messages, we use our bodies, our faces, or our hands to tell people what we are feeling. Nonverbal communication is often used by adults instead of saying how they feel.

Residents who don't see well may miss nonverbal communication. To make sure that the resident understands, stand close, use touch, and talk more. Be careful not to say one thing and communicate something entirely different with your body or face. Remember that nonverbal communication is a natural way of sending messages. Some nonverbal communication is universal—a smile or frown means the same thing in any language. Other forms of nonverbal communication may be used differently in different cultures. For example, in some cultures looking a person in the eyes means you are honest and respectful. In other cultures, looking a person in the eyes is a sign of disrespect.

Review Questions

1. One of the most important parts of being with other people is how we ______________ or exchange messages with them.

2. "Nonverbal" means without ____________.

3. Residents who don't see well may miss ______________ communication.

Answers: 1. communicate, **2.** words, **3.** nonverbal

Verbal Communication

Residents need to have positive communication—someone to talk to and someone to listen. Some things are bridges—they make it easier for you and residents to communicate well. And some things are barriers—they make it harder to communicate. Bridges get you where you want to go. Barriers, like roadblocks, keep you from getting there.

Some examples of barriers and bridges to communication are listed below. Can you think of some others?

Barriers	Bridges
Mumbling	Speaking clearly and slowly
Using jargon—words only certain people use, like medical words	Using simple words

Barriers	**Bridges**
Talking in a very loud voice	Using your voice well—not too loudly and not too softly
Not explaining what you mean	Giving positive nonverbal messages
Using slang	Being respectful—using a resident's title, first and last name, or whatever they want to be called
Using baby talk	Getting the resident's attention
Not saying how you really feel	Looking a resident in the eyes
Interrupting	Sitting at the same level as the resident—so your eyes are at the same level as theirs
Sounding upset or angry	Concentrating on what the resident is saying
Labeling a resident "complainer" or "senile"	Taking time to listen
Being in a hurry	Using physical contact—holding a resident's hand or putting your hand on their arm to keep their attention
Not listening	
Using a language the resident doesn't understand	

Review Questions

1. Residents need to have positive communication—someone to talk to and someone to ________________.

2. ________________ make it easier for you and residents to communicate well.

3. Barriers make it ____________ to communicate.

Answers: 1. listen, 2. bridges, 3. harder

Using Special Communication Skills

Did you know that one of your duties as a nurse assistant is to observe the resident and gather information?

Good communication makes your job easier and more enjoyable. In addition, as a nurse assistant, you must use special communication skills as part of your job.

As a nurse assistant you usually spend more time with residents than other members of the health care team, and your observations are important.

These observations mainly use the senses—sight, hearing, smell, and touch—to take in information about the resident. Being objective—paying attention to the facts and not opinions—is important and will help you make quality observations.

The senses are identified below along with possible observations you might make about the resident's condition. Can you think of any more? Make notes.

- Sight

  The resident's skin looks pale or red.
  The resident has sores in his mouth.
  The resident's hand shakes
  The resident is too weak to hold a glass.
  The resident limps or cannot stand up alone.
  The resident's urine or stool has an unusual color.
  The resident is not eating.
  The resident squints or bumps into things and people.
  The resident's expression is happy or unhappy.

- Hearing

  The resident has a cough.
  The resident makes a noise when breathing.
  The resident complains of pain.
  The resident does not hear well.
  The resident does not speak clearly.

- Smell

  The resident's breath has a funny smell.
  The resident's urine or stool has an unusual smell.

- Touch

  The resident's pulse is very strong.
  The resident's pulse is weak.
  The resident's skin feels warm or cool.
  The resident has a lump under the skin.

As a nurse assistant, you gather information about the resident's condition and then pass it on to other members of the health care team. The more descriptive your information is, the more helpful it will be to those who are hearing or reading it.

Information should be written on the Activities of Daily Living (ADL) Flow Chart. Different facilities use different forms of an ADL Flow Chart. You use it to keep a record of what care a resident receives each day.

Some of the categories included on a flow chart are vital signs and personal care—as you complete these tasks, you should record data on this form.

Review Questions

1. As a nurse assistant you usually spend more time with residents than other members of the health care team, and your ____________________ are important.

2. Observations mainly use the senses of sight, ____________, ____________, and touch to take information about the resident.

3. As a nurse assistant, you gather information about the resident's condition and then pass it on to other members of the health care __________.

Answers: 1. observations, **2.** hearing, smell, **3.** team

Reinforcing Resident's Behavior

Did you know that praise is a verbal reward?

When a care plan is written for a resident, it may include certain behaviors that the health care team wants to increase (for example getting the resident to take part in social/recreational activities.) A special kind of communication called social reinforcement will help increase a resident's desirable behaviors.

People often behave a certain way because they are rewarded or reinforced for that behavior. You can use verbal rewards to help reinforce the resident's desirable behavior. Some examples of verbal rewards are:

Praise—"You did a good job."
Thanks—"Thanks for working with me."
Encouragement—"Come on, you can go another few feet."
Approval—"That is right"
Recognition—"Let us all congratulate Mrs. Roberts."

When you give a verbal reward and add an appropriate touch (like a hug or handshake), it is called social reinforcement.

Review Questions

1. ______________________ reinforcement will help increase a resident's desirable behavior.

2. Two examples of "social reinforcement" are __________________ and __________________.

3. When you give a _________________ reward and add an appropriate touch (like a hug or handshake), it is called social reinforcement.

Answers: 1. social, **2.** praise, thanks, encouragement, approval, recognition, **3.** verbal

Handling Undesirable Behaviors

Did you know that you should always respond to a resident in an appropriate way?

It is easier to help residents increase desirable behavior than it is to deal with undesirable behavior. The health care team may write in the care plan that an undesirable behavior needs to be decreased. Sometimes ignoring an undesirable behavior while continuing to pay attention to the resident will help decrease the behavior. But some things cannot be ignored, such as spitting, hitting, exposing genitals, yelling, swearing, using racist words, etc. You will have your own feelings about these undesirable behaviors but you should always remember:

Most people in nursing homes have illnesses or disabilities and have suffered many losses.

Try to understand residents' feelings and the reasons why they do undesirable things

Regardless of why a resident behaves in an undesirable way, you must respond with appropriate words and behaviors.

Whatever a resident has done to you, your response must always meet the test of the six principles. An appropriate response always allows for safety, infection control, dignity, privacy, independence and communication. And an appropriate response never violates a resident's rights. When a resident does something undesirable, it is okay to feel upset, angry, embarrassed or frustrated. Feelings are always okay. But it is never okay to act the way you feel if that action would be inappropriate.

There are things you can do about your feelings:

- Walk away from the situation
- Talk to someone about what happened
- Go outside and yell or cry.

Some important points to remember when dealing with undesirable behavior are:

1. Try to understand why residents do undesirable things (loss, frustration, anger, confusion).

2. If a resident does something undesirable to you, it is okay to feel upset or angry but do not act the way you feel. You have to change your behavior for the sake of the resident in your care.

3. Always respond to a resident in an appropriate way.

4. Do something to help yourself cope with the undesirable behavior but first be sure the resident is safe.

5. No matter what residents do, they have a right to be treated with kindness, respect, and freedom from abuse or unnecessary restraint.

Review Questions

1. ____________________ resident behaviors need to be decreased.

2. Two examples of behaviors considered undesirable may be ____________________ and ____________________.

3. It is okay to feel upset or angry when a resident does something undesirable, but your behavior must always be ____________________.

Answers: 1. Undesirable, **2.** spitting, hitting, exposing genitals, yelling, swearing, using racist words, **3.** appropriate

Unit 2, Foundation for Caring

Module 5: Principles of Care

Can you think of six principles you should know when caring for a resident?

There are six responsibilities/principles of care that a nurse assistant must know when assisting a resident. These responsibilities/principles should become routine in your daily care of the resident. The responsibilities/principles are:

1. **Safety:** Protect the residents, yourself, and other staff from accidents and injury.
2. **Privacy:** Do not discuss residents' care or condition with outsiders. Respect residents' personal place (room or area of the room) and personal belongings.
3. **Dignity:** Respect the residents as individuals. Remember that not all people in long-term care are alike. Protect the residents from embarrassment. Respect religious and cultural beliefs.
4. **Communication:** Talk with and listen to the residents, their families, and health team members to gain a better understanding of residents' needs.
5. **Infection Control:** Practice methods that prevent spread of infection to residents, yourself, and others.
6. **Independence:** Encourage and help residents to do as much as possible for themselves by allowing time for residents to help with their own care.

Here are some ways you can use these six principles of care:

Principle	You can:
Safety	Use side rails as necessary. Put the call light within reach. Keep the environment free from hazards.
Privacy	Knock on the resident's door before going into their room. Keep the resident covered or close the door when providing care. Always ask permission to provide care. Drape the resident when necessary.
Dignity	Be respectful to the resident. Call the resident by their last name (Mr. or Mrs.).
Communication	Be a good listener. Talk to the resident. Reinforce positive behavior. Observe resident for physical and psychological changes.

Principle	You can:
Infection control	Wash your hands before and after giving care. Use facility disinfectants for cleaning. Keep clean items together and dirty items together. Practice appropriate isolation procedures.
Independence	Ask permission to assist with care. Encourage the resident to do as much of their own care as possible. Pace resident care. Encourage family participation. Encourage the participation of other health care teammembers like the social worker and dietitian.

Review Questions

1. There are ______ responsibilities/principles of care that a nurse assistant must know when assisting a resident.

2. These principles of care should become ____________.

3. The six principles of care are ____________, ____________, ____________, ____________, infection control, and independence.

Answers: 1. six, **2.** routine, **3.** safety, privacy, dignity, communication

Unit 3: Core Skills for Caring

In Unit 2, you reviewed the concepts necessary to build a foundation for caring. This unit reviews the core skills you must master to provide quality care. These core skills are part of your everyday routine in helping the residents. As you review these skills, remember the foundation for caring concepts, especially the six principles of care. The core skills are found within the following seven modules:

Module 1—Infection Control
Module 2—Taking Care of a Resident's Environment
Module 3—Maintaining Mobility
Module 4—Personal Care
Module 5—Nutrition
Module 6—Elimination
Module 7—Vital Signs

Skill sheets for these core skills are found in Part 2. After you read the material and answer the questions correctly, review and practice the skill until you have mastered it.

Unit 3, Core Skills For Caring

Module 1: Infection Control

Do you know how germs are spread?

We all practice some infection control in our daily lives. If we cough or sneeze, we cover our mouths or turn our heads to stop the spread of germs. If we know someone who has a cold or flu, we try to keep our distance from the person so we will not catch their "bug."

All nursing homes have infection control policies and procedures to prevent the spread of germs that cause infections. Because of residents' weakened conditions, constant contact with each other, and exposure to visitors and staff, controlling infection in a long-term care facility is difficult. Therefore, you need to know and practice the infection control policies in your facility.

Some germs are useful and necessary in certain areas of the body. For example, the gastrointestinal (GI) tract needs certain bacteria to aid in digestion, but if those bacteria are present in the urinary tract, infection can occur.

For germs to grow and live, they need warm temperatures, moisture, darkness, oxygen, and food.

The two most common ways that germs are spread in the health care environment are through direct contact and indirect contact. Direct contact means that germs are spread from one person to another person. Indirect contact means that germs are spread from one person to an object and then to another person. Some examples of how germs spread are:

Direct Contact (Person to Person)	**Indirect Contact** (Person to Object to Person)
Touching	Eating contaminated food
Infected body fluids	Handling soiled linen
Coughing, sneezing	Handling soiled equipment
	Drinking or using contaminated water

You can help control the spread of germs in many ways:

- Always wash your hands.
- Know the correct precautions for infection control.
- Keep yourself, the resident, and the environment clean.
- Be aware of the signs and symptoms of infection and report them. (For example, report any of these: vomiting, diarrhea, high temperature, stuffy nose, cough, cloudy or smelly urine, skin rash, break in skin or sores, red and draining eyes.)
- Be aware that there are clean areas and dirty areas in infection control. For example, a clean utility room would have resident supplies and a dirty utility room would have trash containers.

Review Questions

1. If we cough or sneeze, we cover our mouths or turn our heads to stop the ______________ ____ ___________.

2. For germs to ___________ and ___________, they need certain things, including warm temperature, moisture, darkness, oxygen, and food.

3. Indirect contact means that germs are spread from one person to an ___________ and then to another person.

Answers: 1. spread of germs, **2.** grow, live, **3.** object

Hand Washing

Did you know that there are at least seven situations when you should wash your hands?

Hand washing is the most effective way to prevent the spread of infection.

You must wash your hands before and after any activity involving you or the resident. The following are some examples:

- Before and after any contact with a resident
- After going to the bathroom
- After coughing or sneezing
- Before handling any food
- After smoking
- When coming on duty
- Before going home

Remember these three important steps in hand washing:

1. Wet your hands and wrists. Apply soap. If you are using bar soap, rinse the soap before using it.

2. Hold your hands lower than your elbows so that the dirty water runs from the clean area of the forearm to the dirty area of the fingers.

3. To prevent contamination of clean hands from the dirty faucet, use a clean paper towel to turn off the faucet.

Remember to review and practice Skill 1, "Hand Washing," in Part 2.

Review Questions

1. Hand washing is the most effective way to ____________ the spread of infection.

2. Remember to wash your hands ____________ and ____________ any contact with a resident.

3. Hold your hands ____________ than your elbows.

Answers: 1. prevent, 2. before, after, 3. lower

Universal Precautions

Do you know what universal precautions are?

Universal precautions are ways of making sure that every person who has direct contact with body fluids will be protected in case the fluids are infectious or carry a disease. Universal precautions are especially important to prevent the transmission of blood-borne and other infectious diseases.

You should know your facility's policy concerning universal precautions. Examples of the universal precautions that have been adopted by the federal government include:

1. Wear latex gloves according to facility policy. Change gloves after contact with a resident.

2. Wash hands and other skin surfaces immediately after contamination.

3. Wear protective clothing, such as a gown, mask, and gloves.

4. Handle sharp instruments carefully.

5. Do not give care without wearing gloves if you have open cuts or oozing sores on your hands.

6. Clean up blood or body fluid spills promptly.

7. Handle linen carefully.

8. Bag contaminated articles carefully.

9. Be sure waste is put in a leak-proof, air-tight container.

Universal precautions are equally important to everyone. If universal precautions are consistently used, the spread of infection will decrease.

Review Questions

1. Universal precautions are ways of making sure that every person who has direct contact with body fluids will be ________________ in case the fluids are infectious or carry a disease.

2. Do not give care without wearing gloves if you have open ________ or oozing ____________.

3. If universal precautions are consistently used, the spread of infection will _________________.

Answers: 1. protected, **2.** cuts, wounds, **3.** decrease

Isolation Procedures

Do you know why residents are put in isolation?

Additional precautions are used when it is known or suspected that a resident may have a contagious disease, such as infectious diarrhea or tuberculosis. Residents with such diseases are put in isolation to prevent the disease from spreading to other residents and staff, and to keep the infected resident from becoming worse.

When a resident is in isolation, it is important to do the following things:

- Make sure the resident knows why they are isolated.
- Check on the resident often and listen to their concerns. Try to understand their feelings and help care for their needs. Stress that isolation will help speed their recovery.
- Make sure that visitors (if allowed) follow the charge nurse's instructions.
- Know your facility's specific procedures for isolation.
- Keep clean items separate from dirty items.

Different infectious diseases require different precautions to prevent their spread. Review the isolation procedures in your facility. The following is an example of strict isolation, which is the maximum form of isolation. All other levels of isolation are modified forms of strict isolation.

- Resident must be in private (single) room. Door must be kept closed. Everyone who enters the room must wear a mask, gloves, gown, and plastic apron. All articles in the room, including food trays, must be disinfected or thrown away after use, according to the facility's rules.
- Linens must be bagged following universal precaution guidelines and thrown away or washed according to isolation procedures for laundry.
- Everyone must wash their hands before entering and when leaving the room.

Remember to review and practice Skill 2, "Putting on a Gown, Mask, and Disposable Gloves" and Skill 3, "Taking Off Soiled Disposable Gloves, Mask, and Gown," in Part 2.

Review Questions

1. Additional precautions are used when there is evidence or suspicion that a resident may have a ________________ disease.

2. Different infectious diseases require different precautions to ______________ their spread.

3. All other levels of ______________ are modified forms of strict isolation.

Answers: 1. contagious, 2. prevent, 3. isolation

Unit 3, Core Skills For Caring

Module 2: Taking Care of a Resident's Environment

As a nurse assistant, you are responsible for taking care of the resident's environment. This module reviews three parts of that responsibility: making sure the resident's environment is safe; respecting and caring for the resident's immediate surroundings; and knowing how to respond to a fire or disaster.

Promoting Resident Safety

Did you know that the best safety measure is prevention?

All residents need a safe environment. Residents may be physically weak, unfamiliar with their surroundings, not thinking clearly, or unsteady because of medications. These conditions may cause them to have accidents easily. Providing a safe environment for residents is the responsibility of all nursing home employees.

Preventing accidents is the best safety measure. The following is a list of some general safety rules for resident care:

- Do not use defective or broken equipment.
- Never use equipment unless you have been trained to use it and feel sure of yourself.
- Check the temperature of water coming out of faucets. Water temperature should be at or below 120 degrees. If water seems hot to touch, report it to the charge nurse.
- Report any incident to the charge nurse, even if there is no injury.

- Lock brakes on beds, wheelchairs, and shower chairs.
- Put the call light within easy reach of the resident. Answer calls for help promptly (within 3 to 5 minutes) and immediately if you suspect an emergency.
- Never leave a resident alone in the bathtub or shower.
- Handle residents gently. Their skin can be very fragile and injure easily.
- Use raised bed rails to prevent residents who are disoriented from falling out of bed.

Review Questions

1. All residents need a __________ environment.
2. Raising bed rails is a basic, but important way to provide ____________.
3. Lock brakes on beds, ________________, and shower chairs.

Answers: 1. safe, 2. safety, 3. wheelchairs

Sometimes restraints are used as a safety measure:

- Restraints are used as a last resort only after all other options have been examined.
- The reason(s) for a restraint should be explained to the resident and their family.
- A restraint is used only if a physician orders it.
- Using a restraint on a resident violates their legal "right to be free from restraint" and should never be done lightly.

Some conditions under which a resident might be restrained include:

- When a resident is disoriented, extremely restless, or has a balance problem, they may wander, fall, and injure themselves.
- When a resident with a balance problem tends to wake up at night and not know where they are, they may fall and injure themselves.
- When a resident must have a short-term IV or catheter and keeps pulling it out, they may injure themselves.

Residents who are restrained should be checked every 30 minutes and released every 2 hours.

Review Questions

1. Restraints are used as a ________ __________ only after all other options have been examined.
2. A restraint is used only if a __________ orders it.
3. Residents who are restrained should be checked every ________ minutes and released every ________ hours.

Answers: 1. last resort, **2.** physician, **3.** 30, 2

Bed Making

Did you know that a clean, wrinkle-free bed can prevent bedsores?

A resident's bed is part of their personal space. It is important to understand this as part of respecting and caring for the resident's own area.

When making a bed, remember the following key points:

- A clean, neat bed is important for the comfort and dignity of the resident. A clean, wrinkle-free bed also prevents skin irritation and bedsores.

- Beds are usually made in the morning after the resident's bath. You may be making a bed when the resident is out of it (called an unoccupied bed) or when the resident is in it (called an occupied bed).

- To make your job easier:

  Use of good body mechanics prevents back strain as you work. (You will review body mechanics in the next module.)

  Make one side of the bed at a time to save time and energy.

- To control the spread of infection:

  Wash your hands before and after you make a bed.

  Handle linen properly for infection control. Do not shake bed linen. Shaking linen causes air currents that may spread dust and germs around the room. Keep soiled, contaminated linen away from your uniform. Do not allow clean linen to touch the floor.

- When you straighten up the resident's space:

  Clean the over bed table and nightstand as needed. Never move anything without the resident's permission.

Check the bed for dentures, eyeglasses, and hearing aids.

If the resident is in the room, make them comfortable and put the call light within reach (this helps ensure the resident's safety at all times).

Making an Occupied Bed

If a resident is in bed ("making an occupied bed"), be sure to do the following:

- Keep the top sheet on the resident for privacy.
- Check the resident for proper body position and comfort throughout bed making.
- Never leave the resident alone.
- Keep side rail up on side you are not working.
- Lower side rail closest to you, roll the resident toward you, and then raise the side rail. (*Note:* Never roll a resident against the side rail.)
- When you move to the other side of the bed, lower that side rail, and make that side of the bed.

Remember to review and practice Skill 4, "Making an Occupied Bed," in Part 2.

Review Questions

1. A clean, wrinkle-free bed prevents ____________ irritation and ____________________.

2. When a resident is out of bed, you are making an ________________ bed. When a resident is in bed, you are making an __________________ bed.

3. Keep the top sheet on the resident for ________________.

Answers: 1. skin, bedsores, 2. unoccupied, occupied, 3. privacy

Following Safety and Emergency Procedures

Do you know the location of fire alarms and fire extinguishers in your facility?

A disaster can happen anywhere anytime. Nursing homes must always be ready to deal with an emergency.

Where possible, efforts should always be made to prevent the occurrence of an emergency situation like a fire. (Obviously, natural disasters cannot be prevented.) Review the fire prevention rules below:

- Obey the facility's smoking policy (Example: smoke only in designated areas).

- Ask residents to smoke only in designated areas and only when someone is supervising.
- Never empty ashtrays into a container with materials that can burn.
- Post "No Smoking" signs and make sure no one smokes when oxygen is being used.
- Immediately report any fire hazards, such as frayed electrical cords, overloaded electrical outlets, and defective electrical outlets, to the charge nurse.
- Use only battery operated razors in rooms where oxygen is being used.
- Never block fire doors or exits.
- In case of a fire, do not go through fire doors once they have been shut to seal off an area. In the event of a fire, the fire doors close automatically and seal off the area where there is smoke and/or flames. These doors will contain the fire for approximately 20 minutes.
- Know the locations of fire alarms and fire extinguishers and how to use them.

If an emergency occurs while you are on duty, you should take several important steps to ensure your own safety and the safety of residents. The first thing to do is look around to see if the area you are in is safe. If you notice a fire, toxic fumes, or other hazards, you should immediately call the local emergency medical services (EMS) for help. (Example: "Help! I am at __________, and there is a fire in room ______.") The EMS dispatch can contact the fire department, medical care, power company, or other services needed to handle specific life-threatening situations.

It is very important that you know the floor plan of the facility where you work as well as the location of fire alarms and fire extinguishers.

In the event of an emergency, the best way to move a helpless resident to a safe area is in a wheelchair or on a bed. If, for some reason, the resident cannot be moved this way, use one of these methods:

- Blanket carry
- Linen lift
- Two-handed seat carry (for two rescuers)

In case of a fire, remember these important points:

- Never use an elevator during a fire.
- Never go through a doorway until you have felt the door with the palm of your hand.
- Never go through a doorway when the door is hot to touch.
- Call for help. Pull the fire alarm if you are near it, or ask bystanders to pull the nearest fire alarm.
- Help the resident move to a safe area, preferably in a wheelchair or bed. If necessary, use an evacuation carry.

Review Questions

1. If an emergency occurs, the first thing to do is to look around to determine if the area you are in is ________.

2. If you notice a fire, toxic fumes, or other hazards, you should immediately call the local emergency ____________ ____________ for help.

3. In case of fire, never go through a doorway when the door is ________ to touch.

Answers: 1. safe, **2.** medical services, **3.** hot

Unit 3, Core Skills For Caring

Module 3: Maintaining Mobility

Did you know that using proper body mechanics will protect you from back injury?

Correctly moving, positioning, and performing range of motion exercises are important for the resident's comfort, for the maintenance of skin integrity, and to prevent contractures.

A resident's independence is often determined by their mobility. It is your job to help the resident remain as mobile as possible. Three factors to be considered when moving, positioning, and doing range of motion exercises are:

- Your safety (good body mechanics)
- The resident's comfort and safety in moving and positioning
- The resident's level of flexibility

Body Mechanics

When you are helping the resident, remember to use proper body mechanics to help prevent back injury. Body mechanics are the way your entire body adjusts to keep its balance as you move and rest.

The five principles of good body mechanics while lifting are:

1. Use a broad base of support (feet 12 inches apart and one foot slightly in front of the other).
2. Keep the person or object lifted close to your body.
3. Keep your upper body erect.
4. Lift smoothly—don't jerk.
5. Don't lift and twist.

Review Questions

1. Correctly moving, positioning, and performing range of motion exercises are important for the resident's comfort, for the maintenance of skin integrity, and to prevent ________________.

2. Proper body mechanics will help prevent __________ injury.

3. Body mechanics are the way your entire body adjusts to keep its ______________.

Answers: 1. contractures, **2.** back, **3.** balance

Positioning the Resident

Do you know how often you should reposition a resident?

Lack of movement and improper body positioning cause problems in almost all of the body's systems. When residents are always in bed and unable to move on their own, it is important to reposition them at least every 2 hours.

Remember, proper positioning protects the resident from discomfort and deformities.

When positioning residents, specially designed equipment can be used. However, if such equipment is not available, use pillows, rolled blankets, and washcloths. Lack of equipment is not an excuse for improper positioning.

Some examples of positions used in long-term care facilities are:

- Supine—lying flat on back
- Semi-fowlers—head of bed and knee portion of bed are raised
- Prone—lying flat on stomach
- Modified side-lying (lateral)—lying on side with pillow support

Remember to review and practice Skill 5, "Positioning," in Part 2.

Review Questions

1. Lack of movement and improper body positioning causes problems in almost all of the body's ____________.

2. Proper positioning protects the resident from ____________ and deformities.

3. Lack of equipment is not an excuse for ____________ positioning.

Answers: 1. systems, **2.** discomfort, **3.** improper

Moving

Did you know that you may need help from a co-worker when you move a resident?

Before moving a resident, talk to the charge nurse about the resident's level of mobility and independence and check the resident's care plan.

Moving a resident will be easier if you plan ahead. Remember these key points before the move:

- Check to see if you need any special equipment for the move.
- Make sure you have enough room for the move.
- Get help from a co-worker if needed.
- Explain exactly what you are going to do to the resident and any co-worker.
- Position yourself so that you will not hurt yourself.
- Lock the bed and wheelchair brakes.
- Always consider the resident's privacy, safety, and comfort.

Can you think of any other points that will make the move safe and comfortable for you and the resident?

After the move, be sure that the resident is comfortable and safe. Be sure the resident's body is properly aligned.

Remember to review and practice Skill 6, "Moving the Resident from Bed to Chair," in Part 2.

Review Questions

1. Moving a resident will be easier if you ________ ahead.

2. When moving a resident, always consider the resident's __________, safety, and comfort.

3. After the move, be sure the resident's body is properly __________.

Answers: 1. plan, **2.** privacy, **3.** aligned

Range of Motion

Did you know that range of motion exercises can be active or passive?

Exercise keeps muscles and joints working, even if only at a minimum level. For residents, this can mean the difference between being able to help with their care, and not being able to help.

One form of exercise is range of motion (ROM) exercise. Range of motion is the amount of movement in a joint or how far a joint, like the elbow, knee, or shoulder, can comfortably be moved. Range of motion exercises can be active (done by the resident), or passive (done by the nurse assistant). There is a systematic way of doing range of motion exercises. These exercises should be done at least three times a day, repeating each move five times.

Some points to remember when doing range of motion exercises are:

- Move each joint slowly, gently, and smoothly.
- Support each joint during movement.
- Never move the joint beyond its present level of movement.
- If pain occurs, stop the movement and report to the charge nurse. Always watch the resident's face, particularly the eyes, for any expression of pain.
- Always use good body mechanics.
- Always discuss any exercise plan with the charge nurse.

Remember to review and practice Skill 7, "Performing Passive Range of Motion," in Part 2.

Review Questions

1. When moving residents both the nurse assistants' and residents' ___________ must be considered.
2. Range of motion exercises can be active (done by the resident) or ___________ (done by the nurse assistant).
3. One point to remember when doing ROM is: Move each joint slowly, ___________, and smoothly.

Answers: 1. safety, 2. passive, 3. gently

Unit 3, Core Skills For Caring

Module 4: Personal Care

Did you know that assisting a resident with personal care is a 24-hour-a-day job?

In this module, you will review information about assisting residents with personal care, and the importance of personal hygiene, individuality, and cultural differences when providing care.

Personal care is an ongoing, 24-hour-a-day process, beginning with A.M. or morning care to help a resident prepare for breakfast. Morning care gives residents the chance to wash their face and hands, brush their teeth, and go to the bathroom. Fresh drinking water is also given at this time, as well as any other care necessary to make the resident comfortable. A.M. care may be provided by the night or day shift, according to facility policy. Bathing is usually provided by the day shift or the evening shift based on the resident's personal preference. Other personal care skills provided by the day shift are oral hygiene, shaving, skin care, fingernail and toenail care, and hair care.

P.M. or evening care assists the resident to prepare for bed, provides comfort, and promotes sleep. The night shift makes sure the resident is kept clean, safe, and comfortable by changing linens as needed, toileting as needed, and answering call lights immediately to ensure residents get adequate rest. Personal care must be provided by the health care team on all shifts to meet the needs of all residents.

Review Questions

1. A.M. or morning care is done to help a resident prepare for ________________.

2. Bathing is one personal care skill. Other personal care skills provided by the day shift are oral hygiene, shaving, skin care, fingernail and ______________ care, and _________ care.

3. P.M. or evening care assists the resident to prepare for _________.

Answers: 1. breakfast, **2.** toenail, hair, **3.** bed

Complete Bed Bath

Did you know that a bath refreshes and relaxes the resident, gets rid of body odor, removes dirt, and reduces germs?

The complete bed bath involves the bathing of all body parts while the resident is in bed. The bath is important because it refreshes and relaxes the resident, gets rid of body odor, removes dirt, and reduces germs. Bathing a resident, or helping a resident bathe, gives you a chance to notice any physical or psychological changes in the resident. Residents should be bathed on a regular basis. The routine is based on the resident's preference, their level of independence, and the policy of the facility.

On some days, residents may get a partial bath, which involves washing the face, hands, underarms, back, and perineal area. A resident's cultural background may influence their bathing preferences. You should always ask the residents and their families about any special concerns. A back rub is included as part of the bath and P.M. care. A back rub increases circulation to the skin and can be very relaxing.

Some points to consider when giving a resident a bath are:

- Check water temperature. It should be warm to the touch.
- Always wash, rinse, and dry each body part individually to prevent exposure and chilling.
- Use soap sparingly and never leave it in the water. Soap removes natural oils from the skin and can cause drying and cracking. Change the water often during bathing.
- Check the skin for injuries or any changes in condition.
- Put on disposable gloves before giving perineal care to maintain infection control.
- Always wash the perineal area of a female resident from front to back to prevent infection. Be gentle and thorough when cleaning the perineal area.

Remember to review and practice Skill 8, "Giving a Complete Bed Bath," in Part 2.

Tub Bath and Shower

Did you know that a tub bath or shower may be the preferred way to bathe a resident?

Tub baths and showers are better than bed baths for bathing because they let the resident be more independent. Remember the following points when giving a resident a tub bath or shower:

- Maintain the resident's privacy by keeping them fully covered when taking them to the tub room or shower.
- Check the water temperature and always shut the hot water faucet off first, then the cold.
- Remember good body mechanics by keeping your back straight and your knees slightly bent as you help the resident in and out of the tub or shower.
- Never leave the resident alone.
- Be aware of how cultural issues may affect a resident's preferences about bathing.

Review Questions

1. The bath is a good time for the nurse assistant to observe both __________ and __________ changes in the resident.

2. A ________ ________ increases circulation to the skin and can be very relaxing.

3. When shutting off the water in the tub or shower, always shut the ________ water off first.

Answers: 1. physical and psychological, **2.** back rub, **3.** hot

Maintaining Skin Integrity

Do you know why decubitus ulcers form?

The condition of a resident's skin is an indication of the resident's health and a reflection of the nursing care being provided. Good skin care is a continuous process provided by all members of the nursing team.

Regularly checking a resident's skin while giving care and reporting any changes are key to keeping up skin integrity. If a resident's skin is not well cared for, the resident may develop decubitus ulcers (bedsores). Decubitus ulcers develop if the blood supply is reduced in any area of the body. The most common reasons are direct pressure and friction. Decubitus ulcers usually develop in areas where skin is thin, usually over a bone. These areas are sometimes called pressure point areas. Some of the most common pressure point areas are coccyx (tail bone), shoulders, hips, heels, elbows, ears, and ankles.

The following are some causes of decubitus ulcers and ways you can help to prevent them. If you think of others, make a note in the margin.

Cause	What You Can Do
Direct Pressure	Change the resident's position often. Observe and report immediately any reddened, pale, or darkened areas of resident's skin. Make sure resident is in good body alignment, using proper positioning devices. Use special protective devices that ease pressure and protect skin. Some examples of protective devices are air and water mattresses, egg crate mattress, heel and elbow protectors. Make tight, neat, wrinkle-free bed. Check the bed for personal belongings. Remove clips, bobby pins, and barrettes.

Cause	What You Can Do
Moisture	Wash, rinse, and dry skin thoroughly. Check incontinent patients frequently, at least every 2 hours.
Poor circulation	Give mild massaging, including good back and skin care, to promote circulation. Check skin often and report any signs of poor circulation, like change of color or temperature.

Review Questions

1. If a resident's skin is not well cared for, the resident is at risk of developing ____________ ________ or bedsores.

2. Decubitus ulcers usually develop in areas where the skin is thin, usually over a ________.

3. The nurse assistant should observe and report ______________ any reddened, pale or darkened areas of resident's skin.

Answers: 1. decubitus ulcers, 2. bone, 3. immediately

Oral Hygiene

Oral hygiene/mouth care is an important part of daily care and includes care of the mouth, teeth, gums, and tongue. Oral hygiene should be given every morning, every evening, and after every meal. As a nurse assistant, you give oral hygiene to both conscious and unconscious residents. Some important points to remember when giving oral hygiene:

Oral hygiene/mouth care is your responsibility. Mouth care includes brushing and flossing teeth, cleaning dentures, and cleaning the unconscious resident's mouth.

For infection control, you should wear gloves if there is a risk of coming in contact with the resident's blood. This may happen when flossing between the resident's teeth.

When brushing and flossing a resident's mouth, never put floss into the gumline. Gums are sensitive and easily cut. Never use full strength mouthwash because it can harm delicate gums.

Residents should be encouraged to wear dentures to assist in making speech clearer, improve self-image, and prevent gum shrinkage.

Dentures are very expensive and must be handled carefully to prevent any damage. The sink should be lined with a facecloth in case dentures are dropped. Never use hot water because it can change the shape of or warp the dentures. Always store dentures in a cup with enough water to cover them.

Unconscious residents need special mouth care. Their mouths may become dry, resulting in crust forming on their lips, mouth, tongue, and gums. Special mouth care must be given routinely, generally every 2 hours.

Unconscious residents cannot drink or swallow fluids. Therefore, position their heads to the side to prevent choking and aspiration.

Although the resident cannot speak, they may be able to hear. Always tell the resident what you are going to do.

Always report any of the following when providing oral hygiene:

- Dry, cracked, or swollen lips
- Bleeding, swelling, or redness of the gums
- Redness, swelling, sores or white patches in the mouth or on the tongue.

Remember to review and practice Skill 9, "Brushing and Flossing," Skill 10, "Denture Care," and Skill 11, "Mouth Care for the Unconscious Resident," in Part 2.

Review Questions

1. Oral hygiene/mouth care is an important part of __________ care.

2. Never use ________ water when cleaning resident's dentures because it can change the shape of or warp the dentures.

3. Unconscious residents need special ________ care.

Answers: **1.** daily, **2.** hot, **3.** mouth

Grooming

Did you know that having a clean, well-groomed appearance improves a resident's sense of well-being?

Grooming a resident includes brushing and combing their hair, shaving a male resident's face, cleaning feet and toenails, and trimming fingernails. An important part of a resident's self-image is how they look. A clean, well-groomed appearance improves a resident's sense of well-being. For this reason, residents should always be encouraged to brush and comb their own hair and to shave themselves. You should help them as needed. Ask them or a family member what their preferences are (how they wear their hair, what type of razor they use, or do they want to wear makeup, etc.). Remember the following key points:

- Shaving should only be done after talking with the charge nurse. Some residents may have bleeding problems.
- Never share the resident's razor with others.
- Be aware of cultural differences when helping with hair care.
- Never cut a resident's toenails.

Remember to review and practice Skill 12, "Brushing and Combing Hair;" Skill 13, "Shaving," Skill 14, "Cleaning and Trimming Fingernails;" and Skill 15, "Giving Foot Care and Cleaning Toenails," in Part 2.

Review Questions

1. A clean, well-groomed appearance improves a resident's sense of ________-__________.

2. __________ should only be done after discussion with the charge nurse.

3. The nurse assistant should never cut a resident's ____________.

Answers: 1. well-being, **2.** Shaving, **3.** toenails

Dressing and Undressing

Did you know that much of our identity (who we are) has to do with our dress?

Encouraging residents in nursing homes to dress in their own clothes every day helps them to keep their sense of identity. Letting residents choose their clothes helps them to keep control of their own lives. Remember the following points when dressing and undressing a resident:

Help select clothes based on the weather. Remember that elderly residents may need warmer clothes because they may have poor circulation and less body fat and may be less active than younger adults.

Encourage the residents to dress and undress themselves as much as possible to help them feel independent and in control.

If the resident has difficulty moving one side of their body or is paralyzed, take off clothing on the stronger or "good" side first and put on clothing on the weaker side first.

It may be easier to dress residents who need complete help while they are in bed.

Remember to review and practice Skill 16, "Dressing the Resident," and Skill 17, "Undressing the Resident," in Part 2.

Review Questions

1. When a resident is allowed to wear their own clothes, it helps to maintain their sense of __________.

2. Encouraging residents to dress and undress themselves as much as possible helps them feel ______________ and in control.

3. If a resident has difficulty with weakness or paralysis on one side of their body, take off clothes on the __________ side first.

Answers: 1. identity, **2.** independent, **3.** stronger (or "good")

Unit 3, Core Skills For Caring

Module 5: Nutrition

Did you know that aging affects food needs and eating habits?

Helping residents with nutrition is one of your important responsibilities. This module reviews the many parts of nutrition that you need to know: how aging affects our food needs and eating habits, special dietary needs, assisting residents at meal time, and assisting with food intake and waste output.

People must eat the right foods in the right amounts to be healthy. Eating the right kinds of foods is very important for residents in long-term care facilities because they may be weakened by illness and inactivity.

Here are some ways normal aging affects food needs and eating habits:

1. The number of calories needed by any person depends on age, sex, activity, climate, and health.

2. The elderly require fewer calories because they are less active.

3. The body's ability to absorb and use nutrients decreases as you age, so you may require more vitamins and minerals.

4. The sense of taste dulls, causing loss of appetite. It is important to offer food that looks, smells, and tastes good.

5. The loss of teeth and some diseases make it harder to chew and swallow food. An elderly person may need a longer time to eat than a younger person, or a special diet of foods that are easy to eat.

It is important to know the resident's food preferences, especially those based on religious preferences.

Review Questions

1. People must eat the right foods in the right

   ______________ to be healthy.

2. The loss of teeth and some diseases make it

   harder to _________ and ______________ food.

3. It is important to know the resident's food

   preferences, particularly those based on

   _________________ preferences.

Answers: 1. amounts, 2. chew, swallow, 3. religious

Special Dietary Needs and Tray Service

Did you know that another name for a special diet is a therapeutic diet?

Many long-term care residents require special diets because of physical disabilities or diseases. The special or therapeutic diets below are commonly served in long-term care facilities:

- Mechanical, soft, or puree I or II diet. This diet meets a resident's daily nutritional needs but is easier to chew, swallow, and digest than regular diets.

- Clear-liquid diet. This diet may be ordered for one or two days for residents who have a short-term illness, such as flu, where vomiting occurs and digestion is poor. This diet does not provide adequate nutrition because it contains only clear liquids such as broth and jello; juices such as apple, grape, and cranberry; carbonated beverages; and tea. It must be re-ordered by the physician every 48 hours.

- Full-liquid diet. This diet may be ordered for one or two days when a resident has an illness, such as flu, causing a digestive problem. This diet does not provide adequate nutrition because it contains only foods such as ice cream, milk, custards, cooked cereal, and pudding. It must be re-ordered by the physician every 48 hours.

- NAS (no added salt) or 2-gram sodium diet. This diet provides adequate nutrition but limits foods that are high in salt or sodium, such as ham, cheese, canned soups, potato chips, lunch meat, and pickles. Foods are made without using salt, and residents are not allowed to use table salt. The doctor may allow salt substitutes.

- Diets with 1200, 1500, 1800, and 2000 calories. These diets are ordered for residents who have diabetes mellitus or who need to lose weight.

- High-protein diet. This diet is sometimes ordered for residents who have not been eating enough or who need additional protein to build skin or organ tissues. This diet is often ordered for residents with decubitus ulcers.

Review Questions

1. Special or ____________________ diets are commonly served in long-term care facilities.
2. Full liquid diets may be ordered for one or two days when a resident has an ______________.
3. A low _____________ diet limits foods that are high in salt or sodium.

Answers: 1. therapeutic, **2.** illness, **3.** sodium

Did you know that if you don't serve meal trays promptly, food may spoil?

Here are some important things to remember when serving meals to residents:

1. Make meal time pleasant by keeping the atmosphere as cheerful and comfortable as possible and providing adequate lighting.
2. Help the resident to be in a good position for chewing and swallowing.
3. Allow adequate time to get a resident ready for a meal before the trays are served. Always encourage residents to go to the bathroom and wash their hands before a meal.

4. Always check the diet card for resident's name, room number, diet order, food and beverage preferences, allergies, and eating location and make sure all are correct before serving.

5. Serve trays promptly after they arrive from the kitchen to make sure that hot food stays hot and cold food stays cold. Some foods spoil quickly if allowed to stand at room temperature.

6. If a resident is on a therapeutic diet, check with the dietary department or charge nurse before serving any tray. Never give any resident sugar, salt, or butter if it is not included on the tray without checking with the charge nurse.

7. Check tray for any foods listed under allergies or dislikes. If any of these things are on the resident's tray, report to the charge nurse before serving.

8. Never mix pureed foods together.

9. Report to charge nurse any food not eaten by a resident so that a substitute may be offered.

10. Watch residents during meal times to make sure they do not need assistance with eating. Often residents will leave part of a meal because they get too tired to finish feeding themselves. If this happens, you may need to assist the resident to eat more or provide a snack later.

Review Questions

1. Make meal time pleasant by keeping the atmosphere as cheerful and ______________ as possible and providing adequate lighting.

2. Serve trays promptly to make sure that hot food stays hot and cold foods stay _________ .

3. Never give a resident sugar, salt or butter if it is not on the tray without checking with the _____________ _____________.

Answers: 1. comfortable, **2.** cold, **3.** charge nurse

Did you know that the resident may want to eat their food in a certain order?

Sometimes residents need assistance with their meals. When you are helping a resident eat, remember these important points:

- Provide protective covering for the resident's clothing.
- Prepare the food (e.g., cut meat, pour coffee, butter bread, etc.) while talking with the resident about what food is being served. Ask residents if they want to eat their food in a certain order and if they want any seasoning.

- Encourage the resident to feed themselves finger food (bread, cookies, etc.).

- Feed the resident small bites from a spoon, naming each food as you offer it. Allow time between bites for the resident to chew and swallow. Offer liquids between swallows, being careful these liquids are not too hot. Offer food substitutes if needed.

- Wipe the resident's mouth with a napkin after each bite, as needed.

Review Questions

1. Prepare the food while ______________ with the resident about what food is being served.

2. Encourage the resident to feed themselves __________________ food.

3. Slowly feed the resident small bites from a spoon, ____________________ each food as you offer it.

Answers: **1.** talking, **2.** finger, **3.** naming

Assisting With Intake and Output

Did you know that if a resident does not get enough fluid, they may become dehydrated?

Most people need about 1,500-2,000 cc ml (about 1-1/2 to 2 quarts) of liquid each day. Liquids can be anything we drink—water, coffee, juice, milk, soup, etc.—or anything that becomes liquid at room temperature—ice cream, sherbet, or jello. Throughout the day, we must replace liquid that our bodies lose in urine, perspiration, bowel movements, and even talking or breathing. If we perspire a lot, vomit, or have diarrhea, it is especially important to replace these fluids.

Be alert for signs that a resident is not drinking enough fluids. Without enough fluids, residents may become dehydrated. Remember the symptoms of dehydration:

- Confusion
- Constipation
- Drowsiness
- Very dry skin

Dehydration is a very serious condition and should be reported to your charge nurse right away. Here are some ways you can encourage residents to drink the amount of liquids they need:

- Offer liquids that the resident likes.

- Give the resident a pitcher of clean, fresh water every shift, and urge the resident to drink some every time you enter the room.

- Make sure the resident has a clean tumbler or drinking cup within reach. Refill the cup as needed if the resident is unable to do it. Supply a drinking straw if needed.

Review Questions

1. Most people need about __________ to __________ cc of liquid each day.

2. If we perspire a lot, vomit, or have diarrhea, it is especially important to __________ these fluids.

3. Symptoms of dehydration are ______________, __________________, _________________ and very dry _________.

Answers: 1. 1,500, 2,000, **2.** replace, **3.** confusion, constipation, drowsiness, skin

Did you know that a change in a resident's weight may be due to a fluid problem?

Because of special problems, many residents may need an accurate daily record of how much liquid they take in and put out. Accuracy is extremely important in measuring intake and output.

If a resident must have intake and output measured, an "I" and "O" worksheet will be posted on their door or bed.

When keeping track of the fluid intake and output, the resident will also need to be weighed. Some points to remember are:

- Always weigh the resident at the same time of day, since weight can vary at different times of day.

- Always weigh the resident on the same scale, since scale accuracy can vary.
- Always weigh the resident with as little clothing on as possible. If the resident is wearing a brace or artificial limb, try to subtract the weight of these things or record that these things were worn.
- Report any weight loss or gain to the charge nurse.

Not all nursing homes use the same kinds of scales. Some have platform or chair scales to weigh residents in chairs or wheelchairs. Some may have bed scales that allow residents who cannot sit up to be weighed.

If the resident is in a chair, subtract the chair weight from the total weight.

Review Questions

1. ________________ is extremely important in measuring intake and output.

2. Always weigh the resident at the same time of _______.

3. Report any weight loss or __________ to the charge nurse.

Answers: 1. Accuracy, **2.** day, **3.** gain

Unit 3, Core Skills for Caring

Module 6: Elimination

Do you know how to determine the resident's normal elimination pattern?

Eliminating waste from our bodies through urine and fecal material is a natural and normal process. In our society, however, we view elimination as a very personal matter that we are often embarrassed to talk about. It is so private that sometimes we are unable to void or defecate when we are in the presence of someone else. One of your responsibilities is to help residents with daily elimination while respecting their privacy.

What is considered normal elimination is different for every individual. Nurse assistants must learn residents' elimination patterns. This can be done by asking the resident at the time of admission, charting, and routinely checking patterns.

Any change in elimination patterns is important and must be reported to the charge nurse. Remember, it is the change that is most important, so knowing what is normal is the first step.

When helping residents with elimination, remember:

1. Never leave a resident on a bedpan or urinal for more than 5 minutes without checking on them. Pressure sores can develop if they are left longer.

2. Return to the room when the resident signals. If the resident cannot signal, check on them at least every 5 minutes.

3. Help the resident clean and wipe themselves as necessary. Always clean from front to back. Provide perineal care as necessary.

4. Maintain infection control. Wash your hands.

Remember to review and practice Skill 18, "Assisting with a Bedpan or Urinal," in Part 2.

Review Questions

1. Any ______________ in elimination patterns is significant and must be ______________ to the charge nurse.

2. Never leave a resident on a bedpan for more than ______ minutes without checking on them.

3. Maintain infection control by washing __________ ______________.

Answers: 1. change, reported, 2. 5, 3. your hands

Special Urinary Elimination Needs

Do you know the most common problems of the urinary system?

Elderly residents often have urinary problems because of the changes that occur in the urinary system with age. The most common problems are incontinence and urinary tract infections. It is important for you to understand these problems and to assist in providing good care to the resident.

Urinary incontinence is not a normal process of aging. It may, however, be a common problem in a long-term care facility.

Incontinence is the inability to control passage of urine or feces (bowel movement).

The factors that can lead to incontinence are:

- Damage to the brain that keeps the individual from feeling the urge to urinate
- Weakness of sphincter muscles (those muscles that surround the opening of the bladder and help hold urine in the bladder)
- Medications
- Confusion about where to go to the bathroom
- Difficulty in moving, making it hard to get to the bathroom
- Not having a call light answered immediately

Your support and encouragement are extremely important in helping a resident with bladder control problems. The ways that you can assist include:

- Respond quickly to the resident's elimination needs.
- Offer the resident fluids often throughout the day. Less fluid intake will only increase the problem of incontinence. Drinking less fluids may cause dribbling and urinary tract infection.
- Help the resident who has trouble getting up or walking get to the bathroom
- Offer the resident frequent chances to go to the bathroom (particularly confused residents).
- Learn your resident's pattern of voiding to determine how often you should offer assistance in voiding. (For some, their regular pattern may be every hour; for others, every 2 to 4 hours.)
- Be sensitive to the embarrassment a resident may feel about wearing adult briefs to protect their clothing. (Never refer to the briefs as diapers.)

When you are assisting a resident with bladder control problems, always be alert for these signs of a urinary tract infection (UTI):

- Complaints of pain and a burning sensation when urinating
- Increased urges to urinate but little urine produced
- Cloudy, concentrated (dark yellow), and possibly foul-smelling urine
- Milky, mucous shreds in urine

Any of these signs should be reported to the charge nurse. A UTI occurs more often in females due to their short urethra.

When you are caring for a resident with a urinary tract infection; it is important to:

- Offer fluids frequently.
- Allow residents time to completely empty their bladder when toileted.
- Always wipe from front to back when giving perineal care.
- Change adult briefs on incontinent residents often.

Review Questions

1. ________________ means the resident is unable to control passage of urine or bowel movement.

2. Confusion about where to go to the bathroom can lead to ________________.

3. Complaints of pain and a burning sensation when urinating are symptoms of a ________________ ________________ ____________________.

Answers: 1. Incontinence, **2.** incontinence, **3.** urinary tract infection

Sometimes a resident may need an indwelling catheter or tube inserted into the bladder to drain urine from the bladder. A small balloon around the tip of the catheter is blown up to hold the catheter in place. The catheter is attached to a drainage bag to collect the urine. The chance of getting a urinary tract infection is greater when an indwelling catheter is used, so it is used only when it is absolutely necessary. A catheter may be used if the resident has:

- Nerve damage following a stroke
- Spinal cord injury
- Incontinence and is prone to skin breakdown

When you are caring for a catheterized resident, be sure to:

- Offer the resident fluids frequently throughout the day.
- Keep the urinary drainage flow going.
- Protect the resident from injury.
- Give good perineal care.
- See that there are no kinks in the catheter tubing and drainage tubing.
- Position the drainage bag below the level of the bladder to prevent urine from flowing back through the tubing into the bladder.
- Never allow the tubing or drainage bag to touch the floor.
- Move the drainage bag before moving the resident to a chair.

Review Questions

1. An indwelling catheter is a tube inserted into the

   __________ to drain __________.

2. When caring for a resident with a catheter it is

   important to provide good __________ care.

3. Be sure there are no ________ in the catheter

   tubing and drainage tubing.

Answers: 1. bladder, urine 2. perineal, 3. kinks

Special Bowel Elimination Needs

Do you know what information about a resident's bowel movements should be reported?

The bowel is the most important organ for eliminating solid waste products. Solid wastes, also known as feces or stools, are normally brown in color, soft, and formed. Stools are about three-fourths water and one-fourth solid waste products.

The pattern of bowel elimination varies from person to person. Some people have a bowel movement every day and others every two to three days.

Be aware that a change in routine (new environment, illness, medication) can disrupt a person's normal elimination pattern. You should always record a resident's pattern of bowel elimination, including the color, amount, consistency, and odor of the bowel movement. You should tell the charge nurse about any changes.

You can help a resident keep normal bowel elimination. Refer to the list for keeping urinary elimination normal. In addition to this list, remember these important points about elimination:

Report if the resident's appetite has changed. Appetite can be affected by a change in behavior, depression, loneliness, change in bowel habits, nausea, and vomiting.

If the bowel is not emptied regularly of its waste materials, constipation will occur. If constipation is not relieved, stool remains in the rectum too long and fecal impaction can occur.

The resident with constipation may have pain, discomfort, abdominal swelling, and a mucus and water discharge that looks like diarrhea. This occurs because liquid stool is oozing around the hard stool.

The resident with fecal impaction may need an enema or manual removal of stool by the charge nurse. The manual removal is called disimpaction. A nurse assistant does not do disimpaction.

Diarrhea is frequent passage of liquid stools. Continued diarrhea may dehydrate the resident and lead to fluid imbalance and confusion.

Diarrhea may be caused by an infection, a virus, or poor nutritional habits.

Any occurrence of diarrhea should be reported to the charge nurse. Diarrhea can be very contagious. Therefore, principles of infection control must be practiced when handling diarrhea. You can help the resident by:

- Understanding the discomfort associated with diarrhea
- Responding immediately to the call light
- Putting a commode by the bedside
- Offering clear liquids
- Giving good skin care
- A room deodorizer may be needed.

Review Questions

1. A __________ in routine can disrupt a person's normal elimination pattern.

2. If stool remains in the rectum too long, fecal __________ can occur.

3. Diarrhea is __________ passage of liquid stools.

Answers: 1. change, 2. impaction, 3. frequent

Bowel Incontinence

Do you know the causes of bowel incontinence?

Bowel incontinence is not a normal process of aging. Like urinary incontinence, however, it may be a problem to some residents in long-term care.

The following factors can cause incontinence:

- Damage to the brain that keeps the individual from feeling the urge to have a bowel movement
- Limited mobility that makes it hard to get to the bathroom
- Not having the call light answered immediately
- Weakness of anal sphincter muscle (the muscle around the opening of the anus that helps hold the stool in the rectum)

- Medications
- Confusion about where to go to the bathroom
- Diarrhea
- Fecal impaction

You can support an incontinent resident in many ways:

- Respond quickly to the resident's elimination needs.
- Offer the resident fluids frequently throughout the day. Less fluid intake will only make the problem of incontinence worse. Less fluids may cause stool to harden and become an impaction.
- Help the resident who has trouble rising or walking to the bathroom.
- Offer the resident frequent chances to go to the bathroom (particularly confused residents).
- Learn your resident's pattern of defecating to determine how often you should offer assistance. For some, their regular pattern may be daily; for others, every 2 or 3 days.
- Treat each resident based on their individual needs.
- Be sensitive to the embarrassment a resident may feel about wearing adult briefs to protect their clothing. (Never refer to the briefs as diapers.)
- Offer the resident emotional support and encouragement.

Review Questions

1. Bowel incontinence may be a problem to _________ residents in long-term care.

2. Not having the call light answered immediately is a factor that can cause ________________________.

3. Confusion about where to go to the _______________ can lead to bowel incontinence.

Answers: 1. some, **2.** incontinence, **3.** bathroom

Unit 3, Core Skills for Caring

Module 7: Vital Signs

Did you know that vital signs are a measurement of life?

Temperature, pulse, respiration, and blood pressure, abbreviated TPR/BP, are called vital signs. Vital signs are measurements of life. Vital signs tell you if the body is working right. Measuring vital signs is the most common skill used to get important information about a resident's condition. This information often helps decide what treatment or medication the resident may need. Vital signs can give you important information about the resident. Remember, it is your job to measure vital signs accurately and report even the slightest change to the charge nurse.

Taking a Temperature

Do you know the three ways to take a resident's temperature?

Temperature is the measurement that indicates the amount of heat in the body.

Body temperature can be measured three ways—oral, rectal, and axillary. The way temperature is measured depends on a person's condition.

Normal body temperature ranges are:

- Oral—from 97.6 to 99.6 degrees (average = 98.6); can be read in 5 to 7 minutes

- Rectal—from 98.6 to 100.6 degrees (average = 99.6); can be read in 3 to 5 minutes

- Axillary—from 96.6 to 98.6 degrees (average 97.6); can be read in 10 minutes

If body temperature goes higher than normal, it is usually because illness has caused a fever. The common signs of fever are:

- Warm, dry skin
- Chills
- Loss of appetite
- Tired feeling
- Confusion

When taking an oral temperature with a glass thermometer, remember these key points:

- Never take an oral temperature if a resident:

  Has had recent mouth surgery or has mouth disease
  Is getting oxygen
  Is short of breath or having trouble breathing
  Is confused or unconscious
  Is paralyzed on one side of the body/face
  Can only breathe through their mouth

- Put the thermometer under the resident's tongue and slightly to one side.

Remember to review and practice Skill 19, "Taking an Oral Temperature with a Glass Themometer," in Part 2.

- Keep the thermometer in the resident's mouth for at least 5 minutes.

When taking a rectal temperature with a glass thermometer, remember these key points (the use of gloves is optional, depending on facility policy):

- Never take a rectal temperature if the resident has:

  Diarrhea
  A blocked rectum
  Had a recent heart attack
  Had recent rectal surgery or injury
  Has hemorrhoids

- Never put the rectal thermometer in more than 1 inch.
- Never leave a resident alone or let go of the thermometer when taking a rectal temperature.
- Assist the resident to lie on one side with their back toward you. Leave side rail down on side you will be working.
- Hold the lubricated thermometer in place for at least 3 minutes.
- Gently take out the thermometer; clean anal area with tissue and take off thermometer sheath. Throw the tissue and sheath away in disposable bag.

Remember to review and practice Skill 20, "Taking a Rectal Temperature with a Glass Thermometer," in Part 2.

Review Questions

1. There are three ways that body temperature can be measured: ________, ________, ________.

2. Never take an oral temperature if a resident is short of ________ or having trouble breathing.

3. Keep the thermometer in the resident's mouth for at least ________ minutes.

Answers: 1. oral, rectal, axillary, **2.** breath, **3.** 5

Counting a Pulse

Do you know the six most common places to count the resident's pulse?

A pulse is the beat of the heart that is felt at an artery as the blood passes through. A normal pulse rate for an adult is between 60 and 84 beats per minute. A pulse may be regular or irregular, strong (full, bounding) or weak (thready).

The six most common places where a pulse can be felt and counted are:

- Temporal pulse is located on each side of the forehead above the outer corner of the eye.
- Carotid pulse is located in the neck on each side of the Adam's apple.
- Brachial pulse is located at the bend of the elbow and is usually used for taking blood pressure.

- Radial pulse is located on the inside of the wrist at the top of the thumb.
- Femoral pulse is located inside the groin area where the thigh connects with the hip.
- Pedal pulse is located on the top of each foot.

When taking a radial pulse, remember these key points:

- Gently press your first, second, and third fingers over the radial pulse. Never use your thumb, because your thumb has its own pulse.
- Using the second hand on your watch, count the number of beats for 1 minute.
- While you count the pulse rate, note the rhythm and force.
- Write down the pulse rate.

Remember to review and practice Skill 21, "Counting a Radial Pulse," in Part 2.

Review Questions

1. A normal ___Pulse___ rate for an adult is between 60 and 80 beats per minute.

2. The ___radial___ pulse is located on the inside of the wrist at the top of the thumb.

3. Gently press your ___first___, ___Second___, and ___Third___ fingers over the radial pulse.

Answers: 1. pulse, **2.** radial, **3.** first, second, third

Counting Respiration

Do you know the average respiration rate for adults?

One respiration includes breathing in and breathing out. Normal respiration is quiet and easy. Like pulse, it can be regular or irregular. It can also be deep or shallow. Normal respiration rate for an adult is between 14 and 20 times per minute.

You will usually count respiration right after you have counted pulse rate. While you count respiration, you should watch how the resident's chest moves. If a large amount of air is inhaled, it is called deep breathing; a small amount of air inhaled is called shallow breathing. You may notice the following breathing problems:

- Shallow, noisy, or irregular breathing.
- Shortness of breath (dyspnea).
- Bluish or pale color (cyanosis) of lips, skin, nails.

Any breathing problems should be reported immediately to the charge nurse. When counting respiration, remember these key points:

- Count respiration by watching the rise and fall of the resident's chest.
- Use the second hand on your watch, and count respiration for 1 minute.
- Write down the respiration rate.

Remember to review and practice Skill 22, "Counting Respiration," in Part 2.

Review Questions

1. Normal respiration is quiet and _________.
2. If a large amount of air is inhaled, this is called _________ breathing; a small amount of air inhaled is called _________ breathing.
3. Count respiration by watching the _________ and _________ of the resident's chest.

Answers: 1. easy, 2. deep, shallow, 3. rise, fall

Taking Blood Pressure

Do you know what a normal blood pressure reading is?

Blood pressure is the force that blood exerts as it travels through the body.

Measuring blood pressure is very important because it gives the health care team information about the condition of a resident's circulatory system. Treatment and medication are often changed based on blood pressure readings.

When the heart pumps (contracts), it forces blood out into the arteries. The amount of pressure exerted at this time is called systolic pressure. When the heart rests (not pumping), there is still pressure in the arteries. This pressure is called diastolic pressure. Together, systolic and diastolic pressure give a blood pressure reading. Blood pressure readings are written like fractions. The systolic reading is the top number, and the diastolic reading is the bottom number.

Everybody has a blood pressure range that is normal for them. A systolic reading between 90 and 139 is considered normal, and a diastolic reading between 60 and 89 is considered normal.

Many factors influence blood pressure: for example, diet, weight, sex, lack of exercise, smoking, national origin, family history, age, stress, alcohol, and diseases.

Any increase or decrease in a resident's blood pressure should be reported to the charge nurse.

When taking blood pressure, remember these key points:

- Never put a cuff on an arm with a cast.
- Never put a cuff on an arm with an IV (intravenous infusion) in place.
- Never put a cuff on the arm on the side where the resident has had a mastectomy (breast removal).
- Never put a cuff on an arm immediately following venipuncture (drawing blood for testing).
- Avoid putting cuff on the weak arm if resident has had a stroke.

To measure blood pressure, you need to listen for the first pulse which is the systolic pressure; you then listen for the last pulse, or the change in sound, which is the diastolic pressure.

The American Red Cross recommends taking blood pressure using the palpalatory and ausculatory method. This method of instruction is used in the American Red Cross Nurse Assistant Training Course as well as in other Red Cross Programs. If you are interested in information and an explanation of this technique, consult your local American Red Cross.

Remember to review and practice Skill 23, "Taking Blood Pressure," in Part 2.

Review Questions

1. The force that blood exerts as it travels through the body is called __________ ______________.

2. The systolic reading is the ________ number, and the diastolic reading is the ___________ number.

3. The reading when you first hear the pulse sound is the ____________ pressure; the reading when the pulse sound stops or changes is the _____________ pressure.

Answers: 1. blood pressure, **2.** top, bottom, **3.** systolic, diastolic

Unit 4: Special Skills For Caring

Sometimes special skills are needed when caring for residents. This unit reviews how to provide care and give encouragement to residents with special needs. Again, as you review this unit, remember the foundation for caring, particularly the six principles of care.

The three modules review how you can modify care for residents with certain diseases, how you can help residents who are dying, and how you can help residents learn to do things again for themselves.

Unit 4, Special Skills For Caring

Module 1: Modifying Care

Did you know that how you treat residents with special needs can make a difference in how well they recover?

In this unit, you will learn about some of the most common diseases and disabilities the residents in long-term care facilities may have and how to modify or change the care for these residents.

Only the most common diseases are discussed. You may need to refer to Unit II, Module 2, "The Human Body and the Process of Aging," as you review the material on modifying care. These changes may be as simple as giving residents more time to do tasks, such as brushing their hair or walking, or as complicated as working with a resident on reality orientation. The way you treat residents with special needs can make an important difference in how much residents recover from their conditions, or how well they cope with their limitations.

Sensory System

Do you know some of the characteristics of cataracts?

A *cataract* is a clouding of the lens of the eye that causes a gradual loss of sight. Some of the characteristics of cataracts are:

- Distorted sight
- Blurred sight

Some ways you can modify or change care are:

- Stand where the resident can see you.
- If a resident must be fed, describe the food being given in each bite and the temperature of the food.
- When serving food, describe the items on the tray by their place using time on a clock to explain where they are on the tray.
- Remove hot drinks from the tray and serve them separately.
- When helping residents walk, let them hold your arm just above the elbow for support.
- Describe people, places, or events in a way that will help the person picture them.

Review Questions

1. A cataract is a ____________ of the lens of the eye.

2. When serving food, ____________ the items on the tray by their place using a ____________ to explain where they are.

3. Describe people, ____________, or events in a way that will help the person picture them.

Answers: 1. clouding, 2. describe, clock, 3. places

Musculoskeletal System

Did you know that arthritis causes stiffness in joints?

Arthritis is a disease that causes joints to swell. Over many years the tissue around the joints wears away, causing painful friction between bones when they are moved. The remaining tissue around the joint swells, causing stiffness.

Some of the characteristics of arthritis are:

- Stiffness in joints, especially hips and knees
- Pain when moving joints
- Tender and swollen joints
- Depression from not being able to move without pain and thus losing some independence

Some examples of ways you can modify care are:

- Let the resident know that you understand how painful it is for them to move and that you are there to help.
- Plan daily morning care after pain medication has been given.
- Give warm tub baths often.
- Do gentle range of motion exercises to prevent contractures and strengthen muscles.
- Handle joints carefully and support them when moving the resident.
- Always be aware of joints that hurt when helping the resident dress or undress.
- Encourage the resident to exercise those hurting joints on their own.

Did you know that a resident with osteoporosis may have a fear of falling when walking?

Osteoporosis is a disease in which bones become weak and brittle due to a slow loss of minerals, especially calcium.

Some of the characteristics of osteoporosis are:

- Complaints of aching pain, especially in the back
- Rounded or stooped back
- Decreased height
- Fatigue (tired easily)
- Fear of falling when walking
- Depression or irritability due to health change

Some of the ways you can modify care are:

- Use a safety belt when helping a resident to move or walk. *Caution*: Use belt very carefully; remember that the resident's bones are weak.

- Use assistive and prosthetic devices to support resident in activities.

- Encourage the resident to use good posture.

- Assist resident in choosing clothes that do not show off posture changes.

- Encourage the resident to eat their meals.

- Report any changes in the resident's eating habits.

Review Questions

1. Arthritis is a disease that causes joints to become

   ____________________.

2. One way you can help residents with arthritis is by

   giving warm __________ ____________ often.

3. Osteoporosis is a disease in which ____________

   become weak and brittle.

Answers: 1. swollen, **2.** tub baths, **3.** bones

Endocrine System

Did you know that good foot care is important for residents with diabetes?

Diabetes mellitus occurs when the body is not making enough insulin to help it break down, store, and use carbohydrates for energy. There is no cure for diabetes, but it sometimes can be controlled through diet, exercise, and medication used to increase the body's production of insulin. In some cases, people may take insulin injections.

A diabetic needs a special diet, usually one that is low in simple sugars and fats. It is important for a diabetic to eat only foods that have been prepared for them. A diabetic should not have candy, cookies, or other sweets.

Changes in blood vessels that limit blood circulation lead to the complications of diabetes. The complications include poor vision, poor circulation in feet and hands, and even blindness.

Hypoglycemia (too little sugar in the blood) and hyperglycemia (too much sugar in the blood) are two very serious conditions that can go along with diabetes. The charge nurse should be told immediately if there are any physical or psychological changes in the resident.

Some of the ways you can modify care are:

- Provide good skin care to prevent pressure sores.

- Provide good foot care.

- Always make sure the resident has clean socks and wears shoes that fit well.

- Tell the charge nurse when the resident's toenails need to be cut.

- Tell the charge nurse if the resident is not eating or is eating food brought in by friends or relatives.

- Report any unusual amount of exercise, activity, or stress in the resident's life.

- Make sure urine testing for sugar and acetone is done accurately and on time. This test is done to find out how well the body is using sugar; therefore, it is extremely important to do the test on a fresh specimen of urine.

- Encourage the resident to take part in exercise and recreation programs.

Review Questions

1. A diabetic needs a special _________, usually one low in simple sugars and fats.

2. The complications of diabetes include poor ___________, poor _______________ in feet and hands, and even __________________.

3. Provide good skin care to prevent _____________ _________.

Answers: **1.** diet, **2.** vision, circulation, blindness
3. pressure sores

Nervous System

Did you know that a resident may not be able to feel pain in body areas that are paralyzed?

A brain or spinal cord injury can damage the nervous system and cause paralysis or a loss of the ability to move parts of the body. Paralysis can affect one side of the body (hemiplegia), two legs and the lower trunk (paraplegia), or both arms, both legs, and the lower trunk (quadriplegia), depending on where the spinal cord or brain was hurt and how badly.

Hemiplegia is the most common condition and is caused by a stroke. If damage has occurred on the right side of the brain, the left side of the body will be affected. If damage has occurred on the left side of the brain, the right side of the body will be affected.

Some of the ways you can modify care are:

- Supervise residents while they eat. Always put food in the side of the mouth that is not affected and make sure no food is left in their mouth after a meal is over.
- Keep the resident's face clean and dry. Use protective skin cream.
- Supervise residents while they shave.
- Help the resident with walking.

For *paraplegia* and *quadriplegia,* the amount of paralysis depends on where the spinal cord has been injured. An injury in the lower back or waist area will result in paraplegia. An injury in the neck or upper back will result in quadriplegia.

Some of the ways you can modify care are:

- Provide good skin care to prevent pressure sores.
- Be aware that the resident cannot feel pain, temperature, or parts of their own bodies.
- Encourage residents to use any assistive devices they have for eating or walking.

Review Questions

1. For paraplegia and quadriplegia, the amount of paralysis depends on where the ____________ _________ has been injured.

2. An injury in the lower back or waist will result in ____________________.

3. Encourage residents to use any _______________ devices they have for eating or walking.

Answers: 1. spinal cord, **2.** paraplegia, **3.** assistive

Did you know that a resident with Alzheimer's disease may not remember things from one minute to the next?

Alzheimer's disease is a brain disease in which nerve cells in the outer layer of the brain die. A resident with Alzheimer's may not remember things from one minute to the next, and has a short attention span. For this reason, caring for a resident with Alzheimer's may be one of your biggest challenges.

The normal sense of loss felt by an older person when coming to live at a nursing home is even greater when the person is suffering from memory loss. A confused resident feels less secure and is less trusting of people. The way you treat a confused resident, however, can make a difference in how quickly the person gets better or, in the case of someone who cannot be cured, in how hopeful the person feels about life.

Some of the ways you can modify care are:

- Have the same people give care each day—preferably, as few people as possible.
- Have a routine for care that is followed every day.
- Keep the person's environment quiet.
- Supervise confused residents closely because they may wander out of the home and not remember how to get back.
- Do not change the resident's room or bed position in the room.
- Show the person things to help them know where they are.
- Always speak calmly and slowly.
- Give short, simple directions, and when possible, show the person what you are asking them to do.
- Repeat directions often, in a firm but gentle voice.

Review Questions

1. A resident with ________________ may not remember things from one minute to the next.

2. Establish a ______________ for care that is followed every day.

3. Always speak ___________ and ___________.

Answers: 1. Alzheimer's, **2.** routine, **3.** calmly, slowly

---

Did you know that exercise can often delay the progress of Parkinson's disease?

Parkinson's disease is a common neurological disorder of older people. In Parkinson's disease, the parts of the brain that control movement are slowly destroyed. A person with Parkinson's disease has stiff muscles, moves very slowly, and has muscle tremors. As the disease gets worse, greater physical effort is needed to do even the smallest task, and the person easily becomes tired and frustrated. The disease usually appears when a person is in their fifties or sixties. The cause is unknown.

Keeping the resident active in exercise and recreation programs can often delay the progress of the disease. Helping the resident to remain as independent as possible is important in how well a resident copes with the disease.

Some of the characteristics of Parkinson's disease are:

- Muscle tremors
- Muscle weakness
- Shuffling feet
- Difficulty chewing and swallowing
- Poor balance (frequent falls)
- Constipation
- Confusion

Some of the ways you can modify care are:

- Let the resident rest often to keep them from getting too tired or frustrated.
- Do not rush the resident.
- Give warm tub baths and massages to help relax muscles and reduce muscle spasms.
- Encourage the resident to use assistive devices for activities of daily living.
- Encourage the residents to turn themselves in bed and to get in and out of bed by using the bed rails or other aids.
- Encourage the resident to take part in exercise and recreational activities.
- Make sure the resident sits upright while eating.

Review Questions

1. In ______________ __________ the parts of the brain that control movement are slowly destroyed.

2. A person with Parkinson's disease has stiff ____________, moves very slowly and has muscle ____________.

3. Allow the resident to ________ often to prevent them from getting too __________ or frustrated.

Answers: 1. Parkinson's disease, **2.** muscles, tremors, **3.** rest, tired

---

Did you know that mentally retarded residents need an environment where they can learn, grow, and make choices about their life?

Mental retardation results from brain damage and limits a person's ability to learn and act independently. It can range from mild to very severe. Like all other people, mentally retarded residents need an environment where they can learn, grow, and make choices about their life in order to thrive as human beings.

Some of the characteristics of mental retardation are:

- Compared with other people their age, a person who is mentally retarded is more limited in what they can learn, how fast they can learn, and how independent they can be.
- The person may also have a speech problem and/or physical handicaps.
- In a supportive environment, the mildly retarded can usually learn to take care of themselves.
- Moderately retarded residents will take much longer to learn things and need help caring for themselves.
- A person who is severely retarded will be totally dependent on others for care.

Some of the ways you can modify care are:

- Act as an assistant or associate, not as a parent.
- Encourage the resident to make choices about their lives.
- When grooming and dressing mentally retarded residents, treat them the same as any other resident.
- Encourage the resident to take part in social and recreational activities.

Review Questions

1. Mental retardation is a limited ability to learn and act ______________.
2. Compared with other people their age, a person who is mentally retarded is more limited in what they can__________.
3. Encourage the resident to ________ __________ about their lives.

Answers: 1. independently, **2.** learn, **3.** make choices

Did you know that mental illness causes a person to have problems with feelings, thoughts, and behaviors?

Mental illness causes a person to have problems with feelings, thoughts, and behaviors. The person will have trouble thinking clearly and/or realistically, and they may act differently than people usually act in a given situation.

Some of the ways you can modify care are:

- When residents are talking, let them know that you care and are listening to what they are saying.
- Let the residents know that you understand what they have said, or what they are feeling.
- Try to help residents focus on positive things about themselves.
- Talk to residents about familiar objects, people, or events that are important to them to help them keep track of reality—the season, time, place, and people around them.
- If a resident ever becomes loud, angry, or abusive, try to keep your voice calm and your body relaxed. Also, if the person is especially sensitive about other people getting too close, give the person space so they do not to feel threatened.
- Be consistent.
- Keep familiar objects close by and avoid changing the resident's room or bed position in the room.
- Introduce change slowly.
- Help the resident keep a routine of meals, medications, personal care, and activities.
- If a resident ever appears likely to hit someone or become violent, get help to handle the situation. Observe safety precautions by clearing the area, keeping distance and objects between you and the resident, and removing sharp instruments.

Review Questions

1. Mental illness causes a person to have problems with feelings, thoughts and ________________.

2. Talk to residents about familiar objects, __________, or events that are important to them.

3. Help the resident keep a _____________ of meals, medications, personal care, and activities.

Answers: **1.** behaviors, **2.** people, **3.** routine

Unit 4, Special Skills For Caring

Module 2: Death and Dying

Did you know that you, as a nurse assistant, can help the resident come to the end of their life with peace and dignity?

Many people, especially if they are young and healthy, have some fear or feel uncomfortable when talking about death or being with people who are dying. Older people may also fear death. These feelings are normal. Nurse assistants are often the people in a long-term care facility who know a dying resident best. Residents may feel closer to you than to anyone else. Therefore, you have a personal as well as a professional responsibility to care for the dying resident. It is a special privilege to be able to help a resident come to the end of life with peace and dignity and a feeling that someone cares. Often a dying resident has no one else to be with them or they may die in the night before family members or friends can get to the nursing home. No one wants to be alone at the time of their death.

You can help residents who are dying by:

- Sitting by the bed so they know they are not alone
- Telling them you are there and that you care—even those in coma may be able to hear you
- Touching their hand, shoulder, or forehead for comfort so they can feel that you are there
- Asking if they would like you to read the Bible or another religious book

- Doing whatever you can to make them comfortable—changing their position, fluffing pillows, giving fluids or food
- Keeping the room quiet and trying to avoid making noises

Post-Mortem Care

Do you know the purpose of post-mortem care?

Post-mortem care is the name for the care given to the resident's body shortly after death.

Five points to remember are:

1. Even after death, the resident has the right to be treated with privacy and dignity.
2. You have a difficult but very important job to do after the resident's death.
3. You should always think about what a resident's death means to the resident's family and to other residents.
4. After checking with the charge nurse, you should allow the resident's family to view and be with the resident's body if they want.
5. The purpose of post-mortem care is to help put the body in a natural position before rigor mortis occurs.

When caring for the resident's body after death, remember:

- Do not provide post-mortem care until instructed to by the charge nurse.
- Always follow principles of infection control when giving post-mortem care.
- Collect all the resident's belongings, check against the resident's valuables list, and return everything to the resident's family.

Review Questions

1. You can help a resident come to the end of their life with __________ and ______________ and a feeling that someone cares.
2. No one wants to be _________ at the time of their death.
3. Care of the resident's body shortly after death is called _________-___________ care.

Answers: 1. peace, dignity, **2.** alone, **3.** post-mortem

Unit 4, Special Skills For Caring

Module 3: Restorative Nursing

Did you know that you, as a nurse assistant, should not do something for a resident that the resident is able to do?

Restorative nursing is assisting a resident to do something they used to be able to do. It is special nursing care that helps restore residents' abilities and independence.

Remember that assisting the resident to be as independent as possible is one of your most important roles. So, do not do something for a resident that the resident is able to do.

Remember, one of the hardest things for a resident to cope with is the loss of independence. When people lose control of basic functions, such as moving around by themselves or feeding themselves, they often feel humility, grief, and anger and become frustrated and depressed.

When people are functioning as well as possible in all areas of life, they have reached their best overall health. By helping residents to do as much for themselves as possible, you can help increase their self-esteem and help them feel a sense of purpose.

What is involved in restorative nursing?

- Teaching
- Encouraging
- Retraining
- Motivating
- Prompting residents to do for themselves as much as they are physically and mentally able to do.

Often the goals in restorative nursing will be set by members of the health care team, the resident, and the resident's family. Your role is to ensure that the goals are met.

Review Questions

1. Restorative nursing is assisting a resident to regain a ________ of function.

2. Restorative nursing is teaching, encouraging, retraining, motivating and prompting residents to do for ____________ as much as they are physically and mentally able to do.

3. Often the goals in restorative nursing will be set by members of the health care team, the ____________, and the resident's ____________.

Answers: 1. loss, **2.** themselves, **3.** resident, family

Did you know that the plan of care is a vital tool used by the health care team in restorative nursing?

The plan of care is a vital tool used by the health care team in restorative nursing. The charge nurse leads the team. The plan focuses on restoring the resident to their best overall health and increasing independence and self-esteem.

The following example is a plan of care for a resident recovering from a stroke:

Problem	Plan
Right-sided weakness	Provide assistive devices for eating and personal care Progress from a walker to a cane Always use a safety belt when walking
Urinary incontinence	Walk resident to the bathroom on a regular basis Answer call light immediately Offer fluids regularly
Slurred speech	Be patient Encourage resident to complete all statements
Confusion about physical surroundings	Have resident's room close to the nurses' station Orient resident every shift Keep familiar objects in place

Review Questions

1. The plan of care focuses on restoring the resident to their best overall health and increasing their ____________________ and __________-______________.

2. If a resident has a problem with urinary incontinence, the plan of care would be to walk them to the bathroom on a regular basis, answer the __________ _____________ immediately, and offer ______________ regularly.

3. If a resident is confused about their physical surroundings, the plan of care would be to have their room close to the nurse's station, ___________ her every shift, and keep familiar _____________ in place.

Answers: 1. independence, self-esteem, **2.** call light, fluids, **3.** orient, objects

Unit 5: Getting Ready for Your Competency Evaluation

This unit has two parts. First, review the Test-Taking Tips. (Remember to review these tips again right before you take your state competency evaluation.)

Then, take the practice competency test. The test has 25 multiple choice questions. Take your time and remember the test-taking tips. After you finish the test, check your answers. If you have any wrong answers, go back to the correct module and review the information and questions again. If you still have trouble with a question, talk to your facilitator or your supervisor.

Unit 5, Getting Ready for Your Competency Evaluation

Hints to Improve Your Test-Taking Ability*

Stay on top of things!

1. Take your review guide seriously.
2. Read the materials carefully.
3. Make notes and ask your facilitator or supervisor if you don't understand something. Study what you don't know.
4. Review your notes as often as possible before taking the test.
5. Take the review questions in your review guide seriously. If you miss any questions, study the material again.

When it is time to take the test:

6. Get a good night's sleep. Eat wisely. Wear clothing that is comfortable and appropriate for the weather.
7. Be sure you know where you have to go to take the test and what time you have to be there.
8. Wear a watch; be aware of time, but don't think too much about it.
9. Take several sharp pencils and a good eraser.

When you arrive in the test room:

10. If the table-arm chairs are used and if you are left-handed, ask for a left-handed chair or an arrangement that will be comfortable for you.

---

* Adapted from: Dobbin, John E., *How to Take a Test: Doing Your Best*. Princeton, NJ, Educational Testing Service, 1984

11. Be physically relaxed, mentally alert, and feel confident that you will do well. If you feel nervous, take 10 slow, deep breaths to help you relax.

12. Listen carefully to directions that are read to you. Test instructions are very important, so it is important to understand exactly what you are supposed to do.

13. Ask questions immediately if you do not understand the directions.

14. Read directions on the test carefully.

15. Do the practice questions, if there are any.

16. Plan your time. Begin each timed section by checking how long it is and then decide how much time you can take for each question.

While you're taking the test:

17. Don't rush yourself. Work within your time schedule.

18. Read carefully; do not read anything into the test question that is not there. Answer the question as it is being asked.

19. If there is more than one answer, read every answer choice.

20. Work quickly. Don't spend too much time on any one question.

21. On the first pass through the test, answer all the questions that are easy for you; then go back to the hard ones, if there is time.

22. If it is allowed, underline or circle key words, numbers, and definitions in a question.

23. Make sure that any numbered space you use for an answer has the same number as the question you are answering.

24. Take the time to change an answer if you have good reason for doing so. If you change an answer, erase your previous answer completely. Do not make extra marks on the answer.

25. Check to be sure your answers are marked exactly as the instructions require.

26. If time permits, check your answers.

27. If you know a second language, use it to help you make sense out of unfamiliar words in English.

On guessing

28. Ask if there is a penalty for guessing. Always guess when there is no penalty.

29. If you can't decide between two or more answers on a multiple-choice test, guess instead of leaving the question blank.

30. On true-false questions, always guess if you do not know the answer.

Unit 5, Getting Ready for Your Competency Evaluation

Practice Test

IMPORTANT: Read all instructions before starting this test.

INSTRUCTIONS: Mark all answers in pencil on the separate answer sheet. Do not write on this test. Read each question slowly and carefully. Then choose the BEST answer and circle that answer on the answer sheet. If you wish to change an answer, erase your first answer completely. When you are finished, check your answers against the answer sheet. If you have questions, talk to your facilitator or your supervisor.

DO NOT WRITE ON THIS TEST!

1. Which of the following is a good bridge to communications?
   a. Sitting at the same level as the resident.
   b. Speaking very loudly.
   c. Using slang to put the resident at ease.
   d. Talking about your family and home life.

2. Which question is NOT important for a nurse assistant to ask themselves before moving a resident?
   a. Do I have all the equipment I need?
   b. Do I need help?
   c. Have I positioned myself so that I will not injure myself?
   d. Do I have the television turned off.

3. A resident is having trouble hearing what you are saying. Which of the following is a good way to handle this situation?
   a. Write messages if necessary.
   b. Shout to the resident if necessary.
   c. Stop speaking to the resident and continue doing what you have to do.
   d. Ask that the resident be assigned to another nurse assistant.

4. Which of the following can cause bed sores?
   a. Poor blood circulation.
   b. Too much exercise.
   c. Skin lotions.
   d. Changing positions too often.

5. How can a nurse assistant help female residents avoid becoming incontinent?
a. Encourage residents to hold their urine for a few minutes before they eliminate.
b. Wash the perineal area from front to back.
c. Give fluids once a day.
d. Respond quickly to a resident's call to go to the bathroom or use a bedpan.

6. Residents with Alzheimer's disease must be:
a. Restrained.
b. Discouraged from having personal possessions in their room because they cannot keep track of them.
c. Told what to do much like children because they are no longer independent.
d. Supervised carefully to be sure they do not wander away from the facility.

7. When a resident dies, which of the following is an appropriate action?
a. Assume that the family is likely to be relieved by the death.
b. Encourage other residents to attend the memorial service if they can.
c. Discourage other residents from asking questions about the death.
d. Keep your own feelings about the death to yourself.

8. When a resident is using a shower, the nurse assistant should:
a. Stay with the resident.
b. Have the resident call you when finished.
c. Check on the resident every five minutes.
d. Leave the resident alone to bathe in privacy.

9. Temperatures should be taken orally when:
a. The resident is on oxygen.
b. The resident is paralyzed.
c. The resident is alert and cooperative.
d. The resident is having trouble breathing.

10. Which of the following is a nursing home resident's RIGHT?
a. To abuse their own roommate.
b. To harass employees.
c. To have visitors at any hours.
d. To know what their care will cost.

11. What is one of the most effective infection control measures a nurse assistant can use?
a. Using water as a disinfectant.
b. Not touching residents.
c. Washing hands.
d. Shaking bed sheets before putting them in the laundry hamper.

12. Which of the following is a principle of body mechanics? Study body mechanics

a. Keep your knees locked.
b. Keep the person a few inches away from your body.
c. Place your feet about 12 inches apart with one foot slightly ahead of the other.
d. Twist your upper body as you lift.

13. Which of the following is a normal oral temperature?

a. 96.2 degrees
b. 98.6 degrees ✓
c. 99.5 degrees
d. 101.1 degrees

14. Wrinkles in the bed linen should be avoided because:

a. They may cause the resident to sweat.
b. They can cause skin irritations and bed sores. ✓
c. They cause extra wear on the sheets.
d. They can cause wear spots on the mattress.

15. Which one of the following helps germs multiply?

a. Moisture. ✓
b. Light.
c. Temperatures below 40 degrees.
d. Boiling water.

16. When can a resident be restrained?

a. When the resident is being uncooperative.
b. When the resident has threatened a staff member.
c. When a restraint is ordered by a doctor. ✓
d. When the resident is acting in a confused manner.

17. What is the expected normal reading for a <u>rectal</u> temperature?

a. 98.6 ✓
b. 99.6
c. 97.6
d. 96.6

18. Residents who do not drink enough liquids can experience:

a. Dehydration. ✓
b. Decubitus ulcers.
c. Loss of hearing in the higher ranges.
d. Diarrhea.

19. A resident with arthritis complains of feeling stiff and having trouble moving. What can you do to help?
   a. Give a warm tub bath. √
   b. Encourage them to drink more fluids.
   c. Apply ice packs.
   d. There is little a nurse assistant can do to help—a change in medication is needed.

20. Which of the following statements about dietary needs of older persons is true?
   a. The elderly require more calories because they are less active.
   b. As a person grows older, their sense of taste dulls, causing loss of appetite.
   c. As a person grows older, their ability to absorb and use nutrients increases.
   d. The number of calories needed by a person depends only on age.

21. Which of the following statements about incontinence is TRUE?
   a. Only residents who are fully mobile should be allowed to eliminate in private.
   b. Residents will be able to control their elimination better if they are helped to the bathroom promptly. √
   c. All residents should be required to use the toilet on a regular schedule.
   d. Residents who have been in a nursing home for a while will not be embarrassed about needing help with elimination.

22. To comfort a resident who is dying:
   a. Avoid discussing death.
   b. Isolate the resident.
   c. Discuss your feelings about death.
   d. √ Be there and listen.

23. Communicating with residents may be helped by:
   a. Using baby talk.
   b. Always talking in a very loud voice.
   c. Avoiding eye contact.
   d. √ Giving positive non-verbal messages (i.e., smiling, nodding)

24. Which of the following is NOT one of the principles of care?
   a. Dignity.
   b. Privacy.
   c. Communication.
   d. √ Dependence.

25. Which of the following does a resident need to be happy?
   a. Diamond ring.
   b. Love. √
   c. Boat.
   d. Car.

Unit 5, Getting Ready for Your Evaluation

Practice Test Answer Sheet

Name ______________________________ Date ______________

DIRECTIONS: Draw a circle around the best answer for each question.

1.	a	b	c	d	**13.**	a	b	c	d
2.	a	b	c	d	**14.**	a	b	c	d
3.	a	b	c	d	**15.**	a	b	c	d
4.	a	b	c	d	**16.**	a	b	c	d
5.	a	b	c	d	**17.**	a	b	c	d
6.	a	b	c	d	**18.**	a	b	c	d
7.	a	b	c	d	**19.**	a	b	c	d
8.	a	b	c	d	**20.**	a	b	c	d
9.	a	b	c	d	**21.**	a	b	c	d
10.	a	b	c	d	**22.**	a	b	c	d
11.	a	b	c	d	**23.**	a	b	c	d
12.	a	b	c	d	**24.**	a	b	c	d
					25.	a	b	c	d

Check your answers on the next page.

Answer Key

1. a
2. d
3. a
4. a
5. d
6. d
7. b
8. a
9. c
10. d
11. c
12. c
13. b
14. b
15. a
16. c
17. b
18. a
19. a
20. b
21. b
22. d
23. d
24. d
25. b

PART 2: CORE SKILLS

Skill 1: Hand Washing

Name: ______________________________ Date: ______________

Precautions

- Remember to wash your hands:

  Before and after any contact with a resident
  After going to the bathroom
  After coughing or sneezing
  Before handling any food
  After smoking
  When coming on duty
  Before going home

Procedure

Competency check

1. Remove watch, or push it up on your forearm, and roll up sleeves. ☐

   Note: If the watch cannot be worn above the wrist, the watch should be kept in your pocket to prevent contamination.

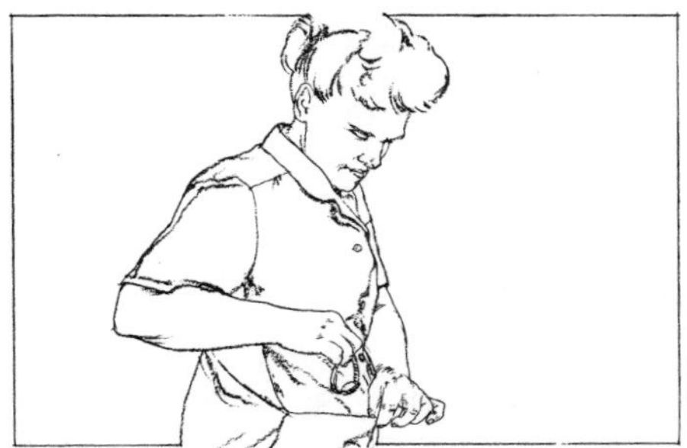

Rationale: Hand washing includes the wrists.

2. Turn on water and adjust temperature. ☐

Note: If the water faucet is the kind you must use your hand to turn on, use a clean paper towel to turn it on.

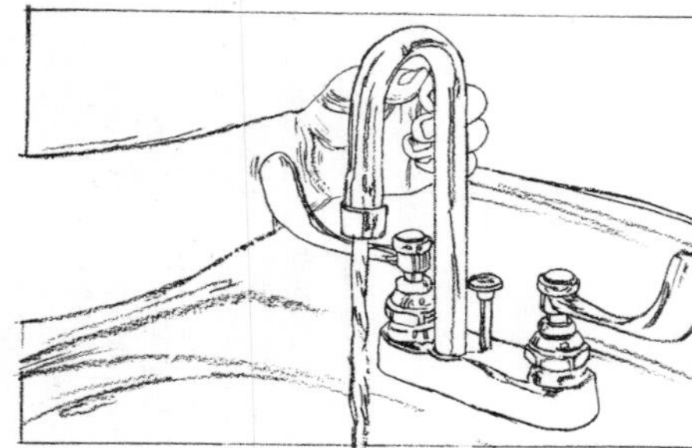

Rationale: Faucets may indirectly transmit germs.

---

3. Wet your hands and wrists. Apply soap. ☐

Note: If you are using bar soap, rinse the soap before using it.

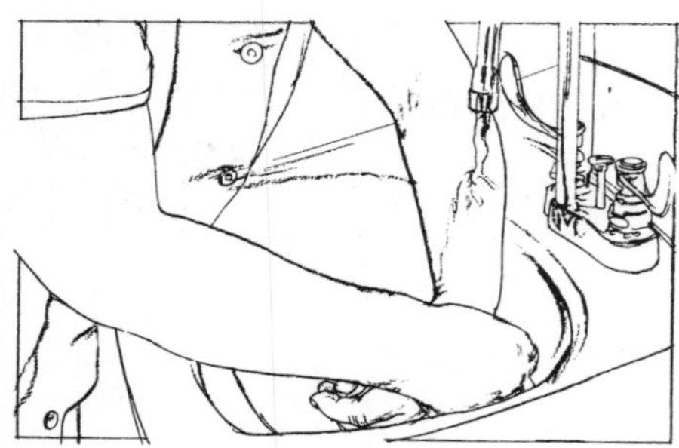

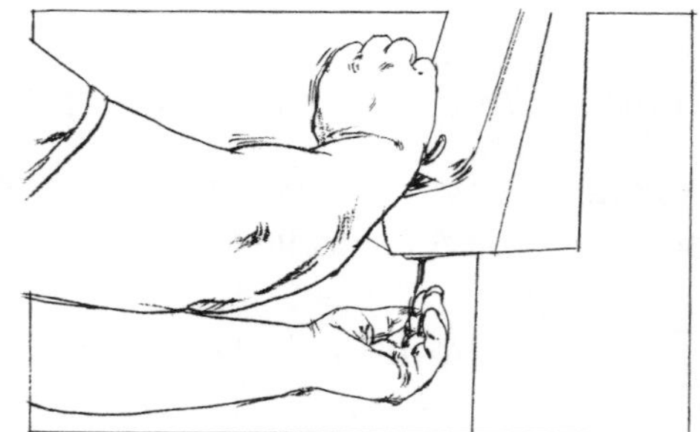

---

4. Hold your hands lower than your elbows and work up a lather.

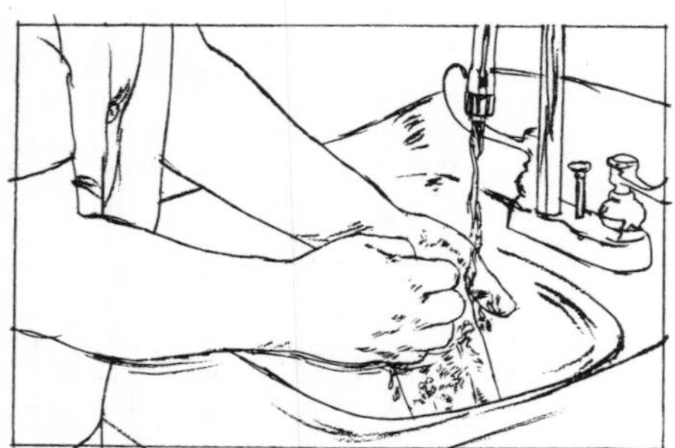

Rationale: This will help water to run from the clean area of the forearm to the dirty area of the fingers. ☐

---

5. Wash:

Wrists (grasping with hand and circling)

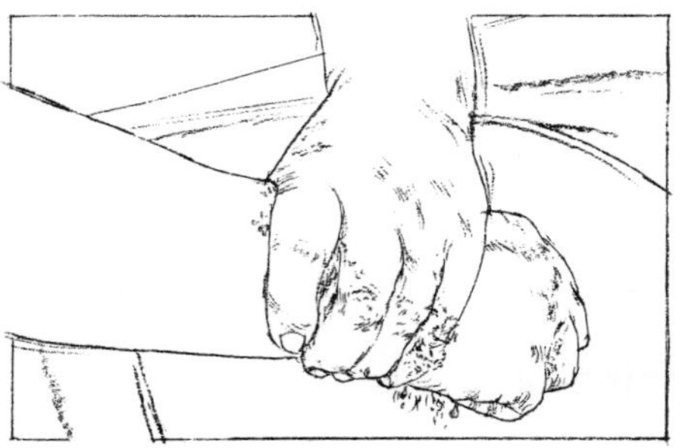

Palms and backs of hands

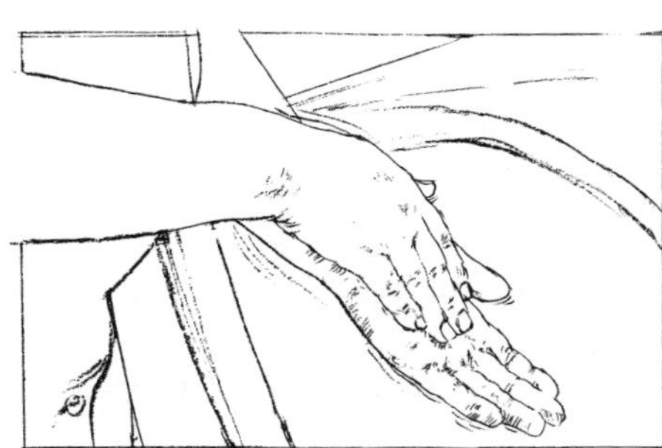

Between fingers

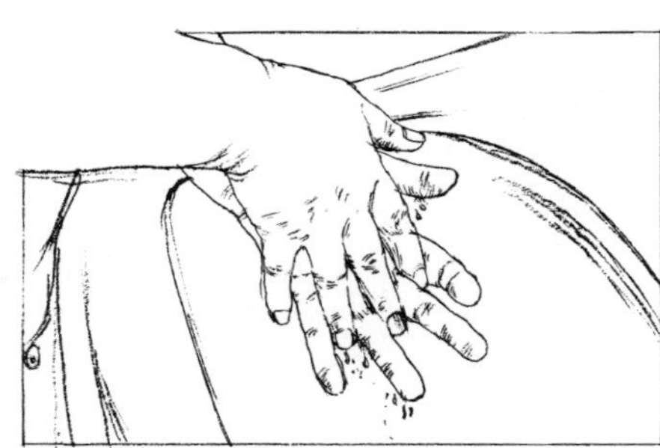

Nails (rub against palms of hands)

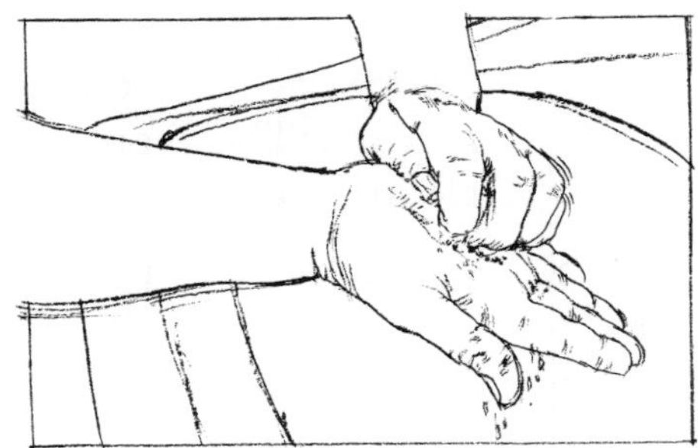

Rationale: Doing this makes sure that all areas are cleaned thoroughly.

---

6. Rinse your hands and wrists, keeping your wrists and hands below your elbows.

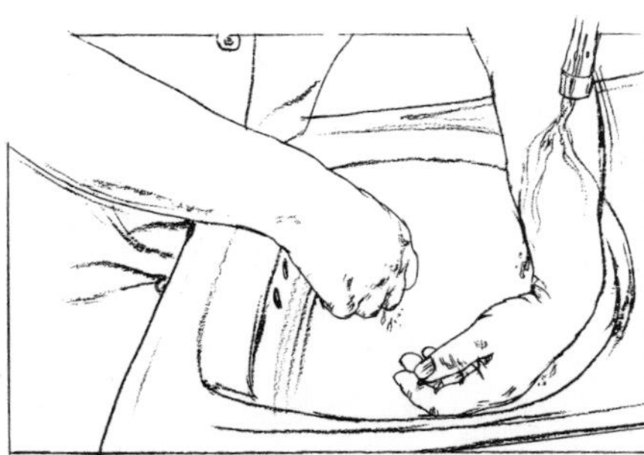

Rationale: Removes and loosens dirt and germs.

7. Dry your wrists and hands thoroughly. ☐

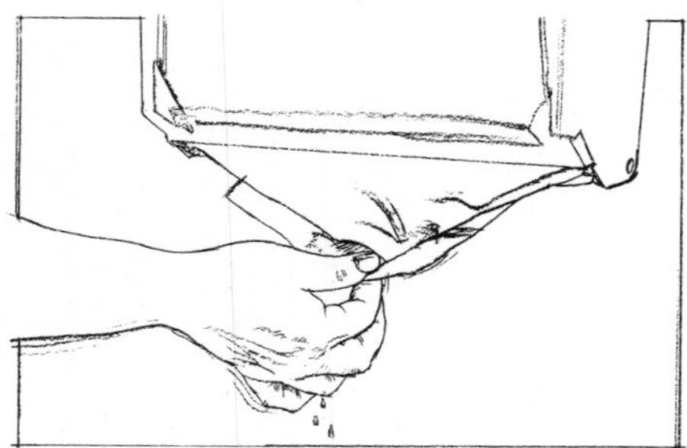

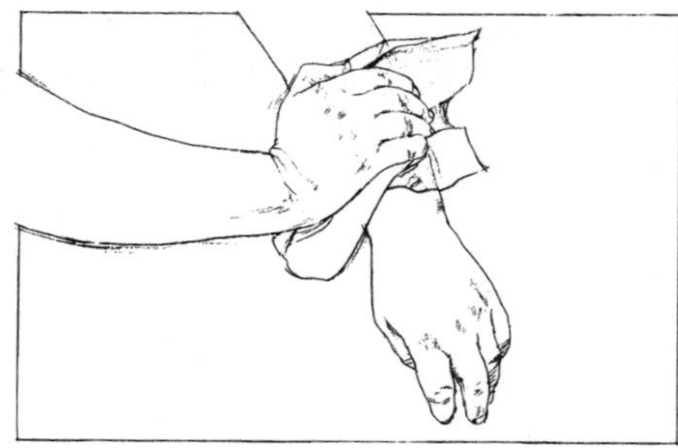

Rationale: Prevents chapping of hands.

---

8. Use a clean paper towel to turn off the faucet. ☐

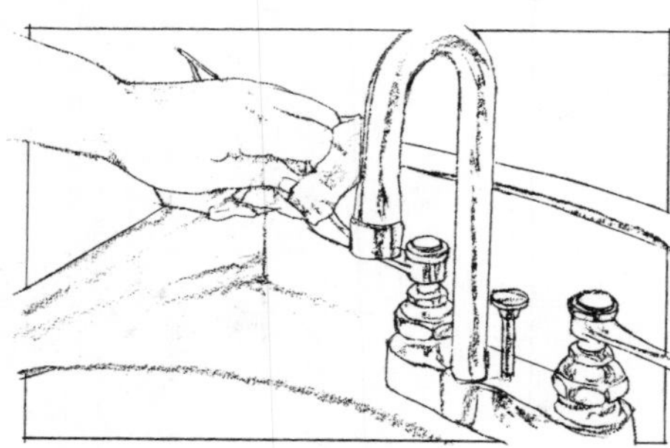

Rationale: Not directly touching the faucet will prevent contamination of clean hands from the dirty faucet.

---

9. Throw towel away. ☐

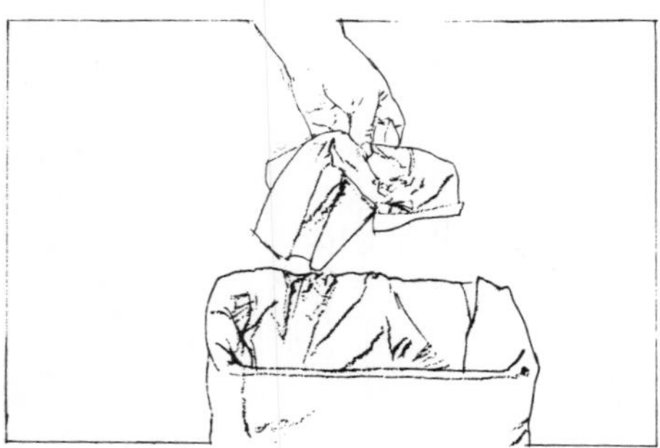

Skill 2: Putting On a Gown, Mask, and Disposable Gloves

Name: ______________________ Date: ______________

Precautions

- Never use gloves with cracks, discoloration, punctures, or tears.
- Never reuse gowns or masks.
- Change a mask if it becomes moist or if it is worn longer than 20 minutes.
- Never wash or disinfect disposable gloves.

Procedure

Competency check

Putting on a Gown

Note: A gown is usually put on outside the resident's room.

1. Put on the gown with the opening in the back. ☐

2. Fasten the ties at the back of your neck and at your waist to cover all your clothing. ☐

3. If gloves are used, pull them over the gown cuff. ☐

Putting on a Mask

1. Put the mask over your mouth and nose and bend the nose wire. ☐

2. Tie the top strings and then the bottom strings. ☐

3. Adjust the mask for comfort. ☐

Putting on Disposable Gloves

1. Discard the gloves if they are damaged and choose another pair. ☐

2. Be sure to pull gloves up over the gown cuffs. ☐

Skill 3: Taking Off Soiled Disposable Gloves, Mask, and Gown

Name: ______________________________ Date: ______________

Precautions

- Never touch the inside part of a soiled glove with the other gloved hand.
- Never touch the front part of the mask which covers the nose and mouth.

Procedure

Competency check

Note: This equipment is usually taken off in the resident's room and discarded as contaminated waste.

Taking off Soiled Disposable Gloves

1. Using the fingers of your left hand, make a cuff of the glove on the right hand, grasp the cuff on the palm side, and pull the glove down toward the fingers of the right hand. ☐

   Note: Do not touch the inside part of the glove with the left hand.

   Rationale: The inside of the glove is clean.

   Note: Do not remove the glove all the way.

2. Using the fingers of your right hand, take off the glove on your left hand by pulling it inside out and rolling it into a ball without touching the bare hand. ☐

3. Hold the glove you have removed in your right hand. ☐

4. Grasp the glove on your right hand touching only the inside of the glove with your left hand. ☐

5. Remove the glove by pulling it down so that the glove you have removed is inside the right-hand glove. ☐

6. Throw away the gloves in a covered trash container. ☐

7. Wash your hands. ☐

Taking off a Mask

1. Untie the bottom strings and then the top strings. ☐

2. Throw away the mask in a trash container. ☐

Taking off a Gown

1. Untie the gown in back. ☐

2. Pull off one gown sleeve by slipping your fingers under the cuff and pulling the sleeve part way over your hand. ☐

   Note: Remember that the end of the sleeve is clean because it was covered by the glove.

3. Grasp the other sleeve with the covered hand and pull it off completely. ☐

4. Fold in outer contaminated surfaces and roll the gown up. Throw the gown away in the linen or trash hamper. ☐

5. Wash your hands. ☐

Skill 4: Making an Occupied Bed

Name: ______________________________ Date: ______________

Precautions

- Check bed for personal belongings like dentures, eyeglasses, and hearing aids.
- Do not shake bed linen.
- Keep soiled, contaminated linen away from your uniform.
- Do not allow clean linen to touch the floor.
- Make one side of the bed at a time to save time and energy.
- Use proper body mecahnics.

Procedure

Competency check

1. Remove and fold reusable linen (blanket, spread) and place over a clean chair. ☐

   Note: Keep the top sheet on the resident for privacy.

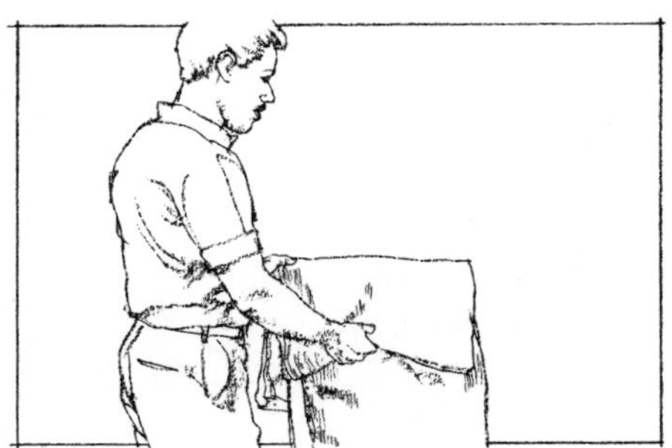

Rationale: Folding the reusable linens at this point will save time and energy when you put them back on the bed.

2. Help the resident roll away from the side where you will begin working, using the procedure learned in Skill 2, turning the resident toward you. Make sure the side rail is up and the resident uses it for balance.

3. Return to the opposite side and lower the side rail where you will be working.

   Note: Lower the side rail only on the side where you will be working to maintain resident safety.

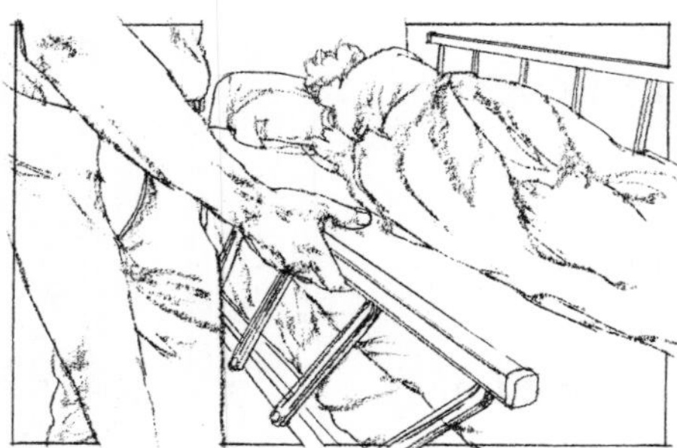

4. Put the pillow under the resident's head to keep them comfortable.

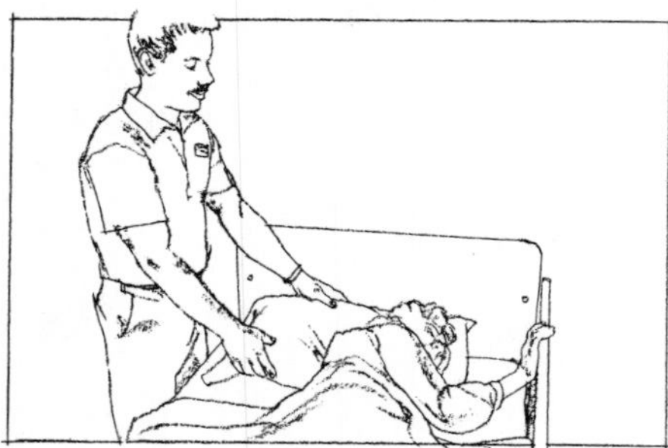

5. Check the bed for personal items, such as eyeglasses, hearing aids, and dentures.

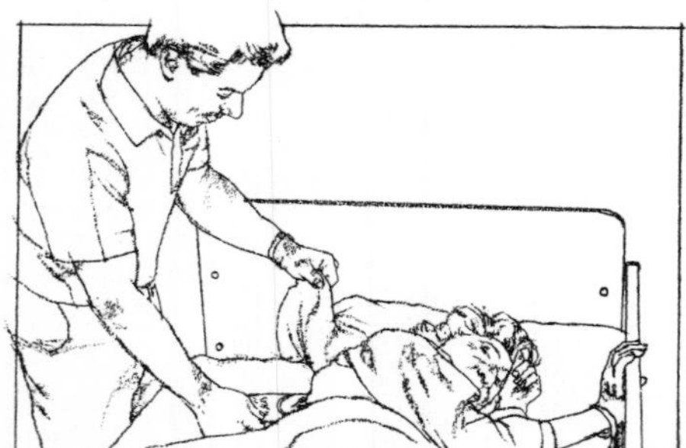

Rationale: Personal items may be costly or impossible to replace if lost or broken.

6. Loosen and roll the dirty bottom sheets snugly toward the resident and tuck them against the resident's back. ☐

Note: If linens are soiled or there is any concern for infection control, put an extra sheet or bed protector between the dirty and clean sheets.

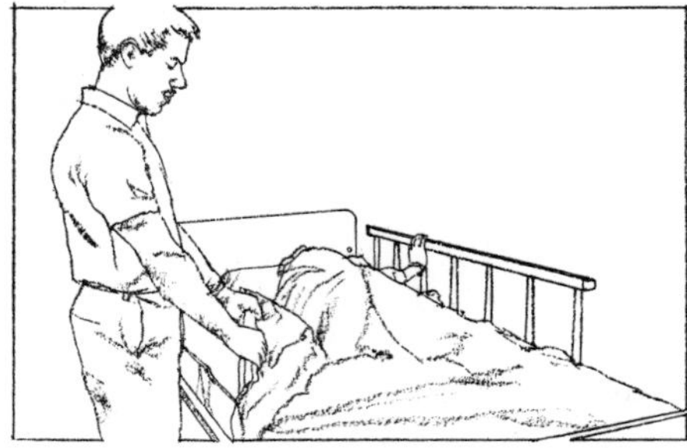
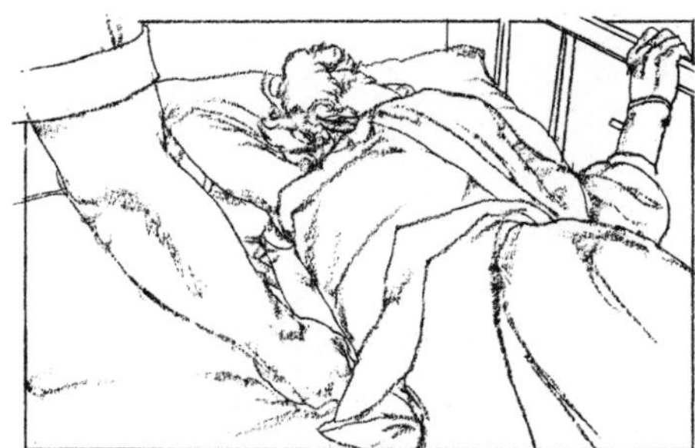

7. Put the clean bottom sheet on the bed and unfold it with the center fold in the center of the bed. ☐

Note: Do not shake the sheets as you open them. This will cause air currents that may spread dust and germs around the room.

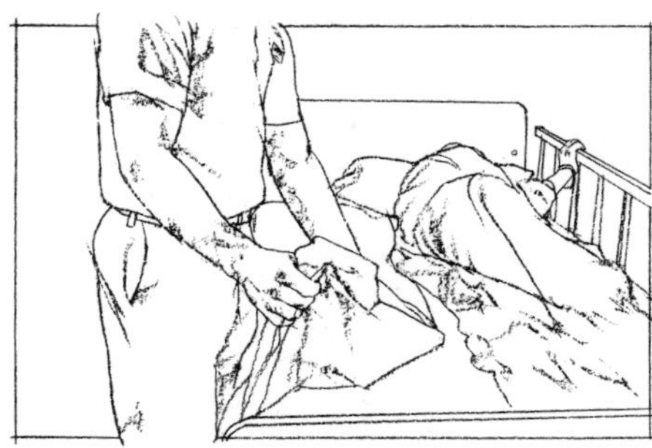

8. Put the narrow hem at the bottom edge of the mattress with the seam on the underside. ☐

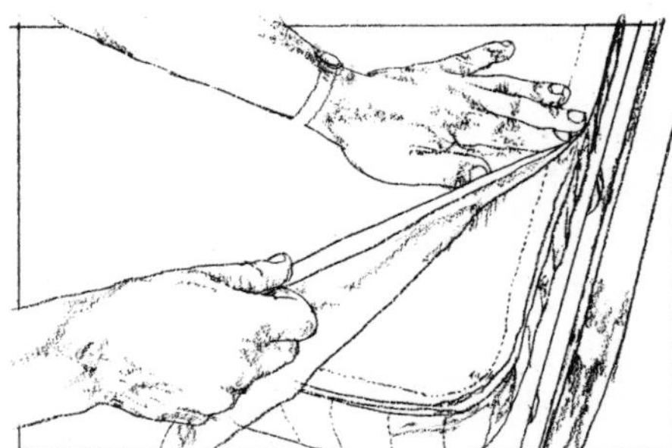

Rationale: This allows for enough fabric to be tucked in at the top and sides of the mattress and prevents the seam edge from irritating the resident's skin.

9. Tuck in the sheet at the top and miter the corners using the following steps:

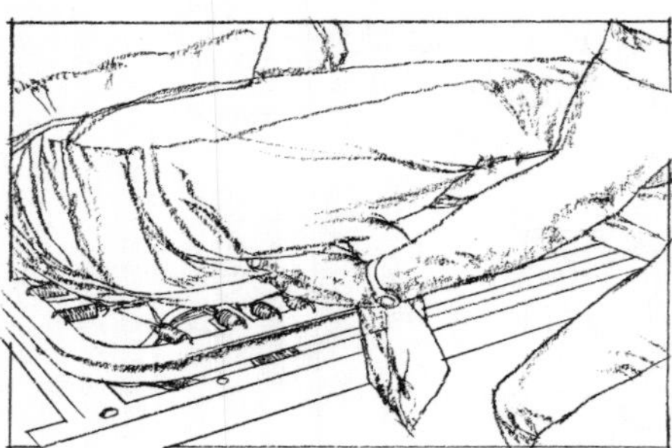

Rationale: Mitered corners make the bed look neat and help prevent the linen from becoming loose and wrinkled.

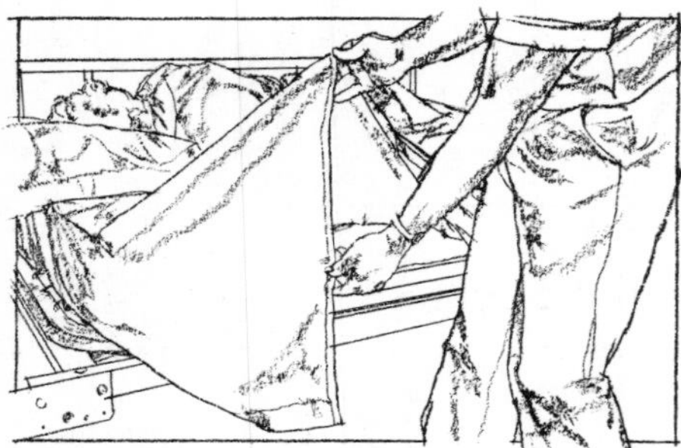

Face the head of the bed. With the hand closer to the bed, pick up the edge of the sheet at the side of the bed about 12 inches from the top of the mattress, making a triangle.

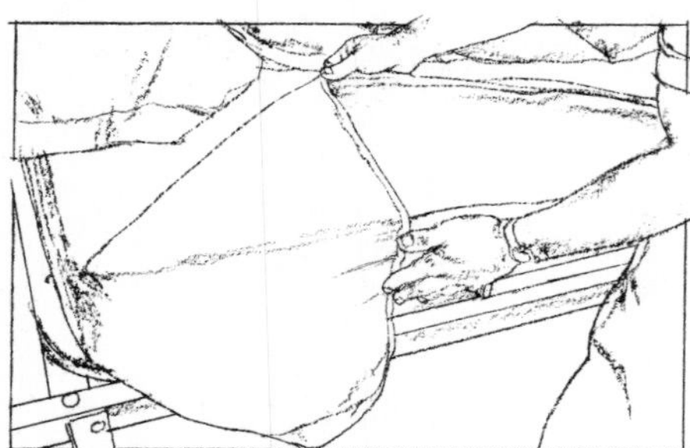

Lay the triangle on top of the bed, holding firmly.

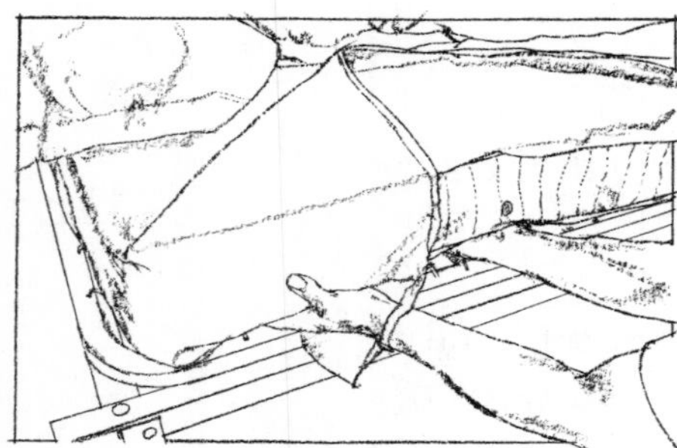

Tuck the hanging portion of the sheet under the mattress.

Bring the triangle down and tuck in. Continue tucking the sheet in all the way to the foot of the bed.

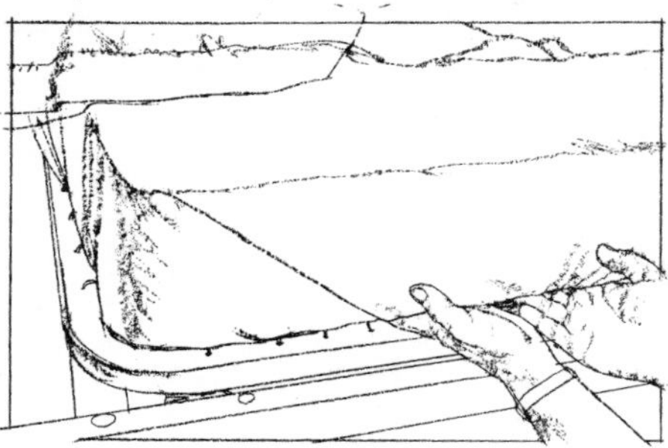
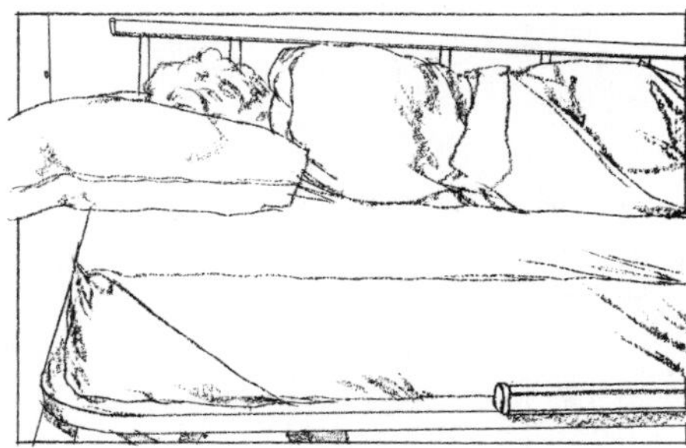

10. Unfold the draw sheet on the middle one-third of the mattress and tuck in the side. ☐

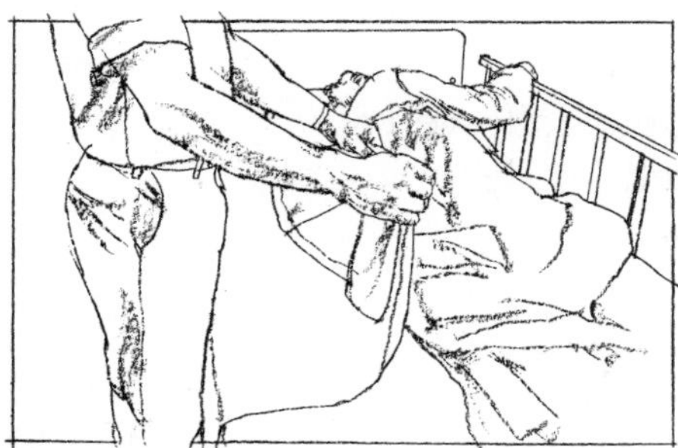
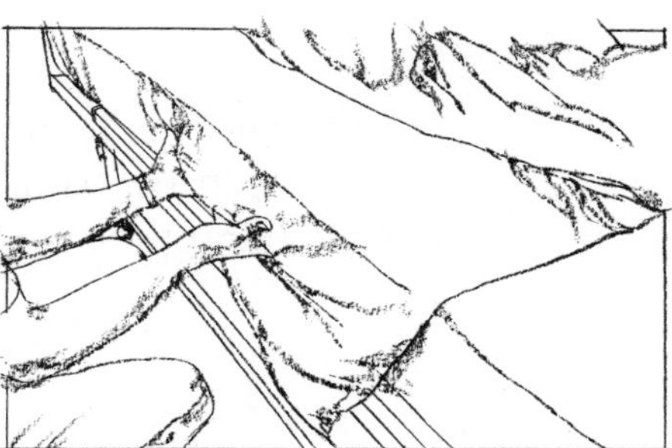

11. Flatten the rolled sheets as much as possible and help the resident to roll over the linen toward you. ☐

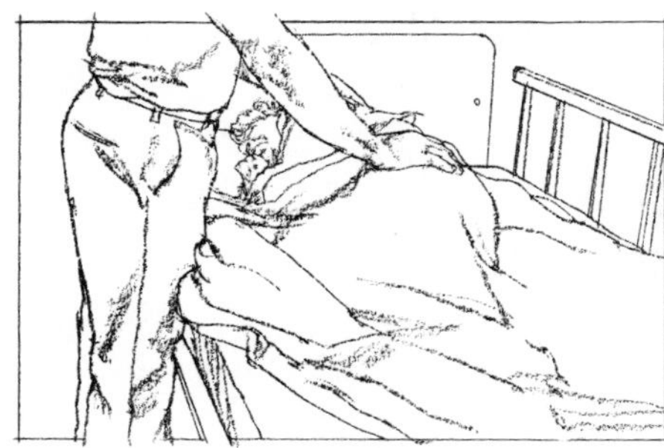

12. Raise the side rail on your side of the bed. Then, go to the opposite side and lower the side rail. ☐

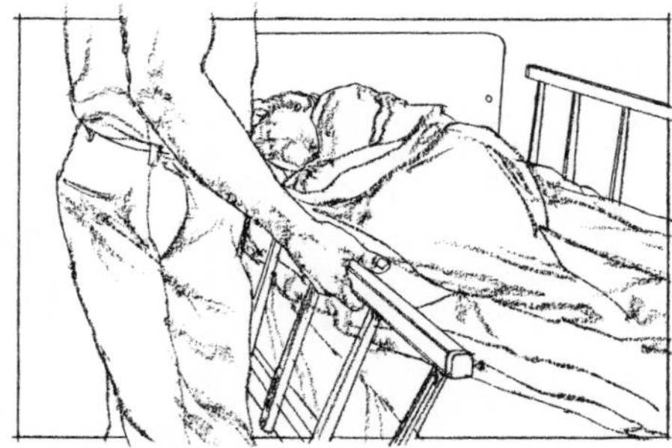

Rationale: Keeping the rail up on one side maintains resident safety and supports resident for balance.

13. Check the bed for personal items.

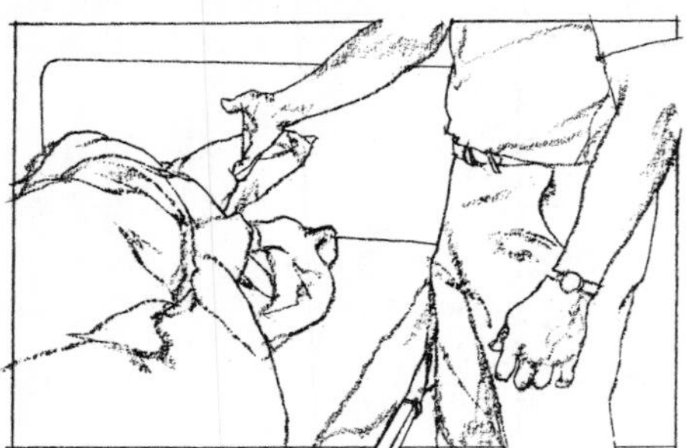

14. Snugly roll and take off the dirty bottom sheets and put them at the foot of the bed between the mattress and the footboard—never on the floor.

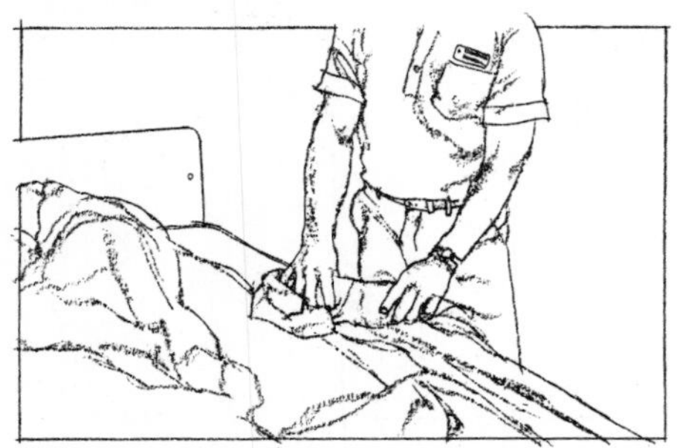

Rationale: This technique is followed so the bed can be completely made without ever leaving the resident

15. Pull the clean sheet toward you until it is completely unfolded, tuck in at the top, miter the corners, and continue tucking in the sheet all the way to the foot of the bed.

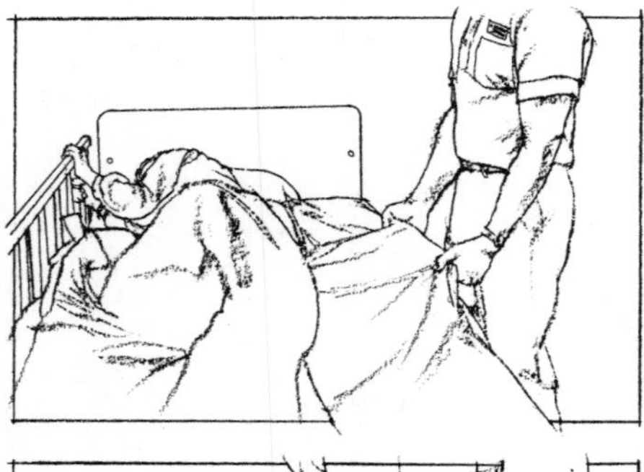

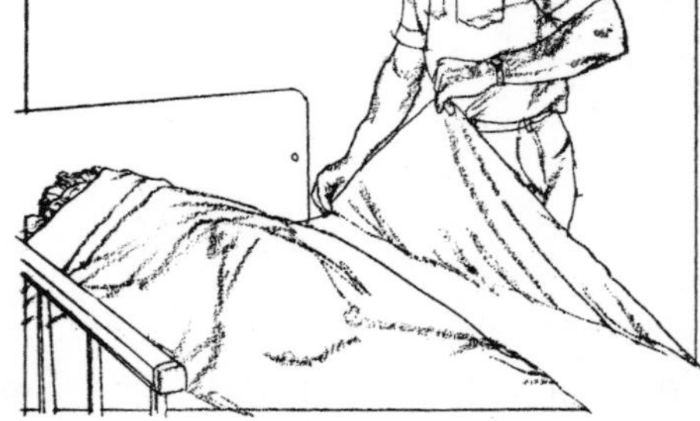

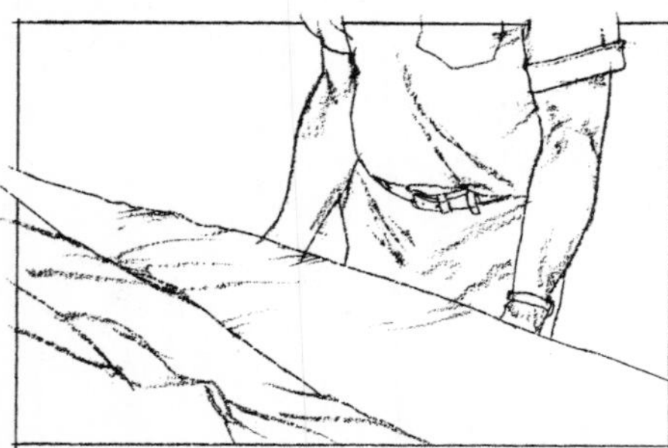

16. Tighten the draw sheet with your palms facing up by tucking in the middle part first, then the top third and the bottom third. ☐

Note: Be sure you move so that you stand in front of the section of the draw sheet you are tucking.

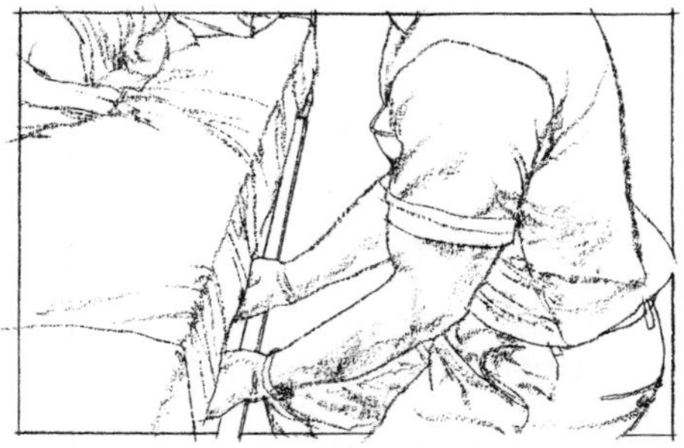

Rationale: Moving as you tuck will prevent you from twisting your upper body. Keeping palms facing up prevents hyperextension of the wrist.

---

17. Help the resident move to the center of the bed. ☐

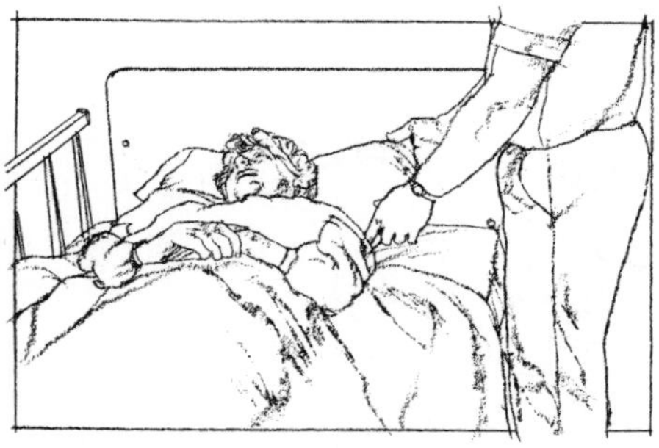

---

18. Raise the side rail. ☐

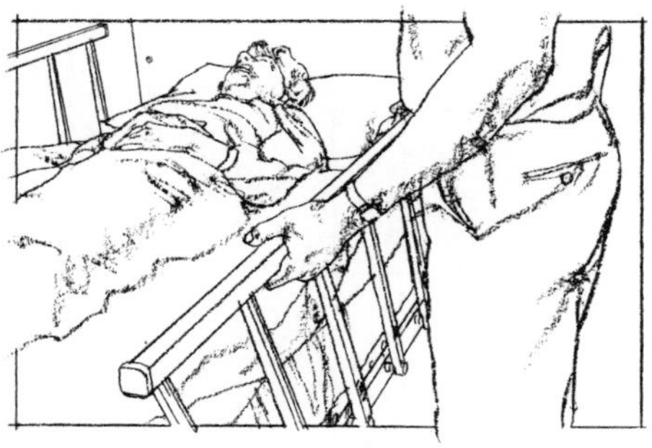

---

19. Put the clean top sheet over the dirty top sheet, if the dirty sheet is not wet, with the wide hem at the top and the seam on the side.

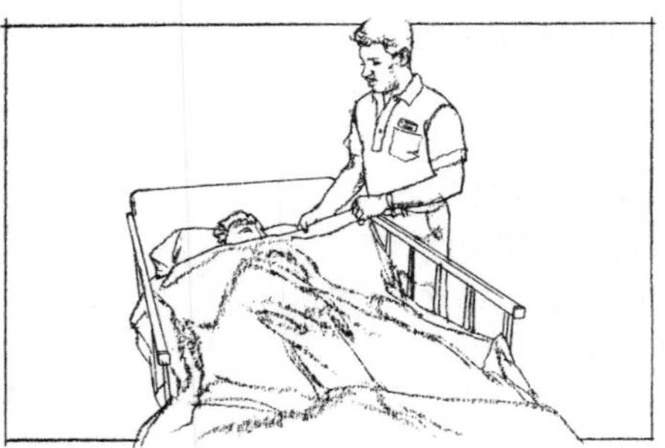

Rationale: This is done to protect the resident's privacy.

20. Have the resident hold the clean top sheet in place while you remove the dirty sheet. Put the dirty sheet with the other dirty linen.

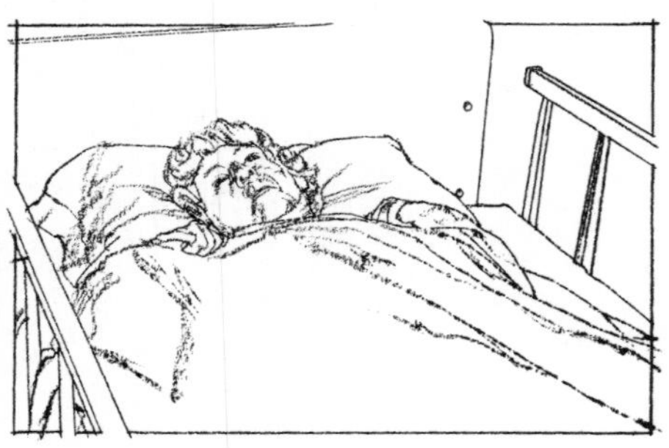

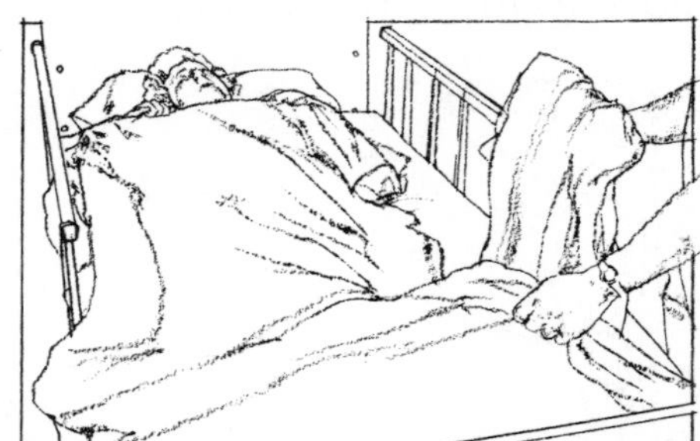

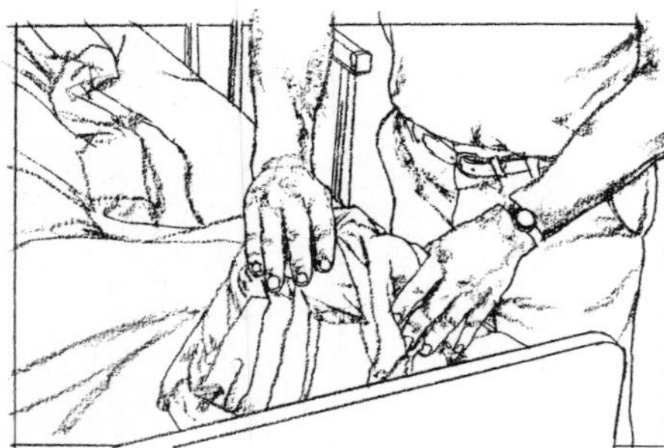

21. Change the pillowcase on the pillow using the following steps: ☐ ☐

Remove the pillow from under the resident's head, and then remove the dirty pillowcase.

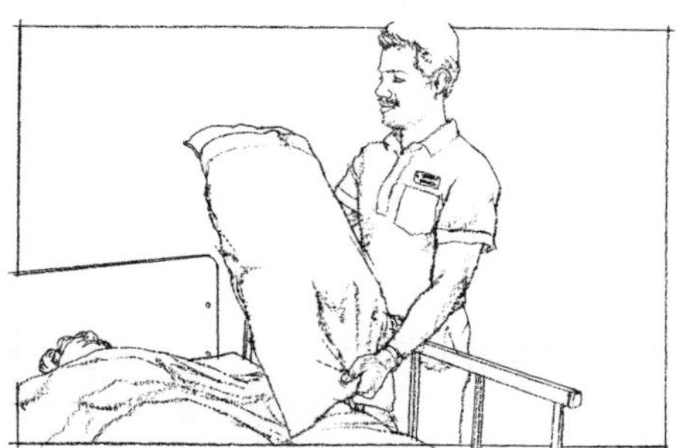

Hold the clean pillowcase at the center of the end seam.

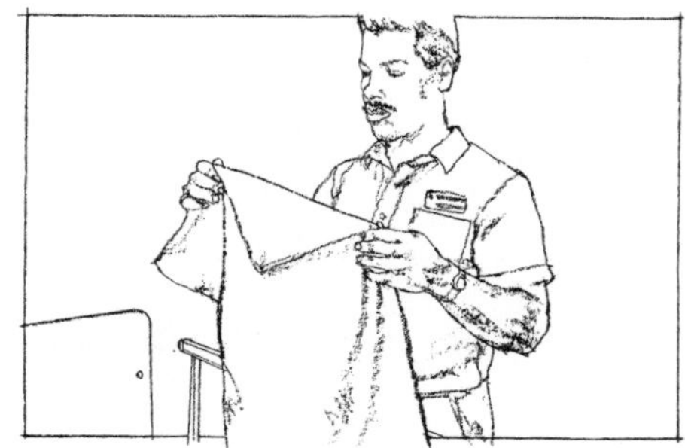

With your hand on the outside of the case, turn the case back over your hand.

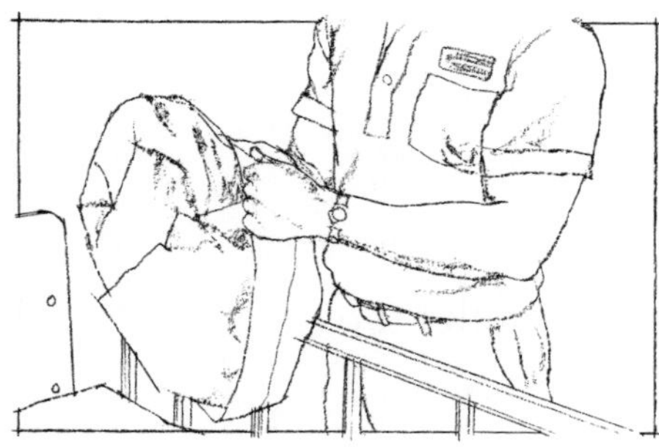

Hold the pillow through the case at the center of one end of the pillow.

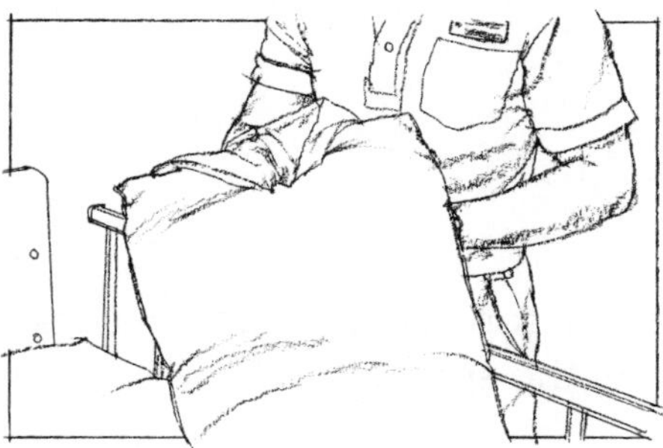

Bring the case down over the pillow.

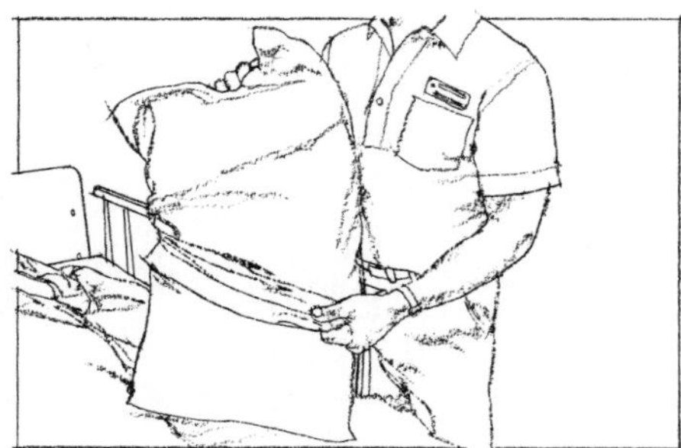

Fit the corners of the pillow into the corners of the pillow case.

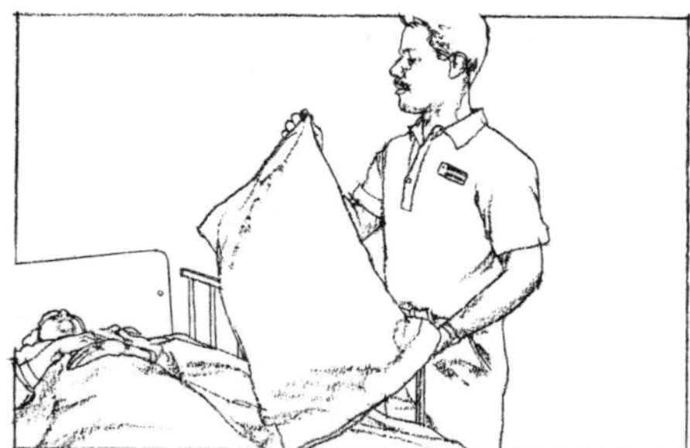

22. Put the pillow under the resident's head. ☐

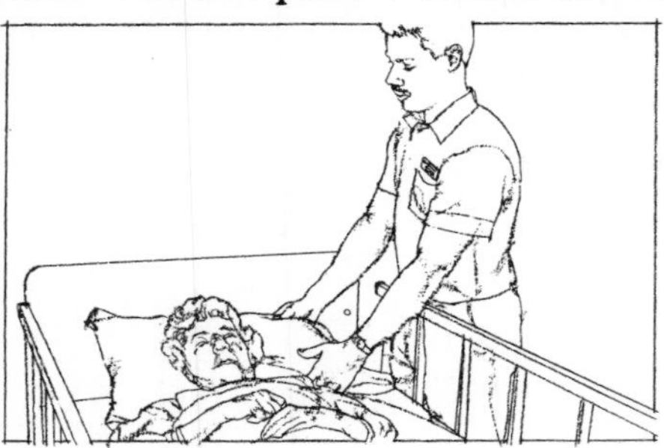

23. Remove dirty laundry from the foot of the bed and put in the laundry hamper. ☐

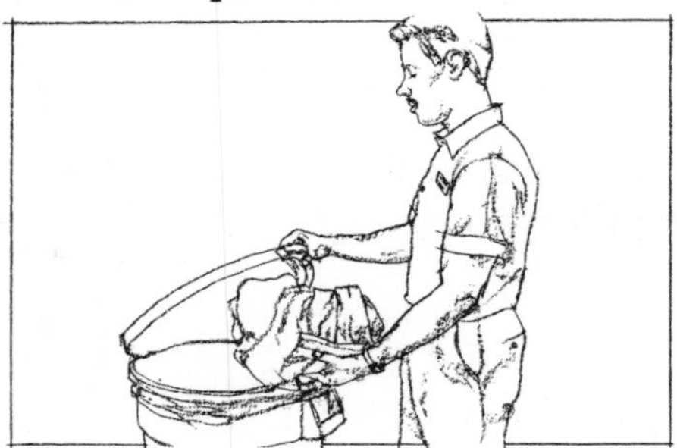

24. Put the blanket over the top sheet about 6 inches down from the top edge, and then put on the spread. ☐

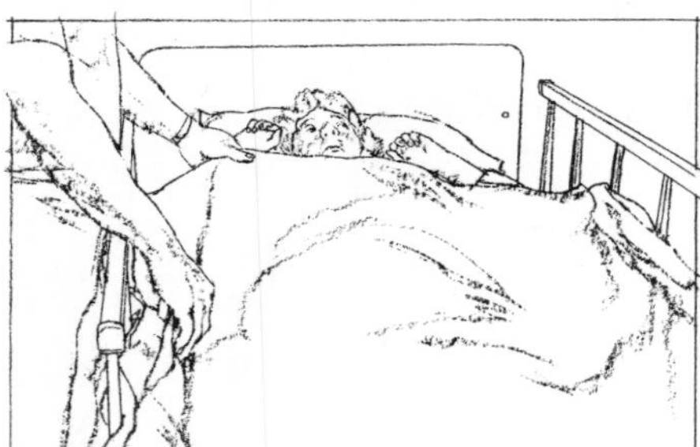

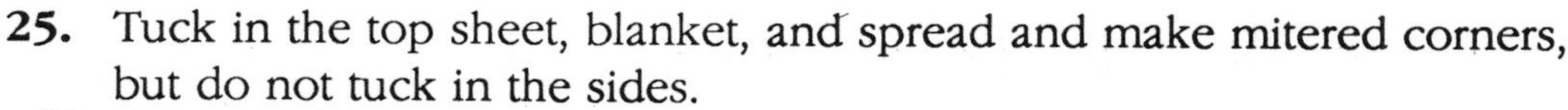

25. Tuck in the top sheet, blanket, and spread and make mitered corners, but do not tuck in the sides.

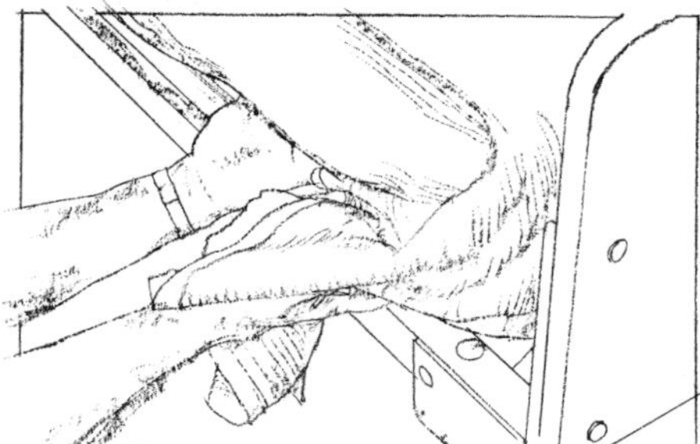

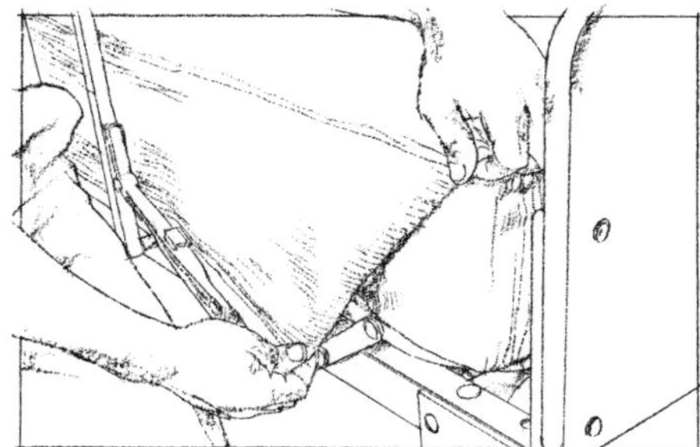

26. Fold the hem of the top sheet down over the blanket and spread.

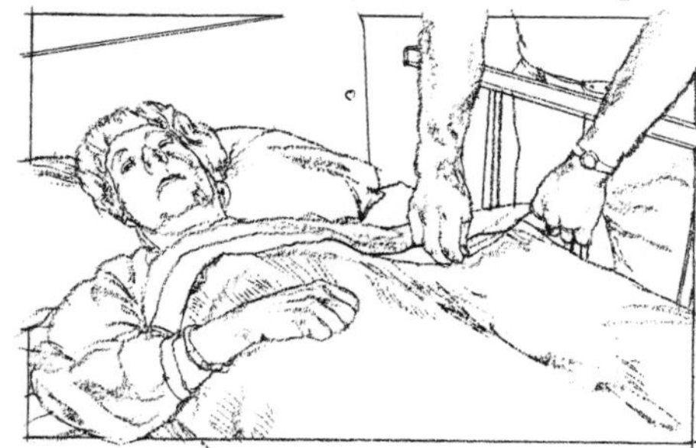

27. Make a "toe pleat" using the following steps:

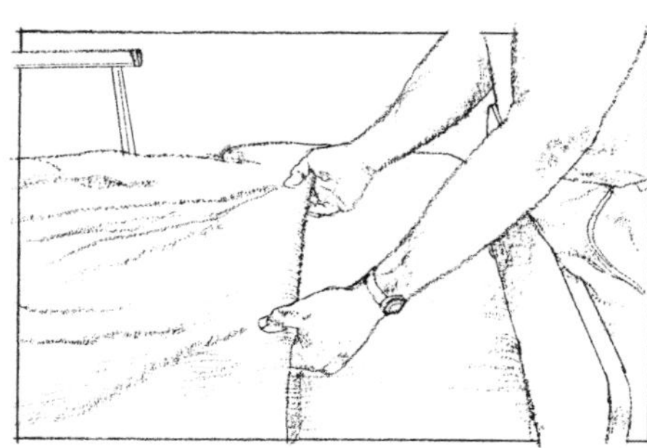

Hold both sides of the top covers at the mitered corners and gently pull the top covers toward the foot of the bed.

Make a 3 to 4 inch fold across the foot of the bed.

Rationale: The toe pleat prevents pressure on the resident's toes from the tight corners.

Skill 5: Positioning*

Name: ______________________ Date: ______________

Procedure

Competency check

Moving the Resident to the Side of the Bed in Order to Position Resident

With Two Nurse Assistants Using a Draw Sheet—
(This is the ideal way to move a resident)

1. Make sure the bed is flat.

   Note: Lower the head of the bed only as much as the resident can tolerate.

2. Stand on opposite sides of the bed.

3. Loosen the draw sheet on each side of the bed and roll it toward the resident with your palms facing up until your hands are close to the resident's body.

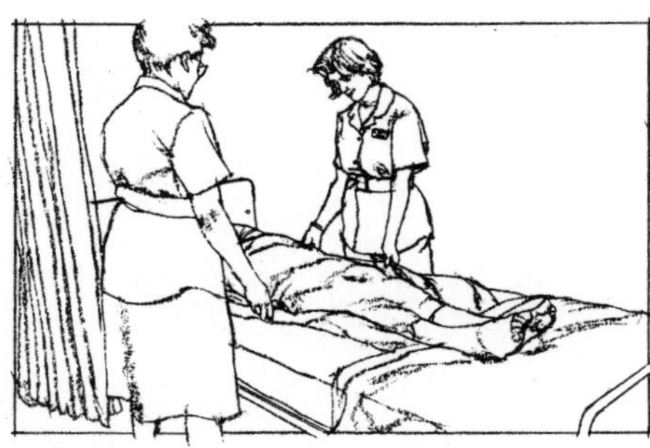

Rationale: Keeping palms up will assist in the nurse assistant's ability to lift.

* Some of the techniques in this skill have been adapted from Beverly Enterprises, *Lift With Care*, Visucom Productions, Inc., 1987.

4. Hold onto the rolled up draw sheet.

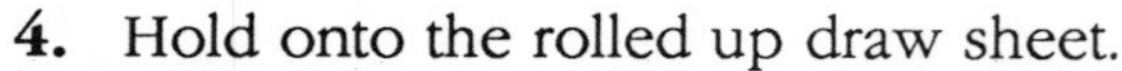

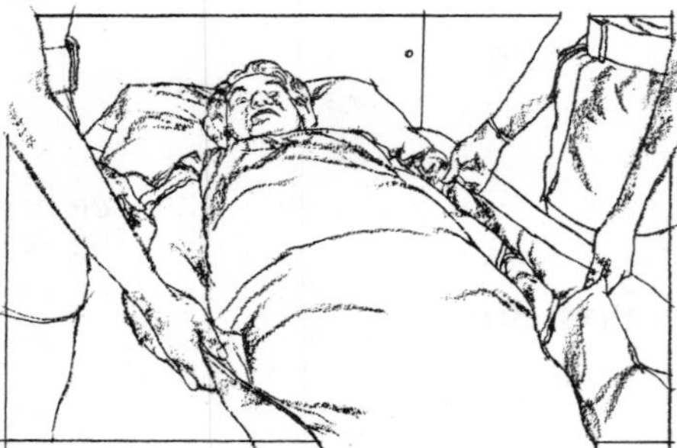

5. If the resident is to be moved toward you, position your feet about 12 inches apart with one foot slightly behind the other and keep your knees slightly bent.

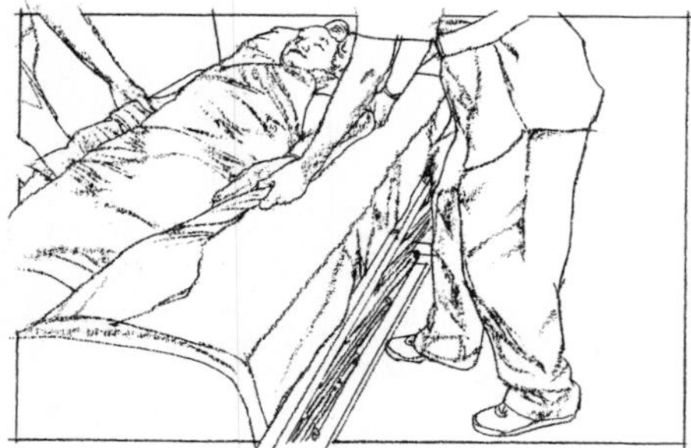

6. If the resident is being moved away from you, put one knee up on the bed.

Note: If there is a risk for contaminating nurse assistant clothing, place bed protection on bed

Note: Be sure the bed is in a lower position than working height so you can keep one foot firmly on the floor.

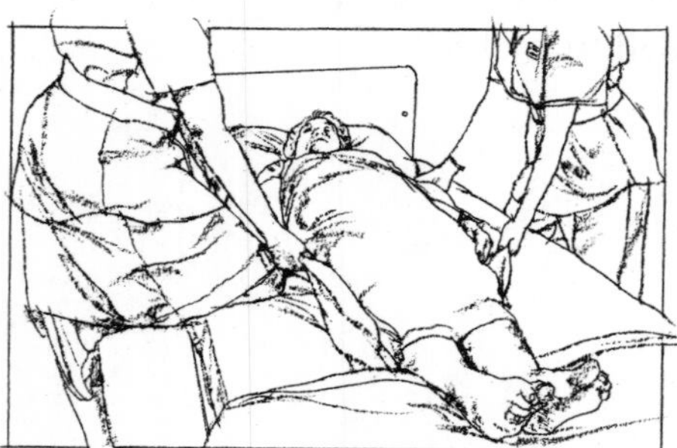

7. At the count of three ("1 - 2 - 3"), gently lift/slide the resident to the side of the bed using the draw sheet to support most of the resident's body. ☐

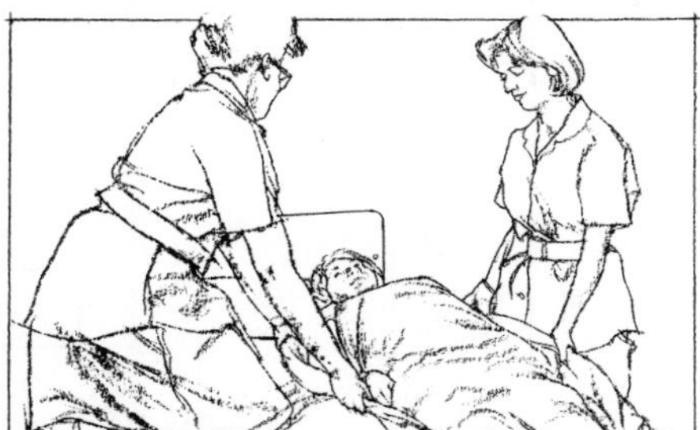

8. Make sure the resident's body is properly aligned. ☐

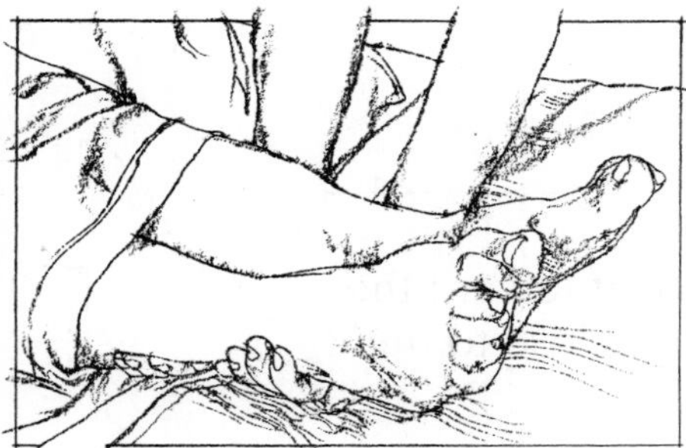

Moving the Resident Up in Bed

1. Take away the resident's pillow and place it against the headboard. ☐

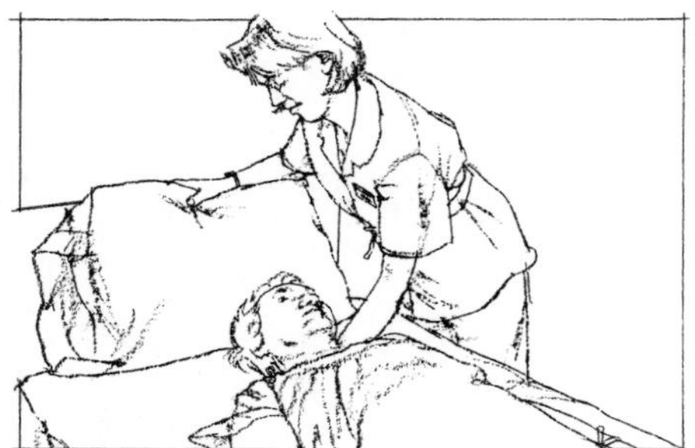

2. Check for placement of any drainage tubes.

Note: These tubes are often not visible. Therefore, it is important to always check before moving the resident so nothing is pulled out.

With Two Nurse Assistants Using a Draw Sheet—

1. Stand on opposite sides of the bed.

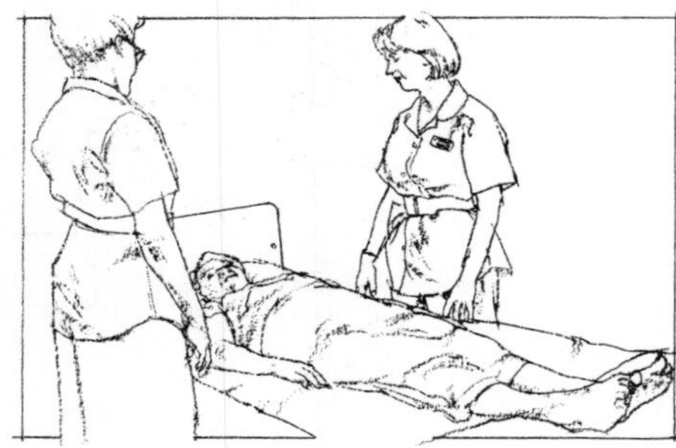

---

2. Loosen the draw sheet on each side of the bed and roll it toward the resident with your palms facing up until your hands are close to the resident's body.

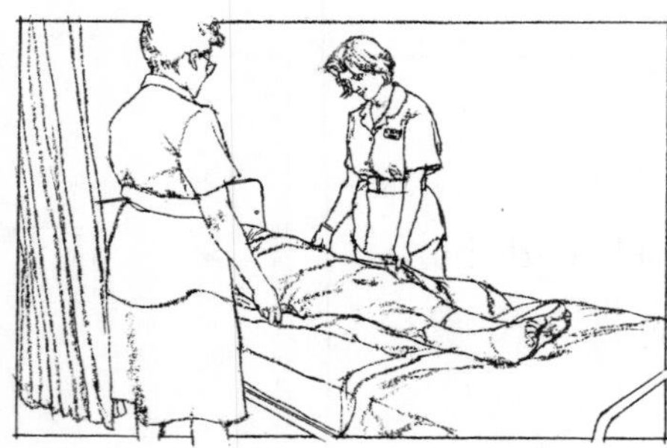

---

3. Hold onto the rolled up draw sheet. ☐

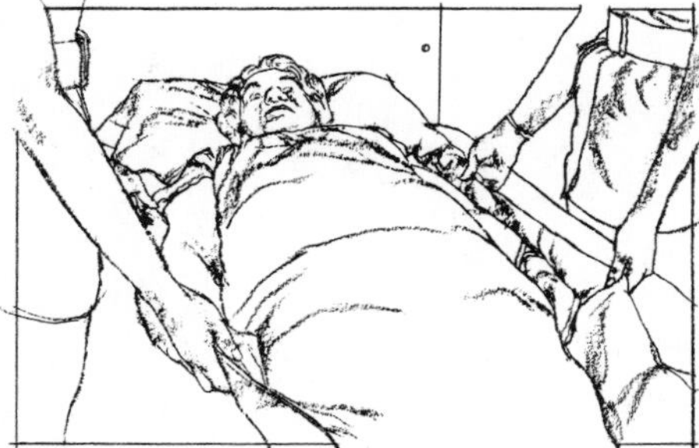

---

4. Stand as close to the bed as possible and put your knee closest to the headboard on the bed. ☐

Note: Be sure the bed is in a lower than working height position so you can keep one foot firmly on the floor.

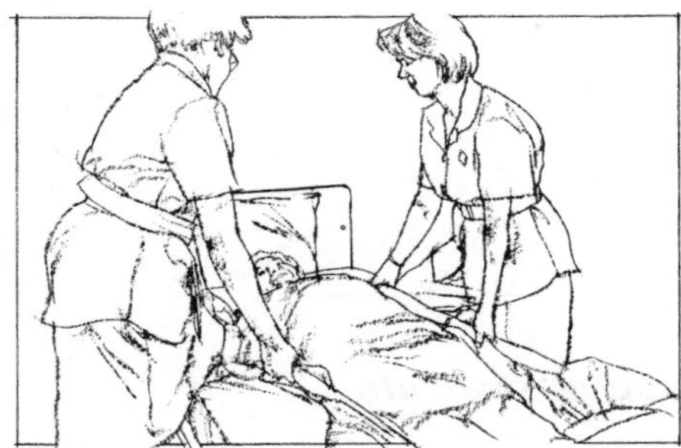

---

5. At the count of three, move the resident to the top of the bed. ☐

Note: Lift the resident smoothly (don't jerk).

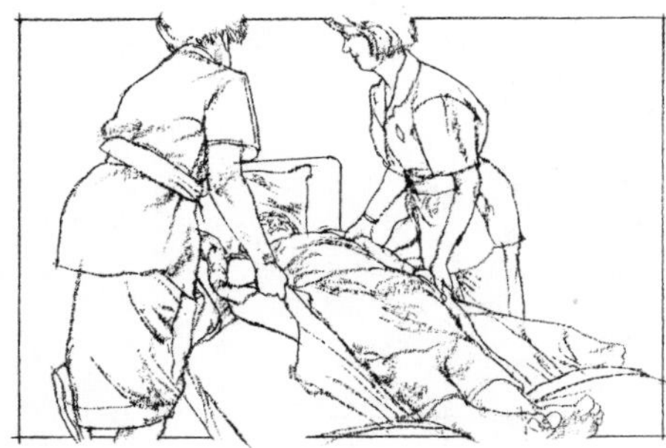

---

6. Retuck the draw sheet and replace the resident's pillow. ☐

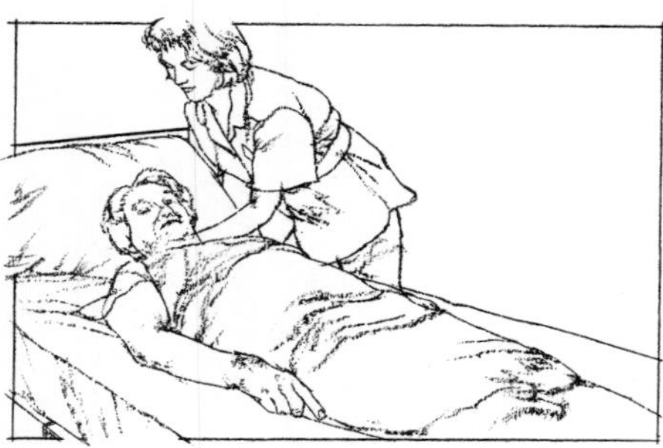

7. Make sure the resident's body is properly aligned. ☐

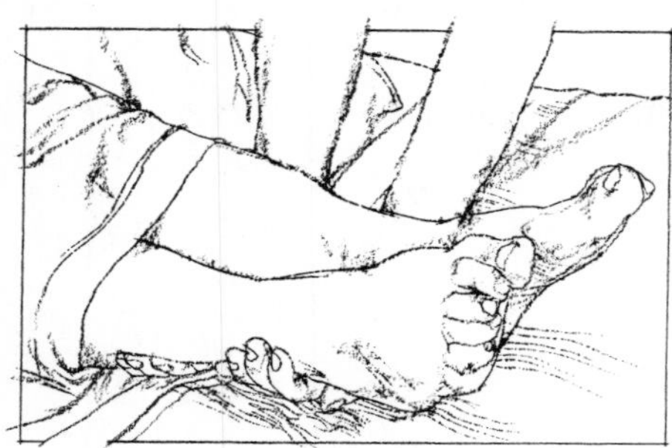

Turning the Resident For Personal Care with Two Nurse Assistants and a Draw Sheet—

1. Begin by lowering the siderails and check the placement of any drainage tubes. ☐

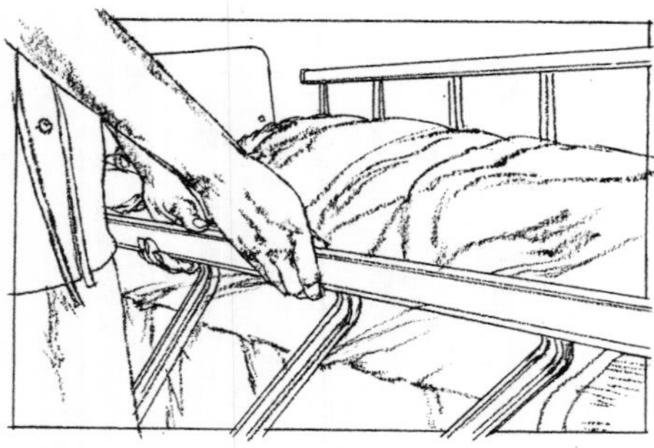

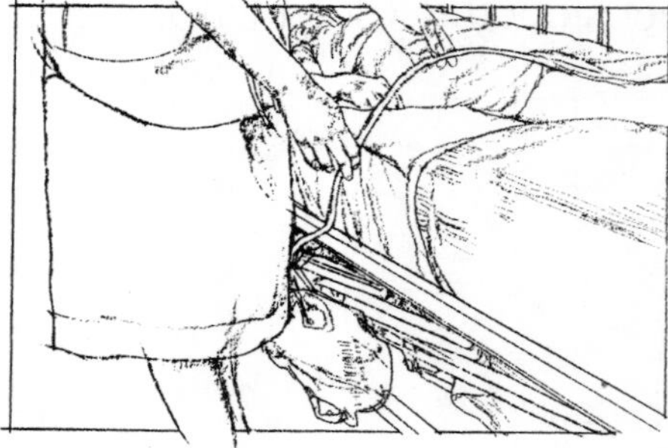

2. Have the resident cross their arms over their chest and cross their ankles toward the direction you are turning them. ☐

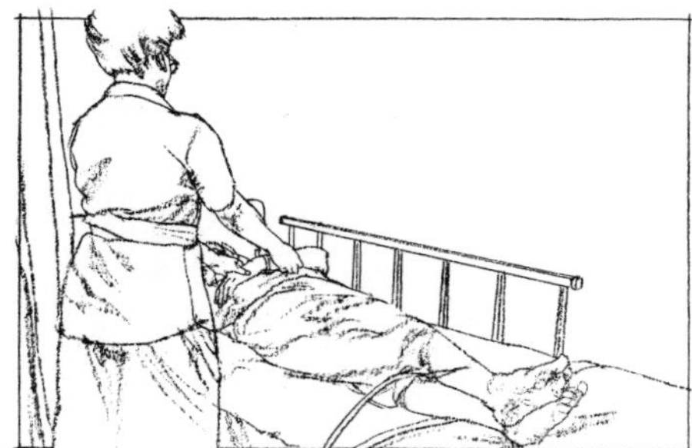

3. The nurse assistant on the side toward which the resident is turning should place one hand on the resident's shoulder and the other hand on the resident's upper thigh. ☐

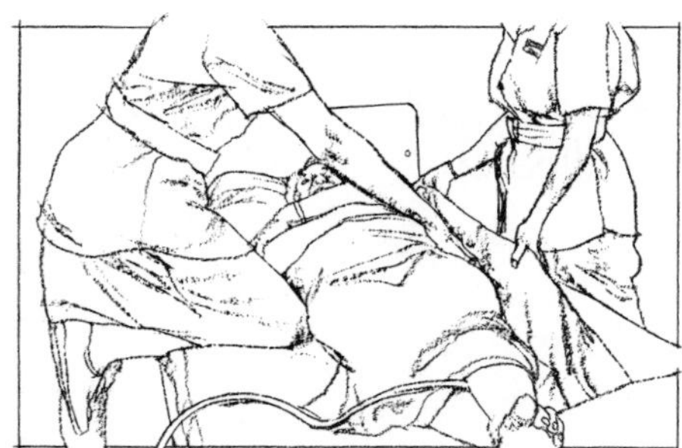

4. The other nurse assistant rolls the draw sheet close to the resident's body with palms up. Be sure to use a broad base of support and lift the draw sheet rolling the resident onto their side. ☐

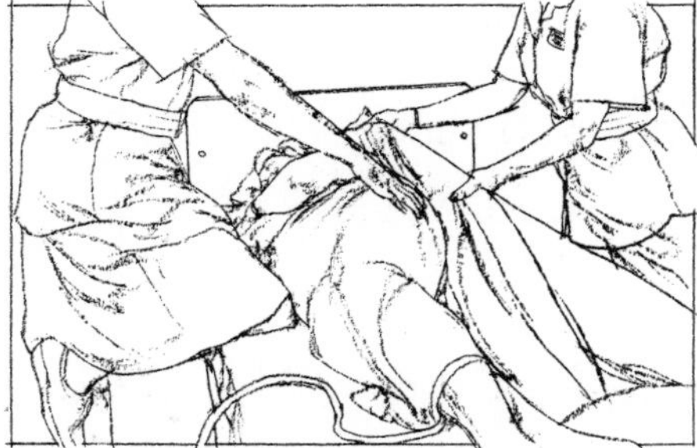

5. Retuck the draw sheet and raise the side rails. ☐

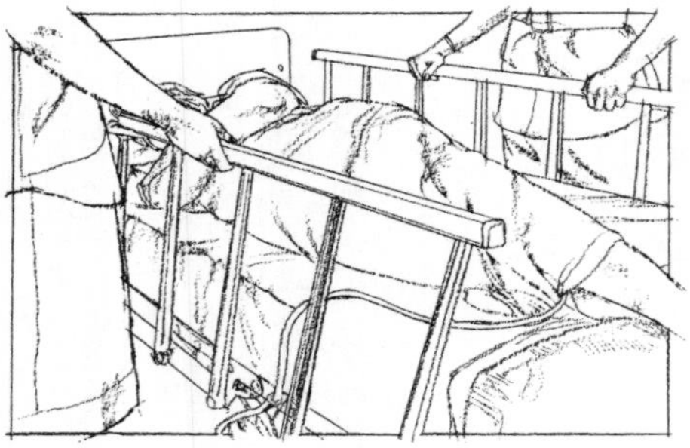

Turning the Resident for Personal Care

Lower side rails

1. Check for placement of any drainage tubes. ☐

Note: These tubes are often not visible. Therefore, it is important to always check before turning the resident so nothing is pulled out.

---

2. Have the resident cross their arms over their chest and cross their ankles toward the direction you are turning. ☐

---

3. Put one hand on the resident's shoulder and the other on the resident's upper thigh. ☐

---

4. Roll the resident onto their side toward you. Raise the side rail. ☐

Note: You may also untuck the draw sheet and use it as a turn sheet.

Positioning

Supine position

1. Put a pillow under the resident's head just to the top of the shoulders. ☐

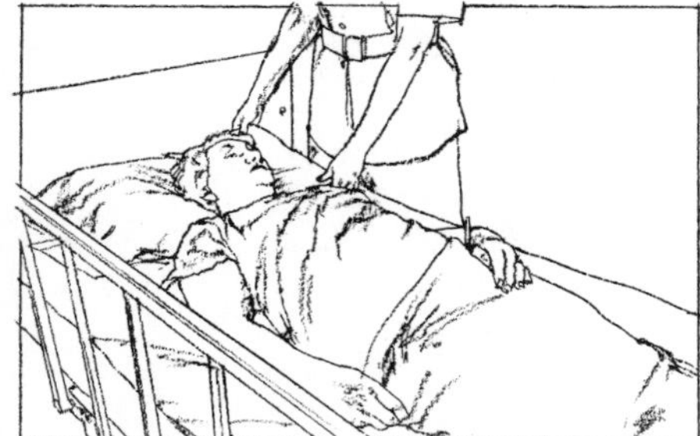

2. Put resident's arm alongside but not against their body. ☐

Note: If the resident has a paralyzed arm, place a pillow under the arm with the wrist slightly higher than the elbow, the elbow slightly higher than shoulder, and a hand roll in place.

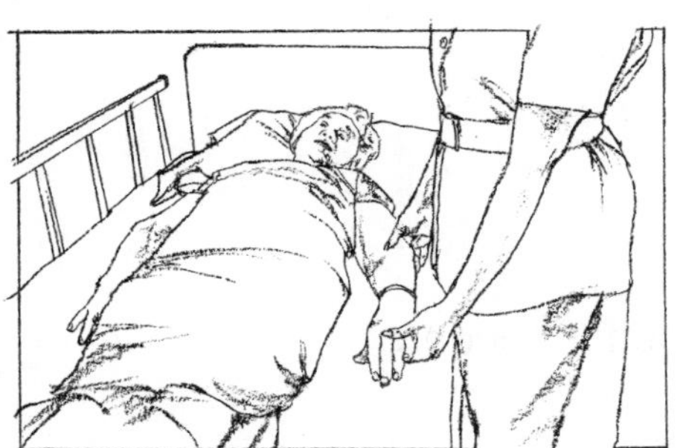

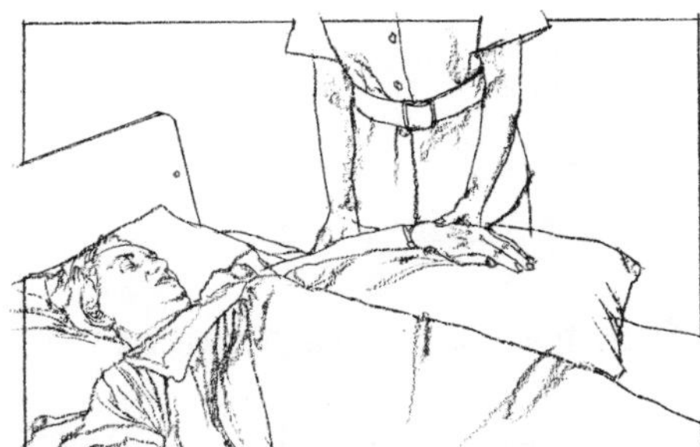

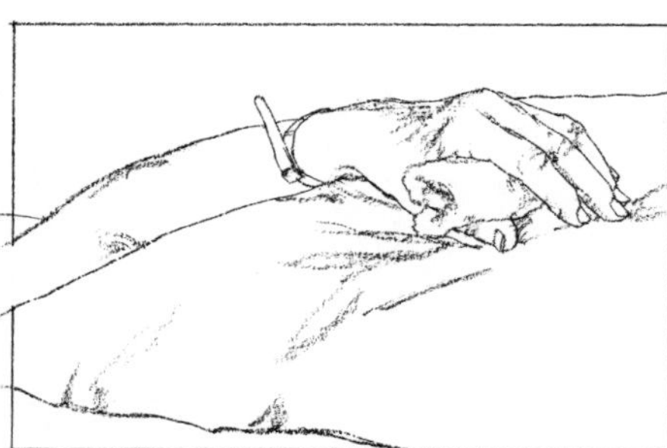

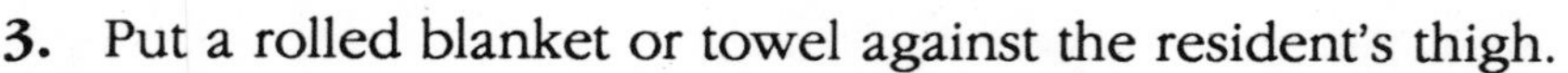

3. Put a rolled blanket or towel against the resident's thigh.

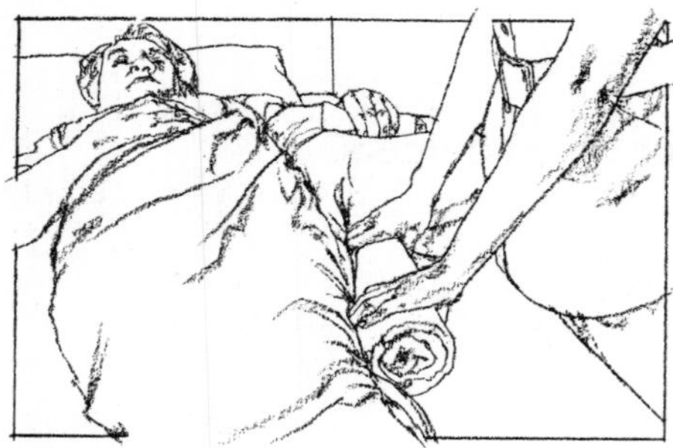

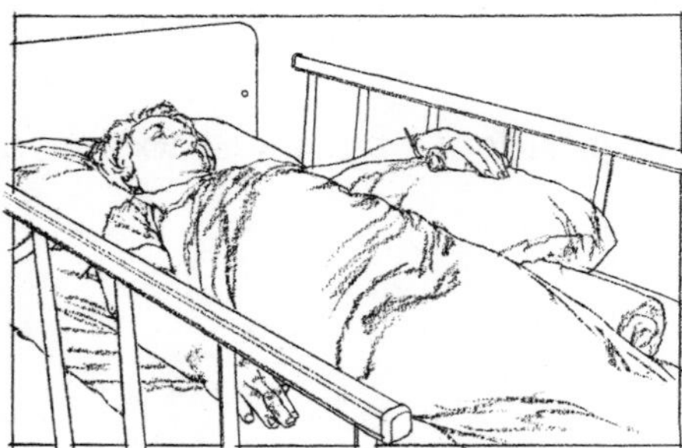

Fowler's position

1. Make sure the bed is flat and the resident is lying down. Take away all pillows and devices.

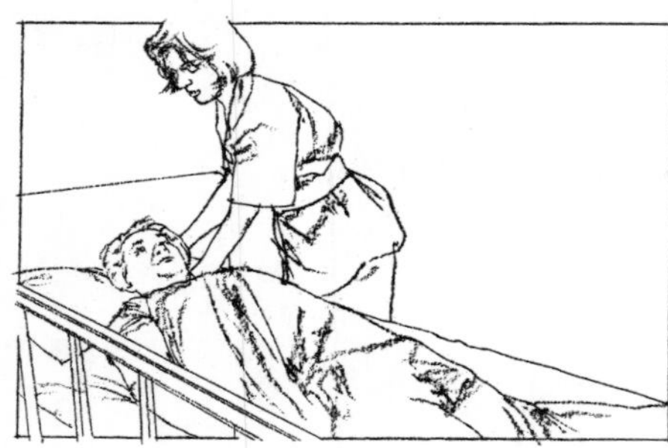

---

2. Following the procedure for moving a resident up in bed if needed.

Note: Make sure the resident is in the center of the bed.

---

3. Raise the head of the bed 30 to 45 degrees.

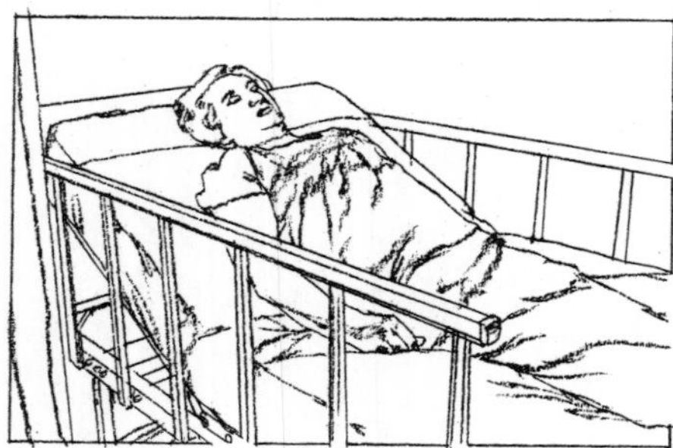

---

4. Elevate the foot of the bed just enough to prevent the resident from sliding down in bed. ☐

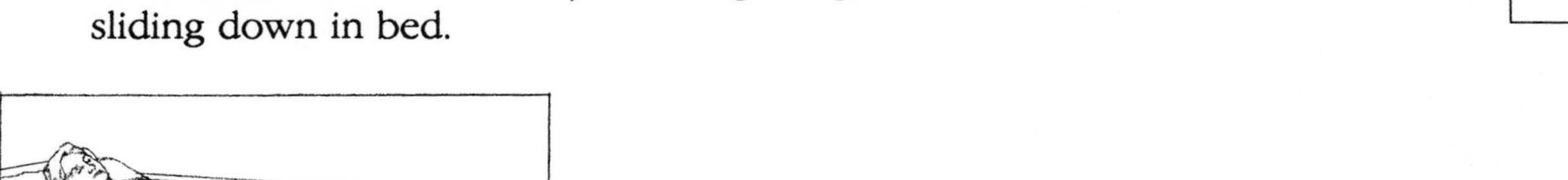

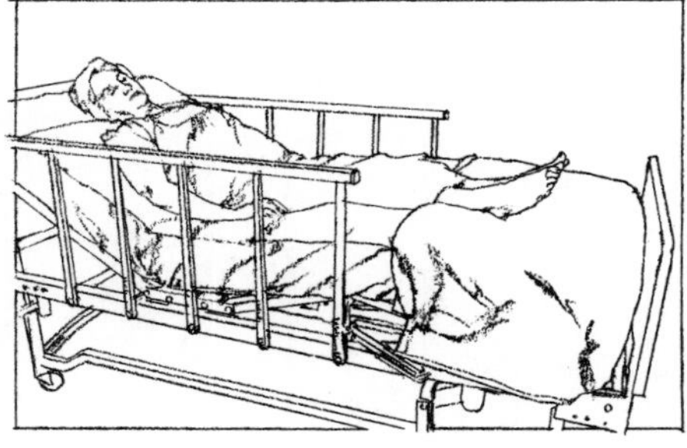

---

5. Put a pillow behind the resident's head for comfort. ☐

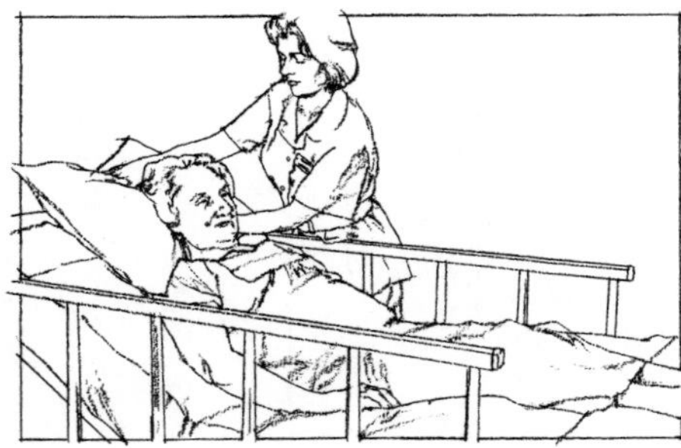

---

6. Support the resident's forearm and wrist with pillows, keeping the wrist higher than the elbow, if needed. ☐

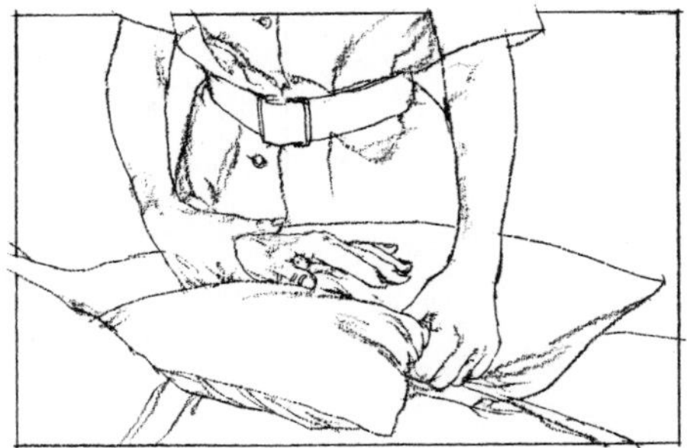

---

7. Place a foot support, if needed. ☐

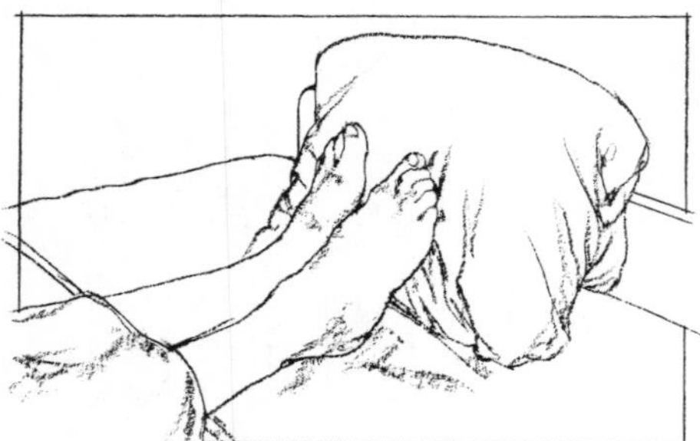

Prone position

1. Make sure the bed is flat. ☐

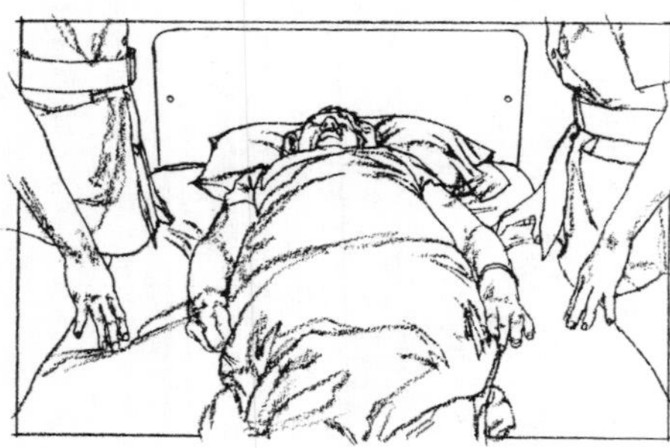

---

2. Follow the procedure for moving a resident to the side of the bed. ☐

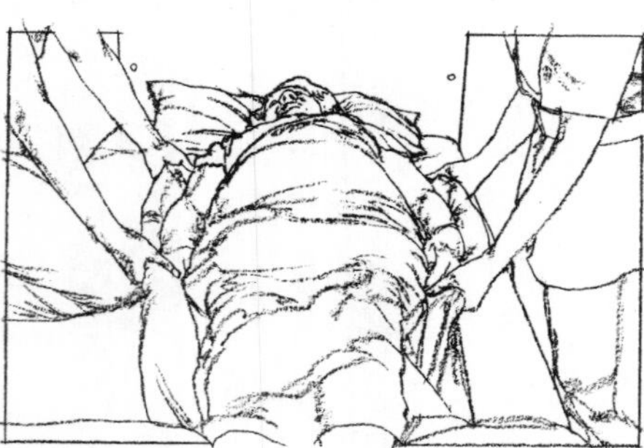

---

3. Put one hand on the resident's shoulder and one on their hip. ☐

Note: Be sure the arm away from you is tucked close to the resident so it will not be trapped or caught under the body when rolled over.

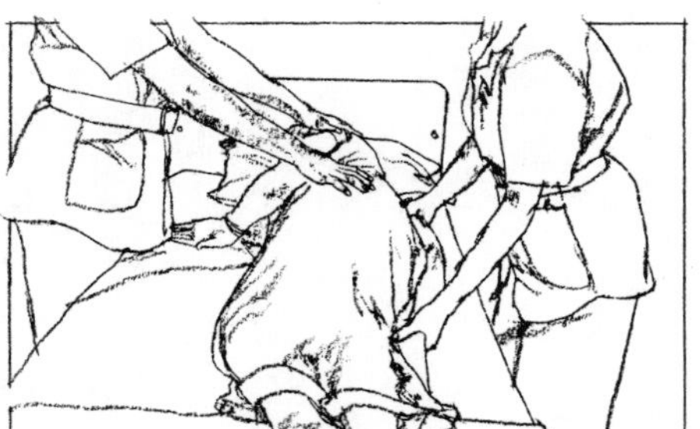

4. Gently turn the resident onto their stomach with their head turned to the side. ☐

5. Help the resident to move down slightly so their feet are over the end of the mattress, or place a pillow under the resident's shins. ☐

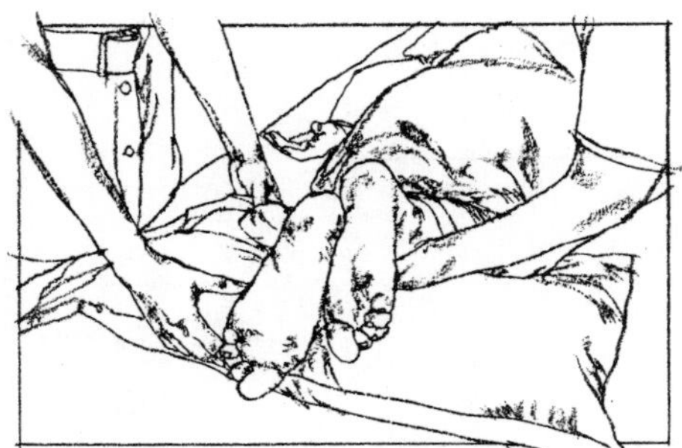

6. Place a small pillow or folded bath blanket under the resident's head and one under the upper abdomen. ☐

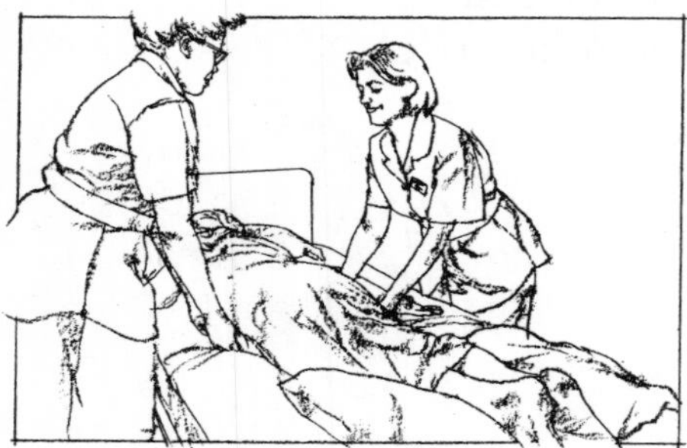

7. Place one of the resident's arms with the elbow bent at a 90 degree angle at their side and the other arm straight along the other side. ☐

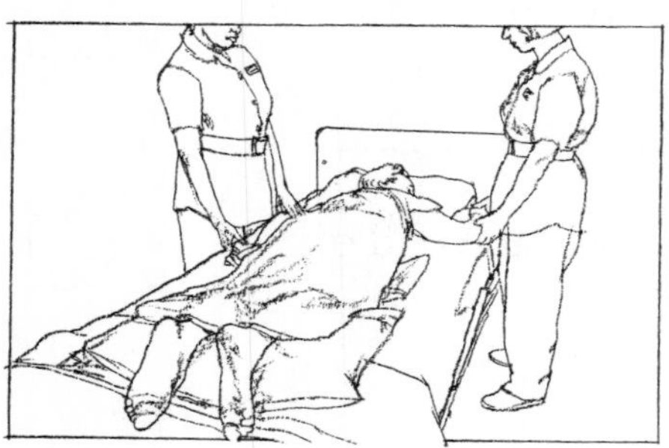

Modified side-lying (lateral) position

1. Make sure the resident is flat in bed. ☐

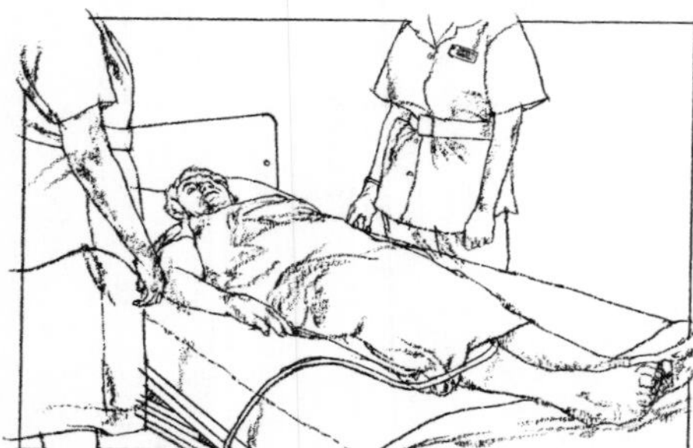

2. Cross the resident's arms and ankles toward the direction you are turning. ☐

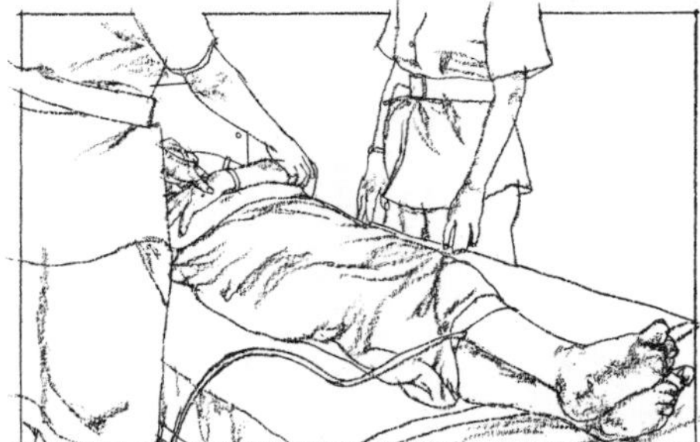

3. Following the procedure for moving a resident to the side of the bed, move the resident to the opposite side of the bed to which they will be turning. ☐

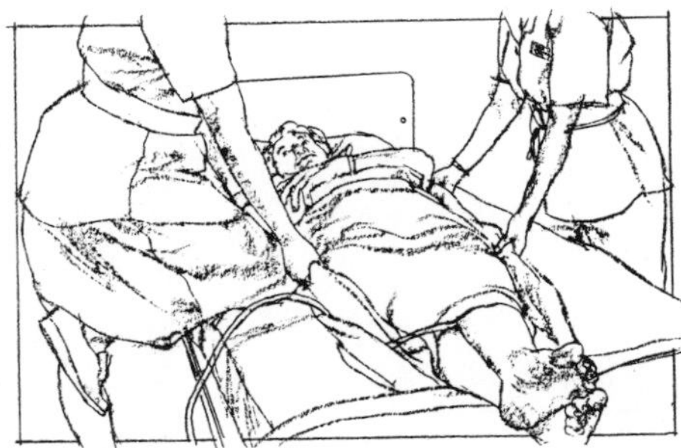

4. Turn the resident onto their side so that they are off the coccyx (tail bone), but not directly on the hip. To do this, the nurse assistant on the side to which the resident is turning should place one hand on the resident's shoulder and the other on the resident's upper thigh. The other nurse assistant rolls the draw sheet close to the resident's body with palms up. Be sure to use a broad base of support and lift the draw sheet and roll the resident onto their side. ☐

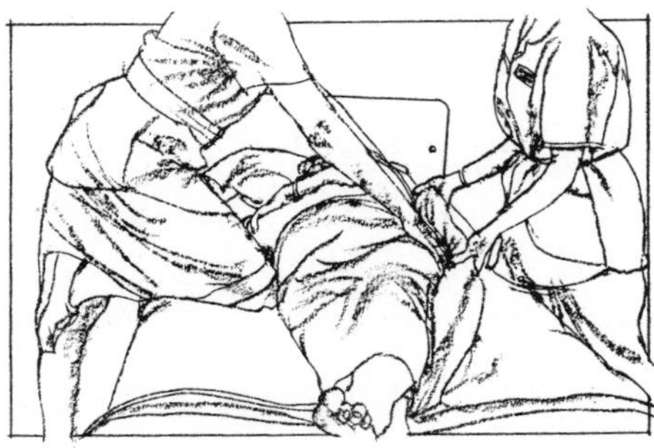

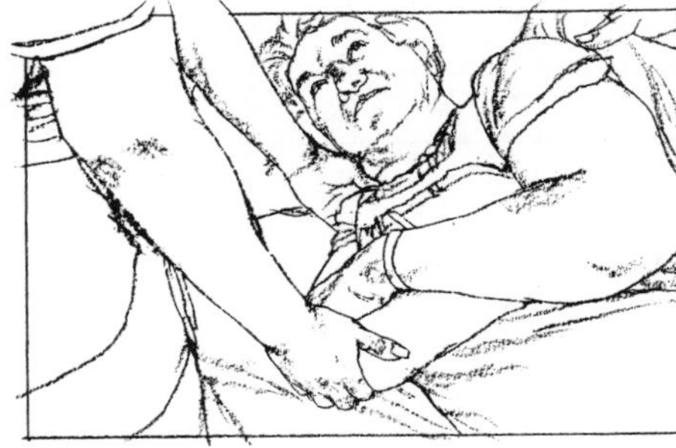

5. Adjust the resident's shoulder so that they are not lying on their arm. ☐

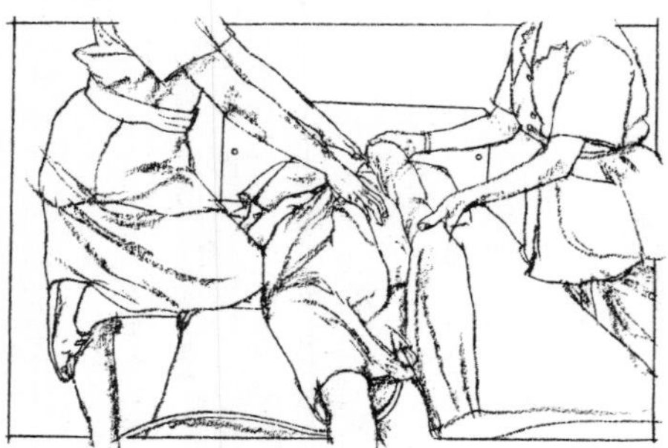

---

6. Support the resident's back with a rolled blanket or towel to keep them in proper position. ☐

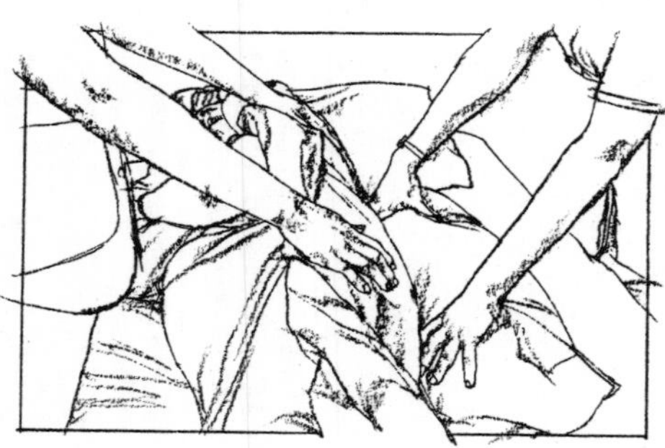

---

7. Support the resident's top arm with a pillow, and put a hand roll in place, if needed. ☐

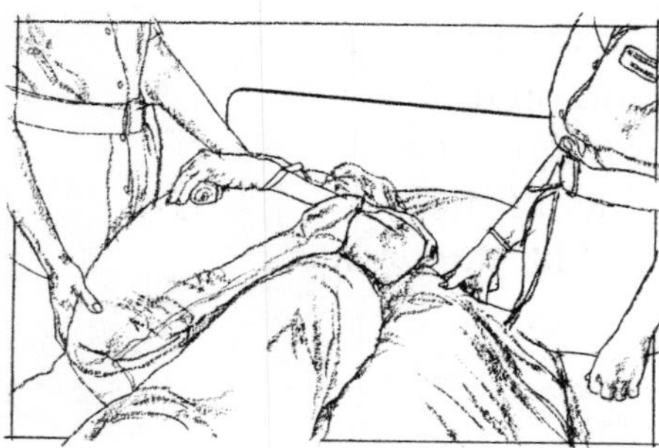

---

8. Place the resident's top leg forward and support it with pillows so that it does not rest on top of the lower leg. 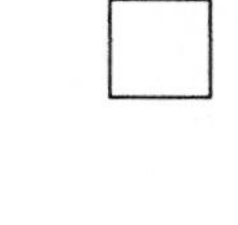

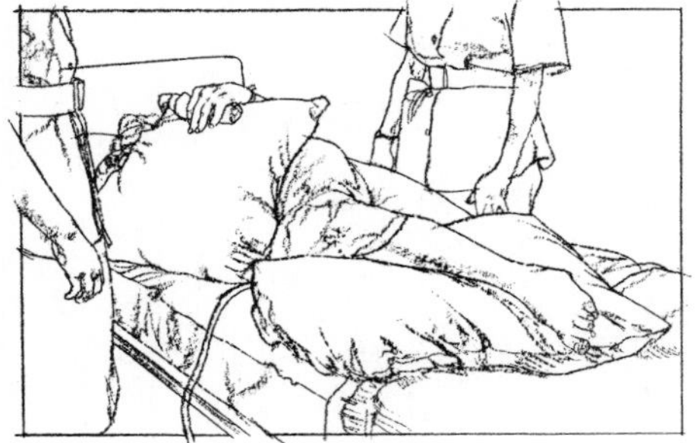

Skill 6: Moving the Resident From Bed to Chair*

Name: ______________________________ Date: ______________

Procedure

Competency check

Without Safety Belt When Resident Can Help

1. Place chair or wheelchair at a slight angle against the bed on the resident's stronger side. ☐

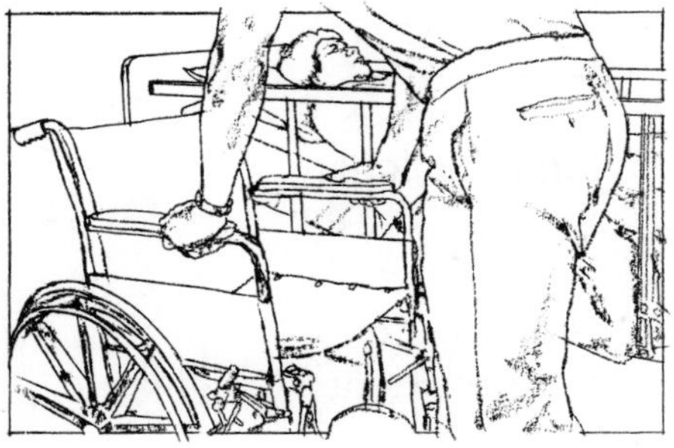

Rationale: This angle will allow a smooth, safe transfer and prevent resident from hitting sidearm.

2. Remove, or fold back, the wheelchair footrest and lock bed and wheelchair brakes. ☐

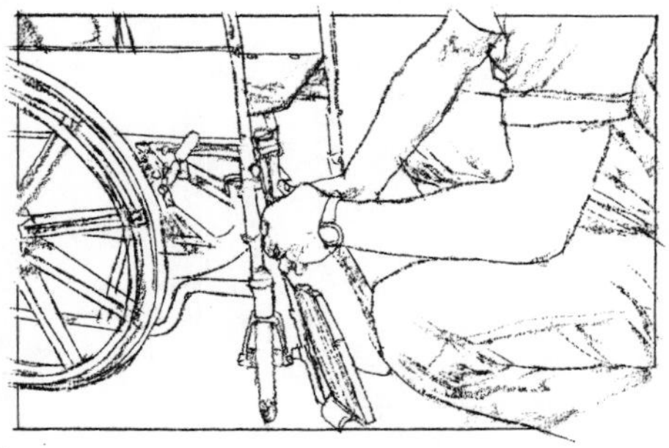

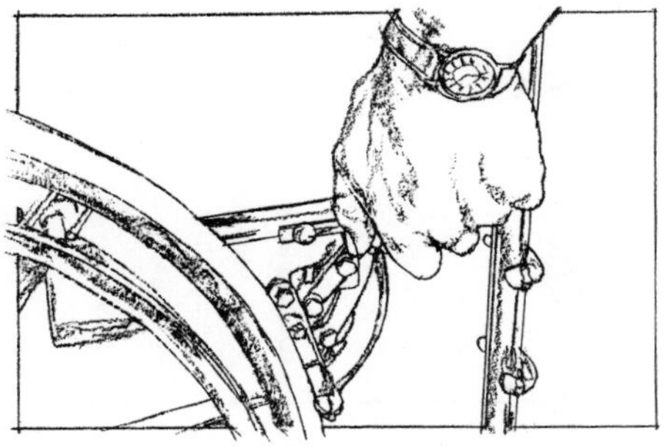

3. Raise the head of the bed and lower the side rail. ☐

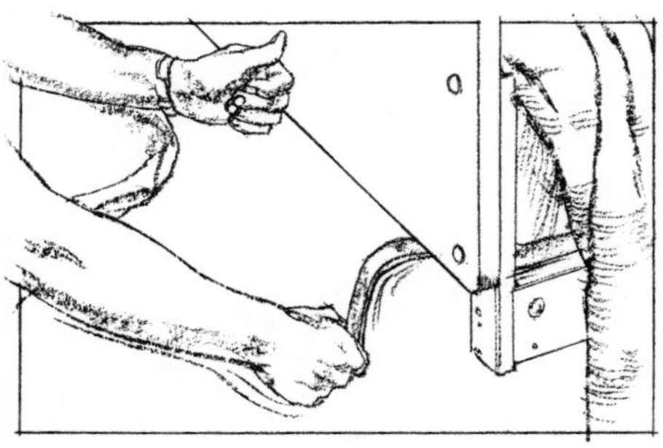

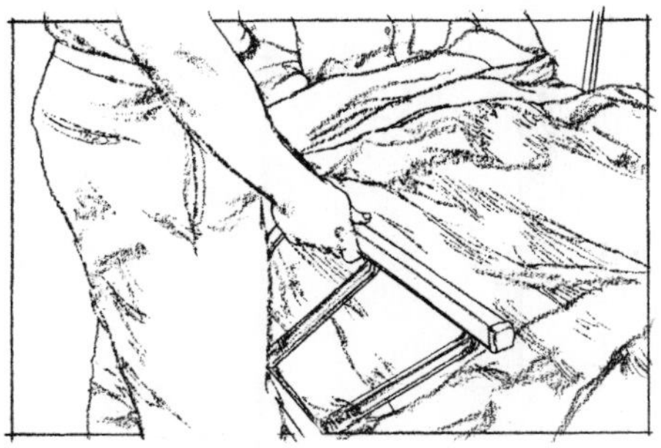

* Some of the techniques in this skill have been adapted from Beverly Enterprises, *Lift With Care*, Visucom Productions, Inc., 1987.

4. Put one of your arms under the resident's shoulders and the other arm under their thighs. ☐

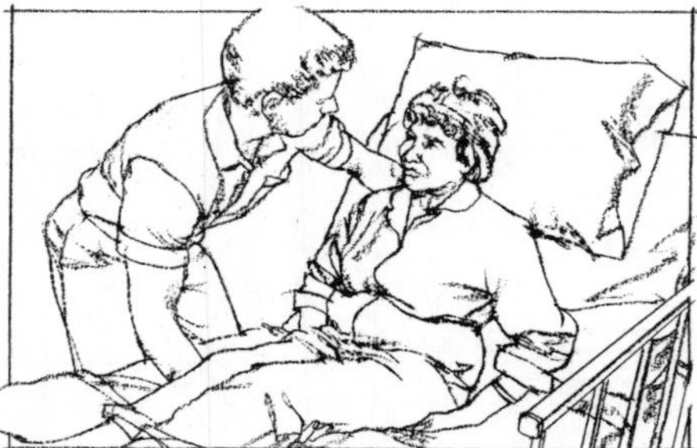

5. Turn the resident toward you into a sitting position bringing their legs into a dangling position over the side of the bed. ☐

Note: Stay with the resident and allow them to sit on the side of the bed for 2 minutes before going on with the procedure. If the resident becomes dizzy, sweaty, short of breath, or is in any pain, lay them back down and report to the charge nurse.

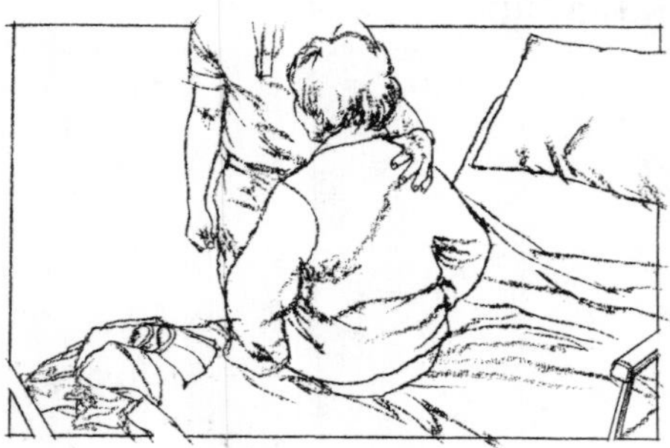

6. Help the resident put on their clothing, including footwear. ☐

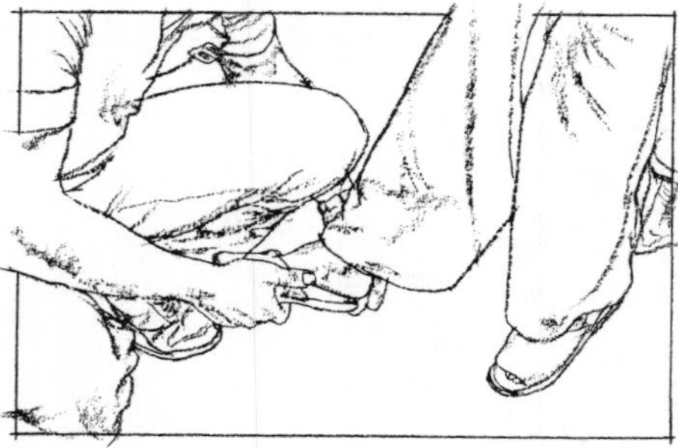

7. Place your arms under the resident's arms, holding on to the resident's shoulders, and have the resident place their arms around your waist or shoulder while leaning forward. ☐

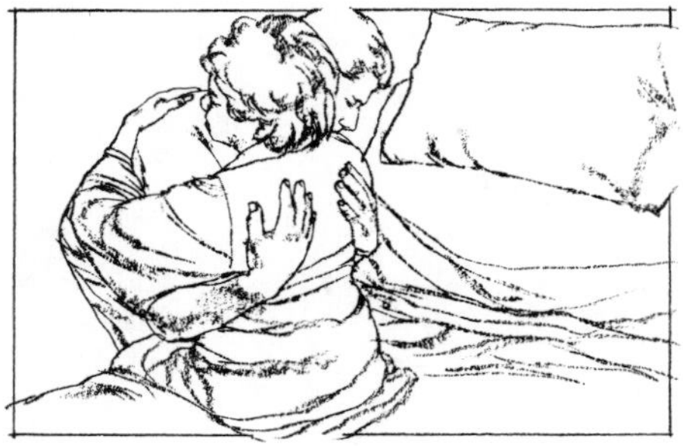

---

8. Put your knee (the one further from the chair) between the resident's knees. ☐

---

9. On the count of three, raise the resident to a standing position. ☐

Note: Get as close as possible "Hugging Position". Remember to use good body mechanics—use a good base of support; keep the resident close; keep your upper body erect; lift smoothly; and don't jerk.

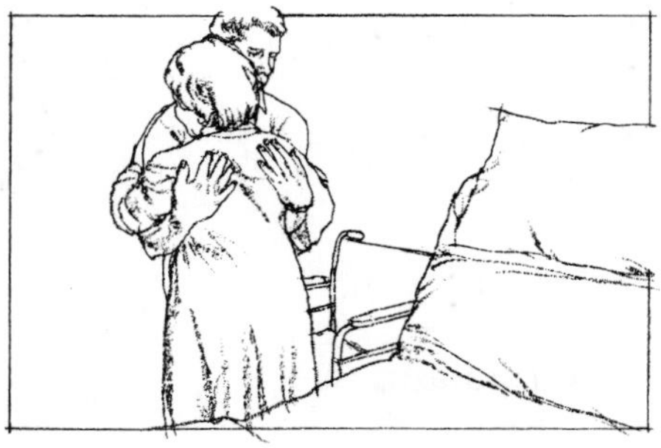

---

10. Turn your body with the resident until the resident is right in front of the chair. ☐

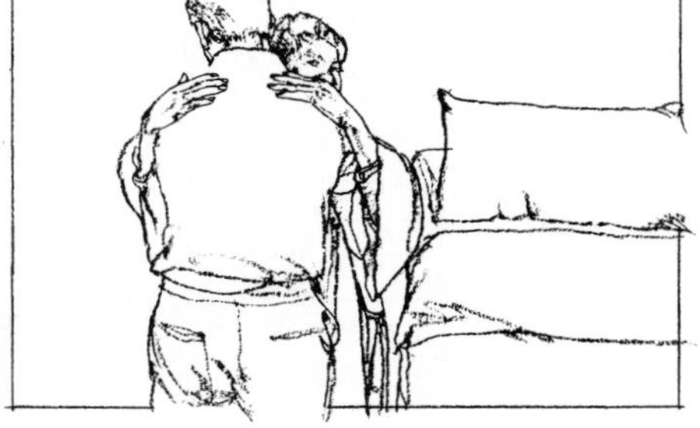

---

11. Lower the resident into the chair. ☐

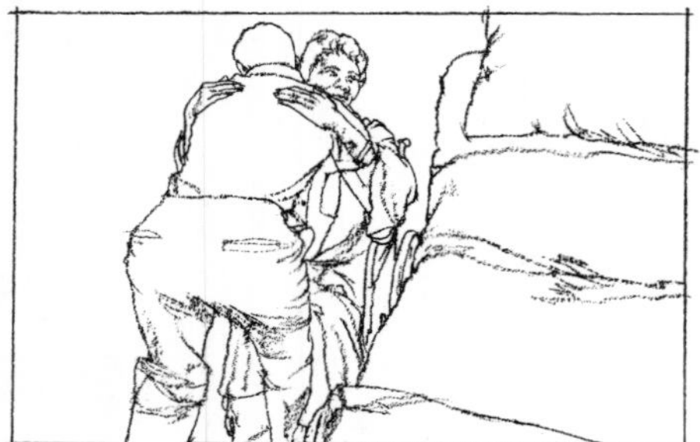

Reverse these steps to move the resident from a chair to their bed.

With a Safety Belt

1. Place the wheelchair at a slight angle against the bed on the resident's stronger side. ☐

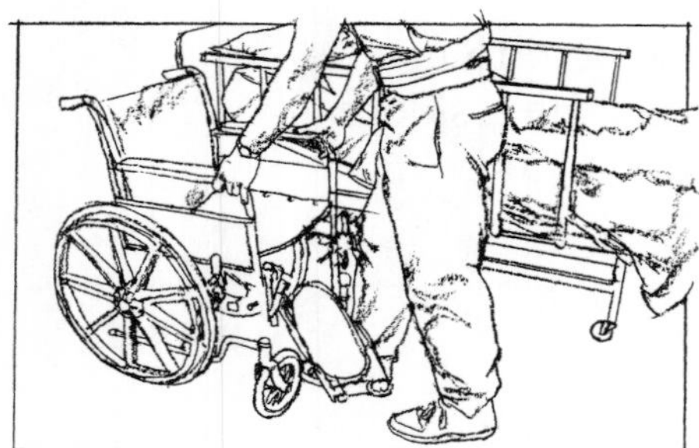

---

2. Remove, or fold back, the wheelchair footrest and lock the bed and wheelchair brakes. ☐

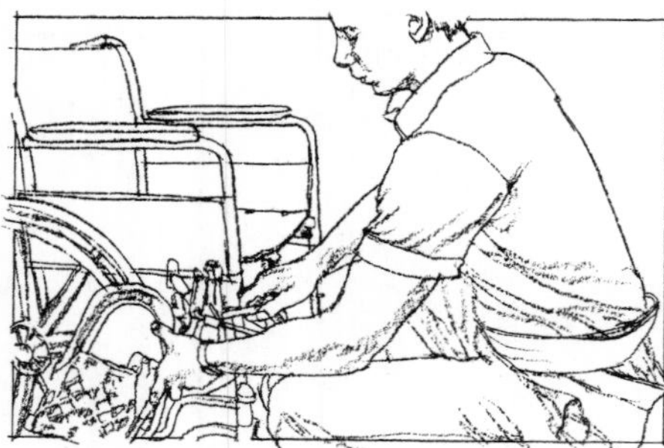

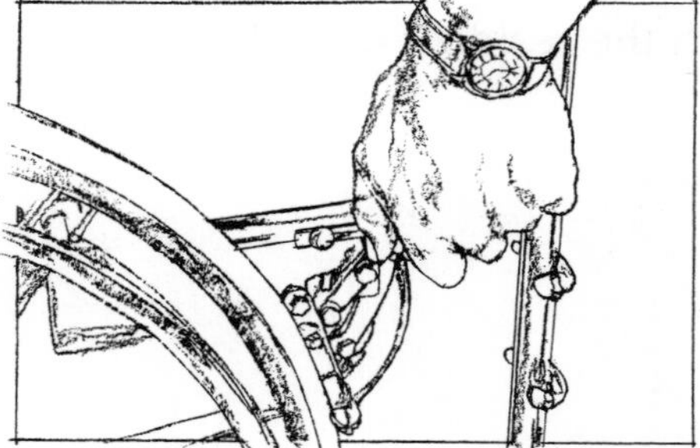

---

3. Raise the head of the bed so that the resident is almost in a sitting position. ☐

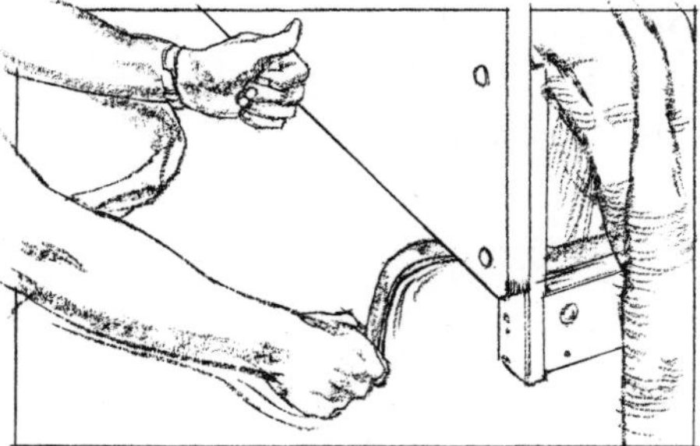

4. Lower the side rail nearest to the chair. ☐

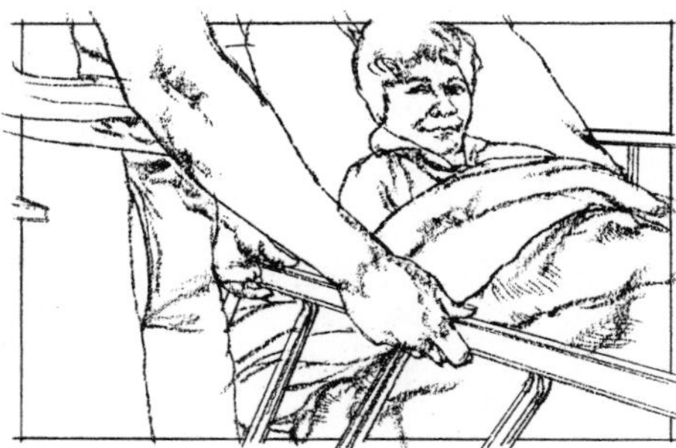

5. Put one of your arms under the resident's shoulders and the other arm under their thighs. ☐

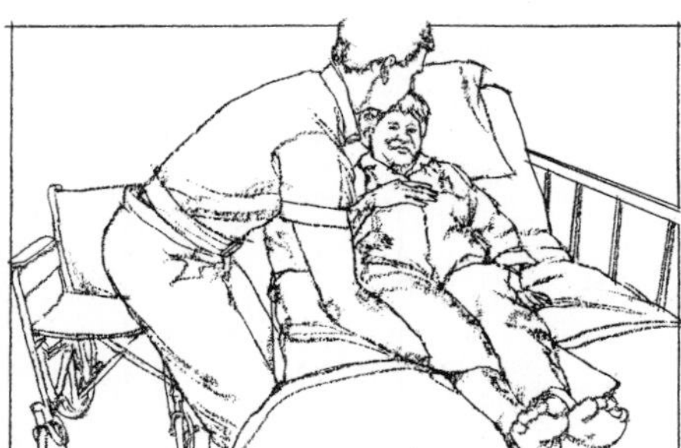

6. Turn the resident to a sitting position with their legs dangling over the side of the bed.

   Note: Stay with the resident and allow them to sit on the side of the bed for 2 minutes before going on with the procedure. If the resident becomes dizzy, sweaty, short of breath, or is in any pain, lay them back down and report to the charge nurse.

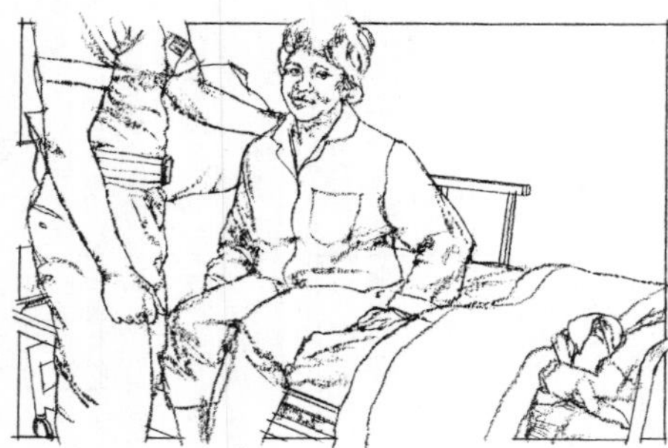

7. Help the resident put on their shoes and clothing.

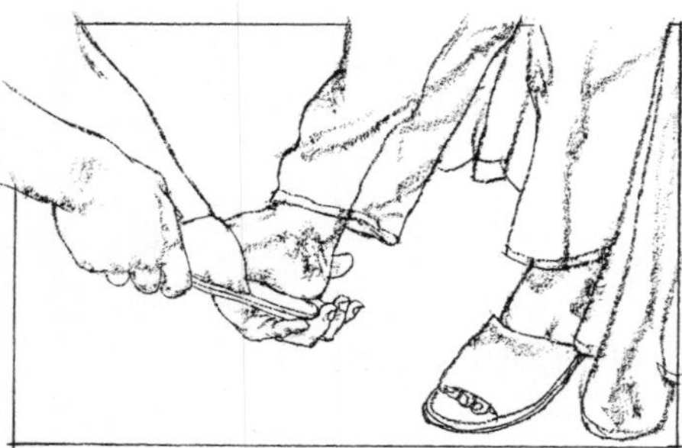

8. Help the resident put on a safety belt.

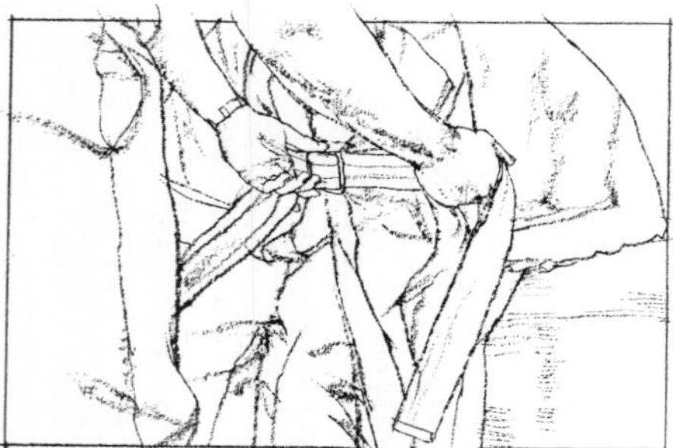

9. Grasp the safety belt on the back sides of the resident's waist and have the resident hold around your shoulders. ☐

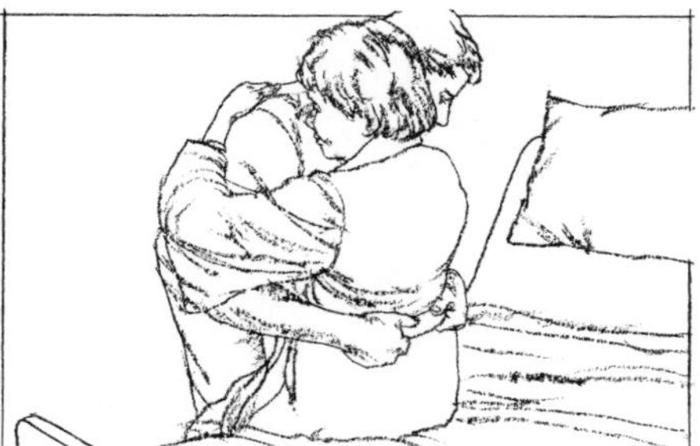

10. Put the knee farthest from the wheelchair between the resident's legs. ☐

11. On the count of three, raise the resident to a standing position. ☐

Note: Remember to use good body mechanics—use a broad base of support; keep the resident close; keep your upper body erect; lift smoothly; don't twist.

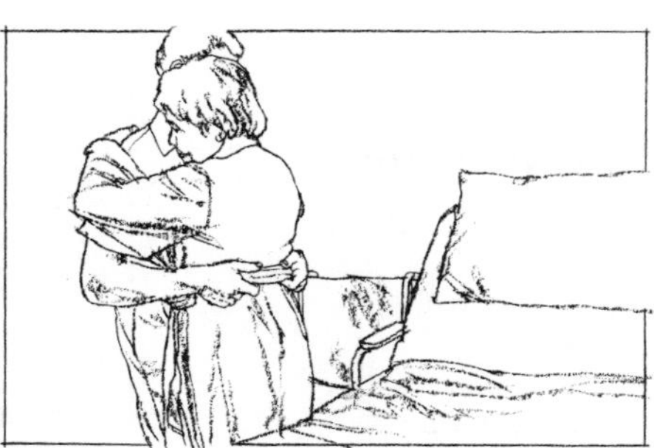

12. Turn your body with the resident until the resident is right in front of the chair. ☐

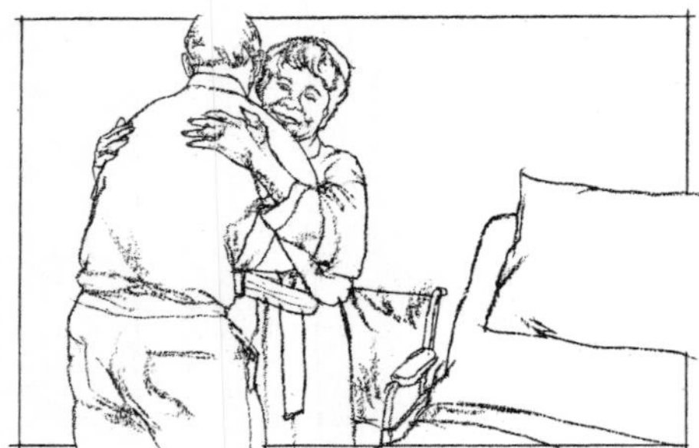

13. Lower the resident into the chair. ☐

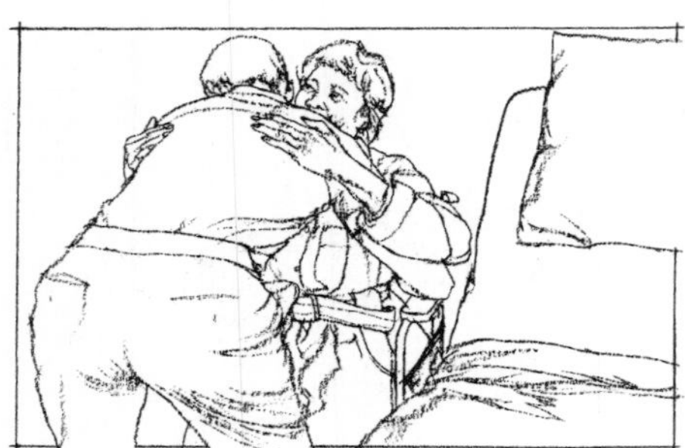

Reverse these steps to move the resident from a chair to their bed.

With Two Nurse Assistants and Safety Belt

1. Put the chair next to the side of the bed but leave a space between the chair and the bed. ☐

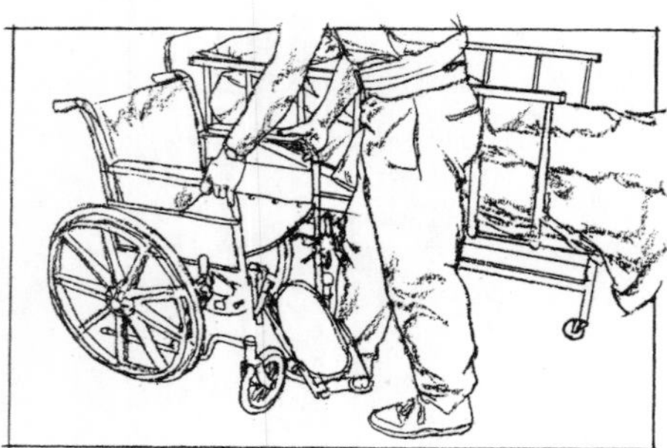

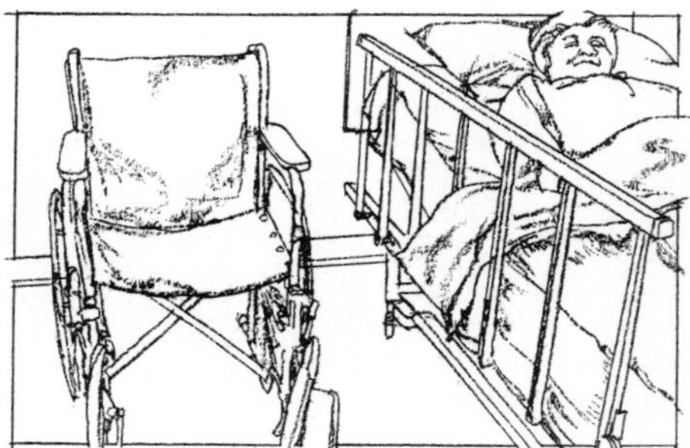

2. Remove or fold back the wheelchair foot rest and lock the bed and wheelchair brakes. ☐

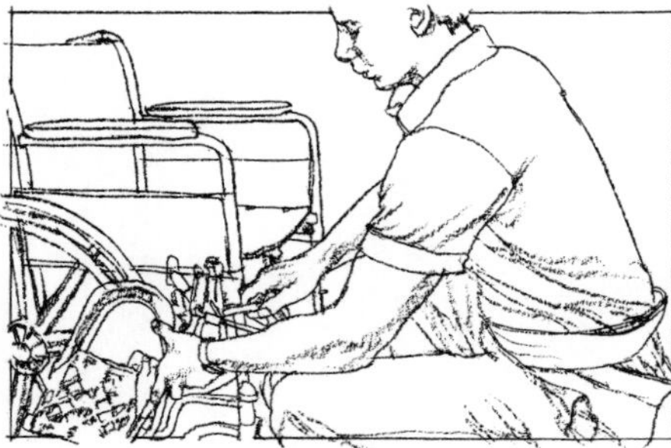
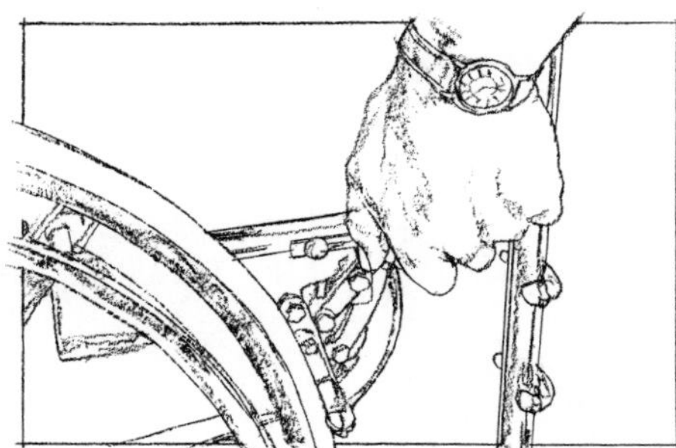

---

3. Raise the head of the bed so the resident is in a sitting position and lower the side rail. ☐

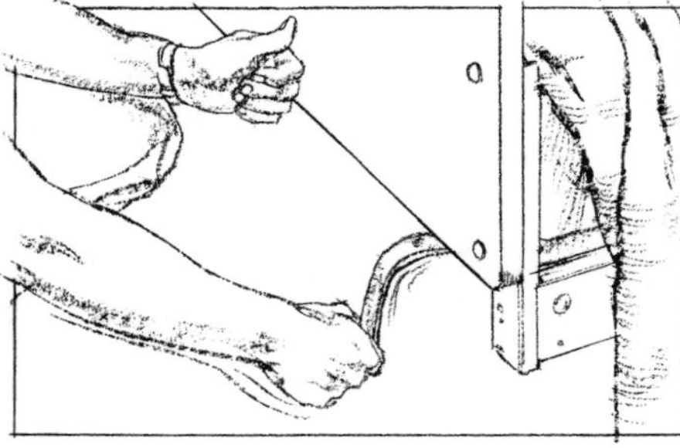
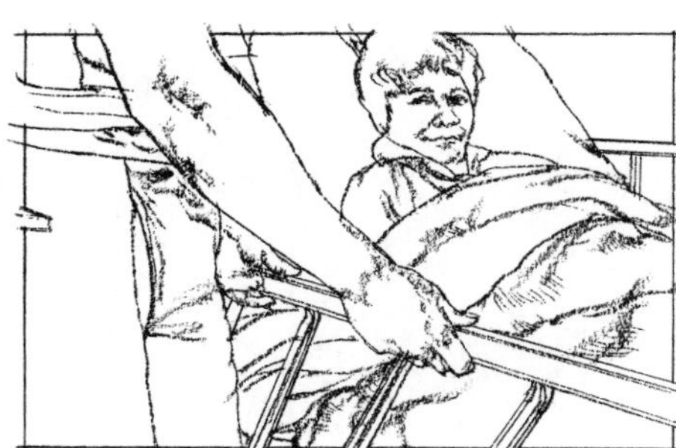

---

4. One nurse assistant puts their arm around the resident's shoulders and the other nurse assistant puts their arm under the resident's thighs. ☐

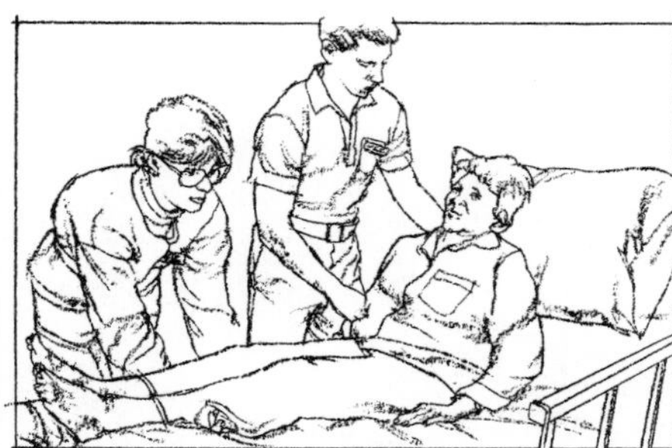

---

5. Turn the resident toward you into a sitting position bringing legs into a dangling position over the side of the bed. ☐

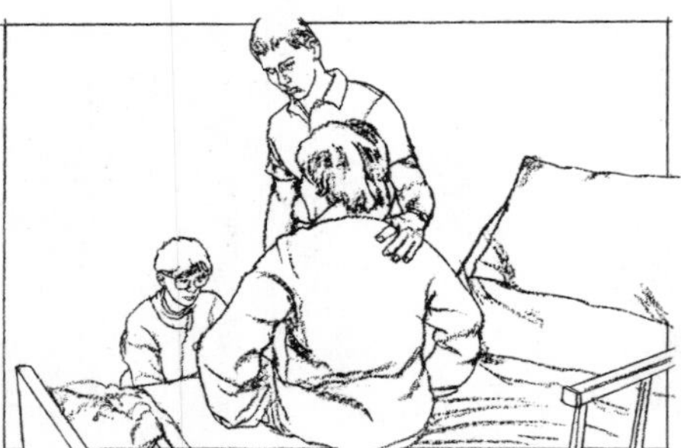

6. Help the resident put on their clothing including foot wear and safety belt. ☐

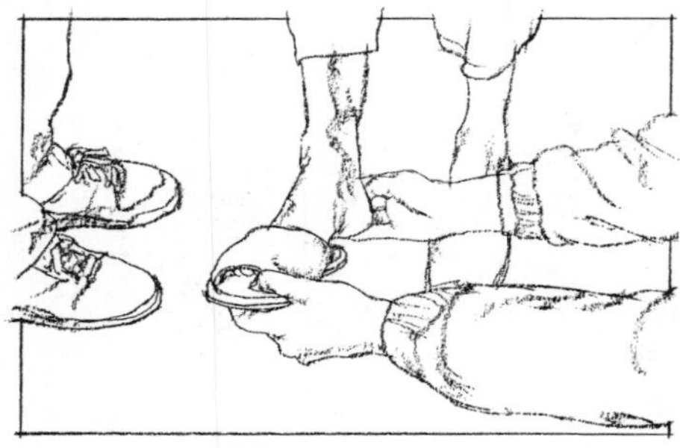

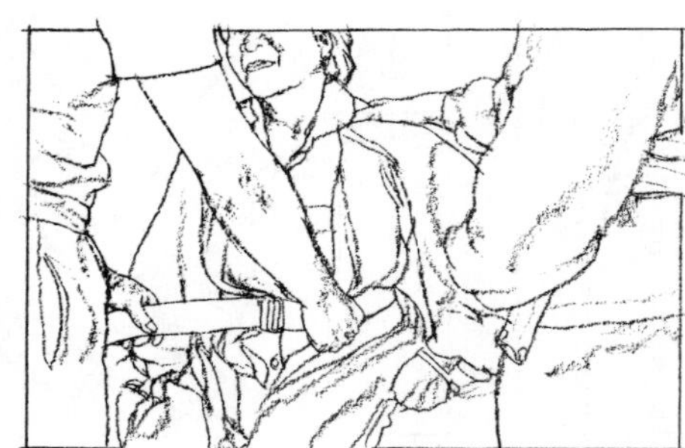

7. Each nurse assistant should put their arms nearest the resident under their resident's underarm and grasp the resident's safety belt. ☐

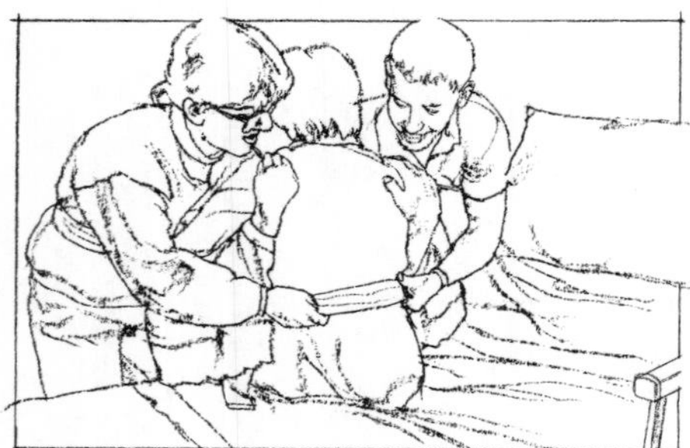

8. On the count of three, raise the resident to a standing position. Remember to use good body mechanics. ☐

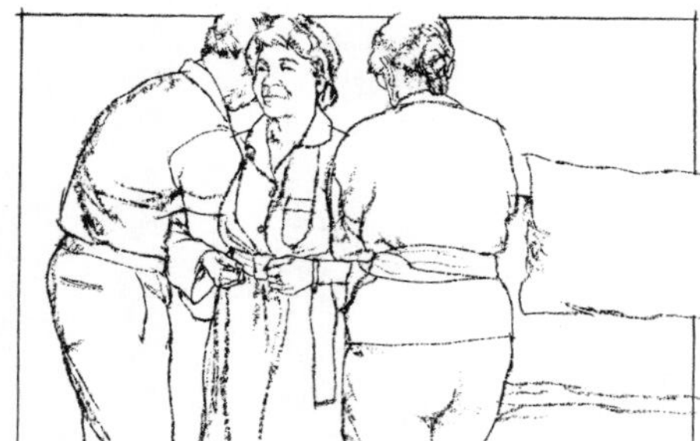

9. Turn the resident. Each nurse assistant should move to the sides of the wheelchair and lower the resident into the chair. ☐

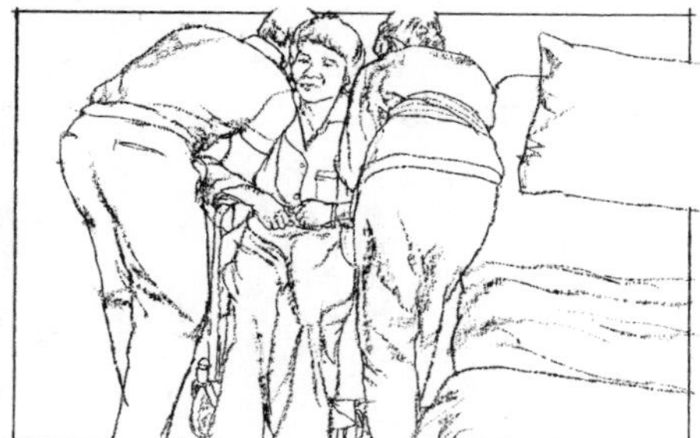

Positioning the Resident in the Chair

1. Lock wheels of wheelchair and check safety belt. ☐

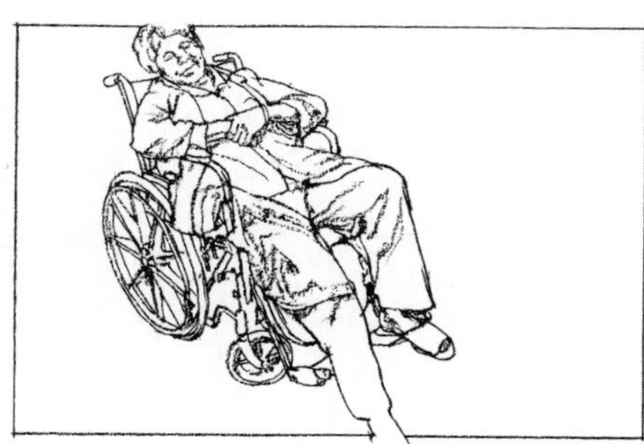

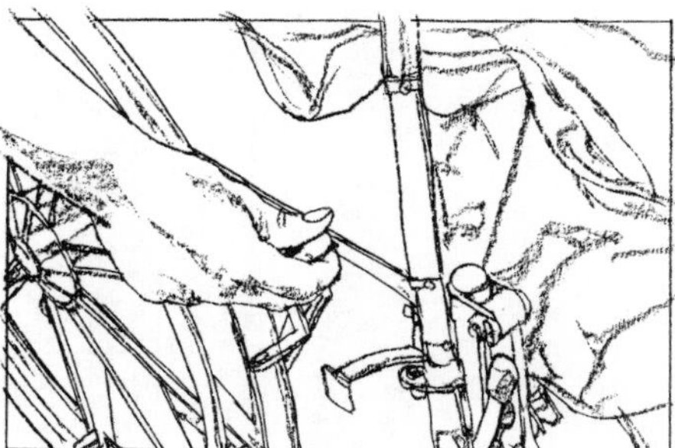

2. Stand as close as possible to the back of the wheelchair facing the back of the resident. ☐

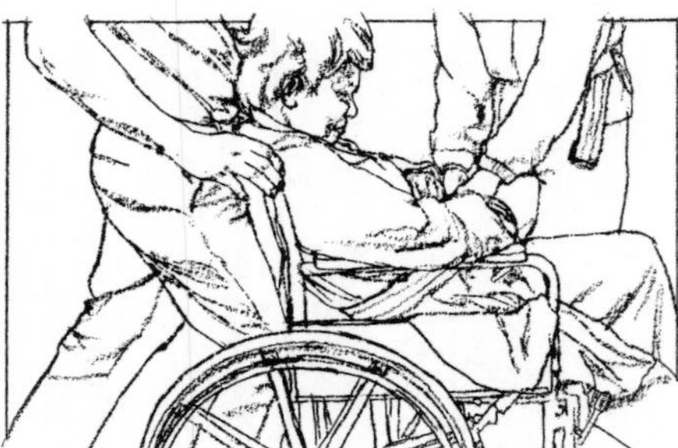

3. Using a strong base of support, position one knee against the back of the wheelchair, bend knees and position other foot "shoulder width" and slightly in back of the first foot. ☐

4. A teammate assists by kneeling on one knee close to the resident's legs and placing an arm under the resident's knees. ☐

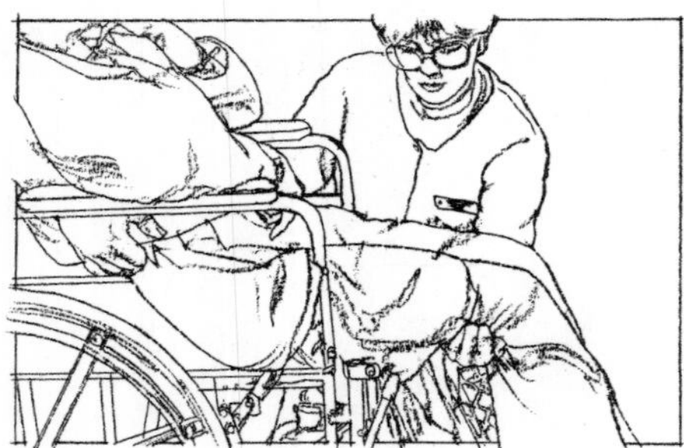

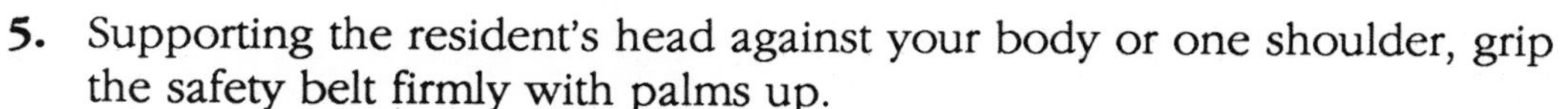

5. Supporting the resident's head against your body or one shoulder, grip the safety belt firmly with palms up. ☐

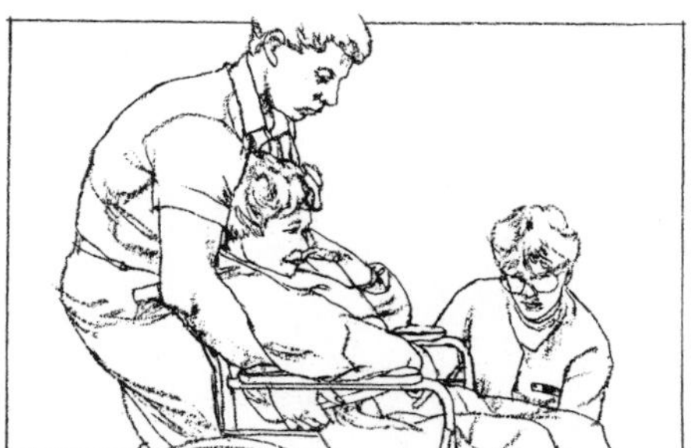

6. Communicating and counting to three, a teammate slides the resident's legs and hips to the back of the chair at the same time you lift the resident by slowly straightening your legs. ☐

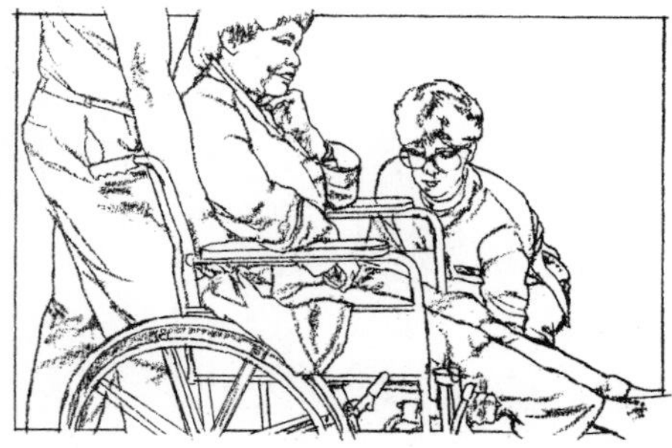

7. Place foot rests under the resident's feet. Cover knees with blanket or afghan as needed and give the resident personal items such as newspapers, kleenex or other items. ☐

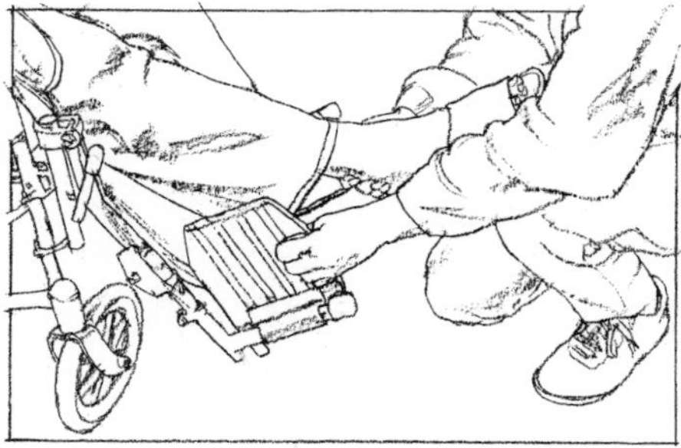

Skill 7: Performing Passive Range of Motion

Name: ______________________________ Date: ______________

Precautions

- Move each joint slowly, gently, and smoothly.
- Support each joint during movement.
- Never move the joint beyond its present level of movement.
- If pain occurs, stop the movement and report to the charge nurse. Always watch the resident's face, particularly the eyes, for any expression of pain.
- Always use good body mechanics.
- Always discuss any exercise plan with the charge nurse.

Note: You should perform range of motion on one side of the resident's body at a time and they should move each joint five times at least three times a day.

Procedure

Competency Check

Shoulder

Hold the resident's wrist with one hand and put your other hand under the resident's elbow.

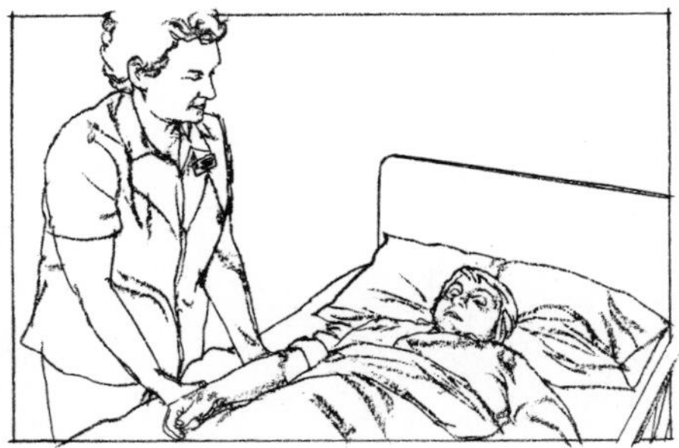

____

1. Raise the resident's arm straight alongside their ear and lower their arm to the side. (**flexion** and **extension**) ☐

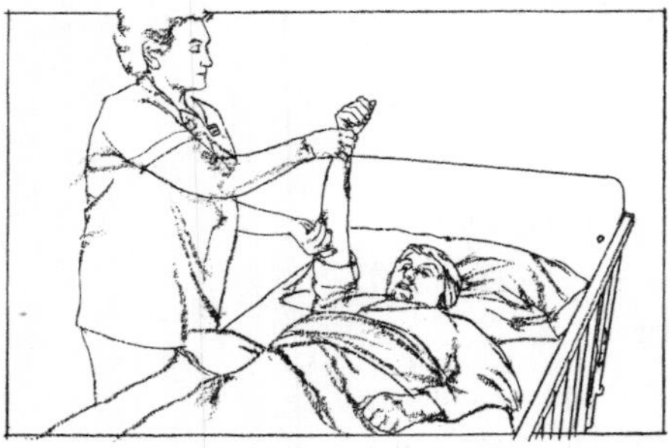

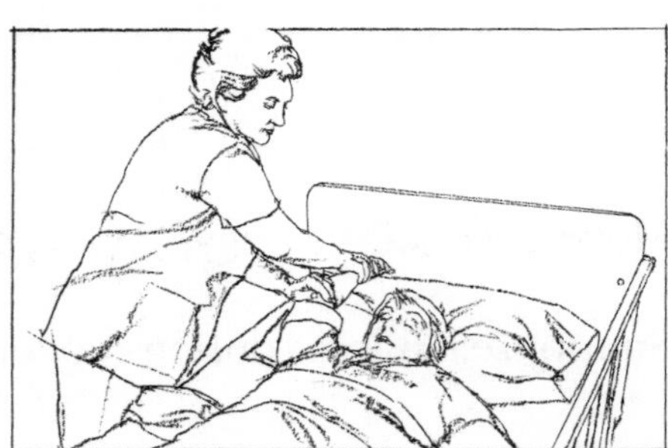

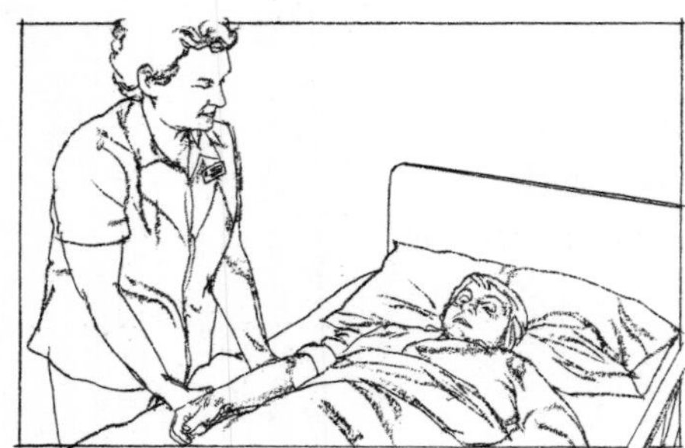

2. Move the arm out away from the resident's body and return it to the resident's side. (**abduction** and **adduction**) ☐

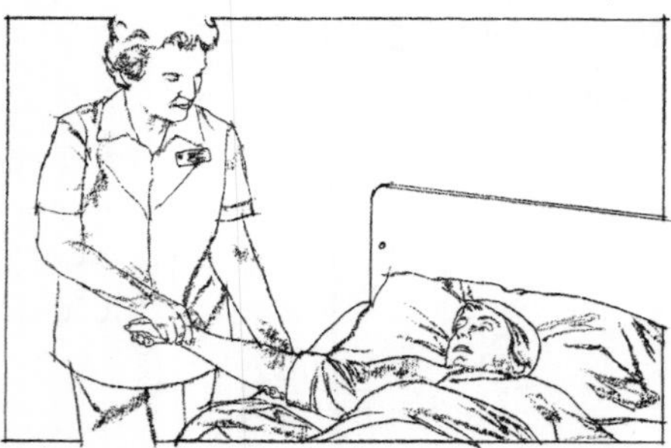

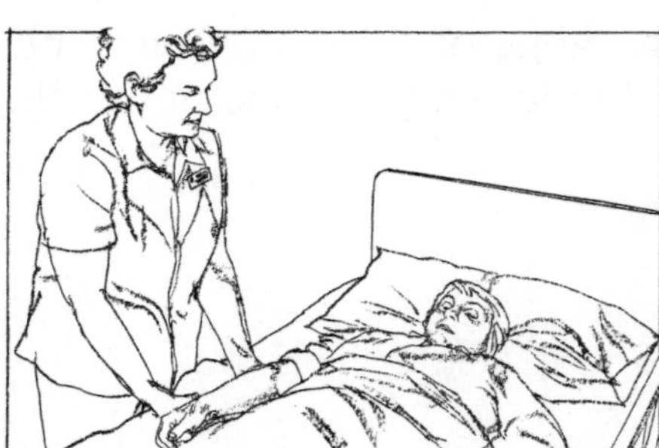

3. Carry the resident's hand to the opposite shoulder, then back out to shoulder level. (horizontal abduction and adduction) ☐

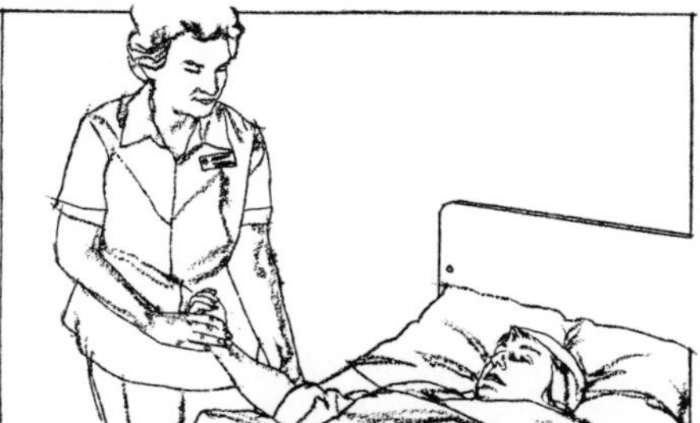

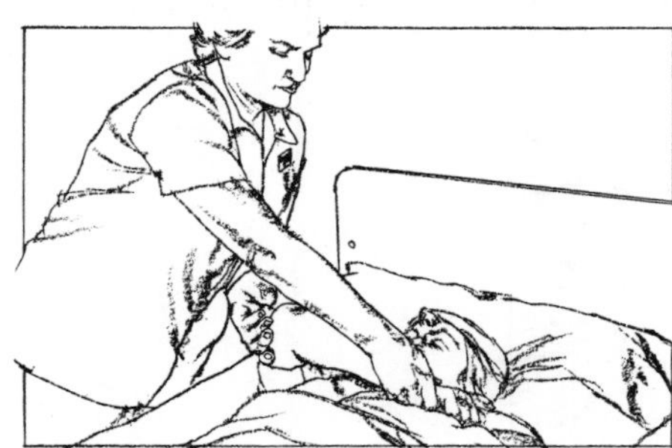

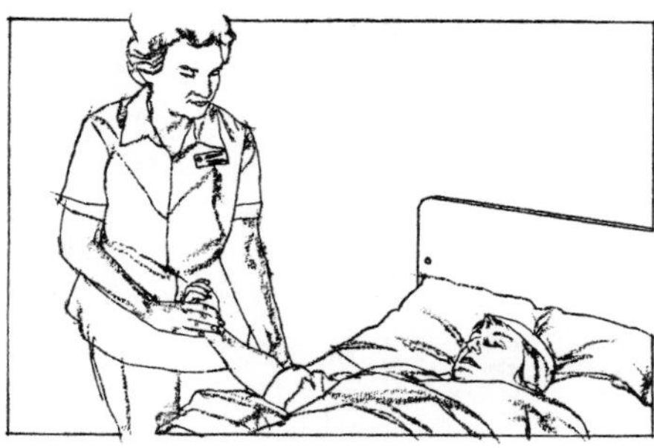

---

4. Raise the resident's elbow so it is at the same height as the shoulder. Move the resident's forearm up and down, as in giving a hand signal or a policeman saying stop. **(rotation)** ☐

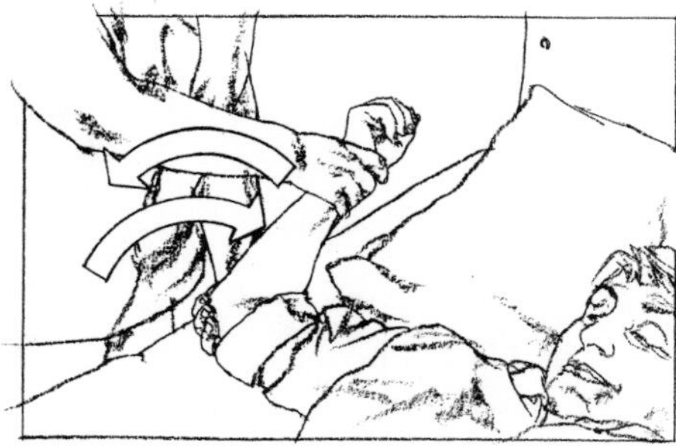

Elbow and Forearm

Hold the resident's wrist with one hand and put the other under the resident's elbow.

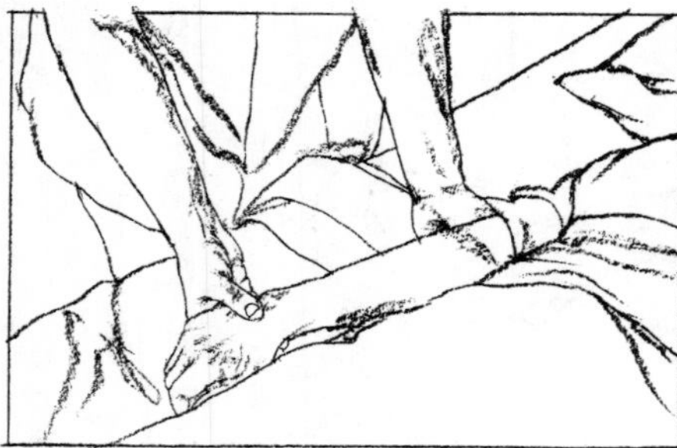

1. Bend the arm at the elbow. (flexion)

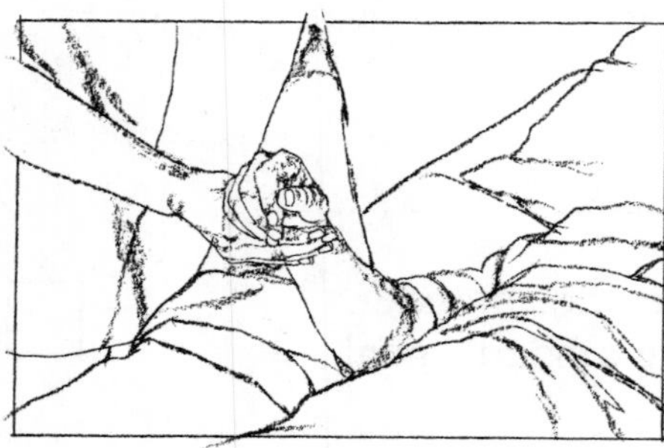

2. Straighten the arm. (extension)

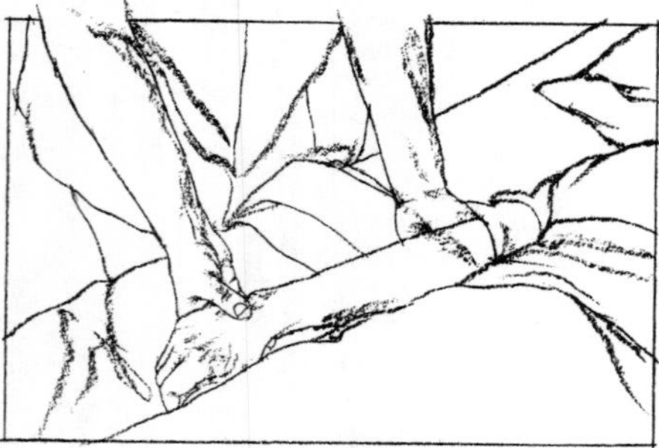

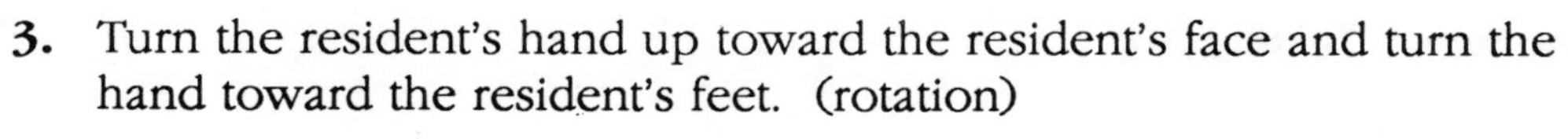

3. Turn the resident's hand up toward the resident's face and turn the hand toward the resident's feet. (rotation) ☐

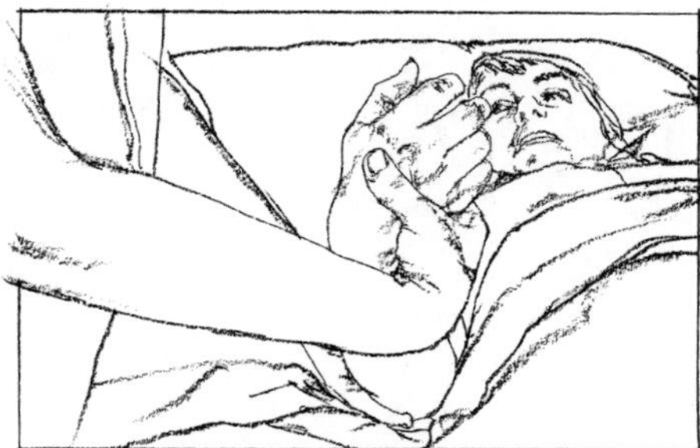

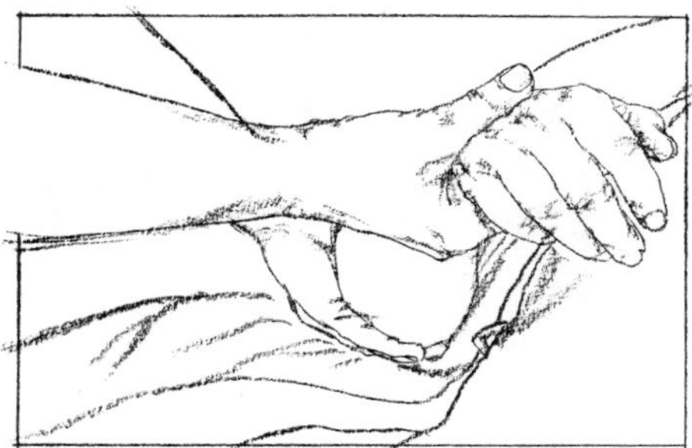

Wrist

Hold the resident's wrist with one hand and the resident's fingers with the other. ☐

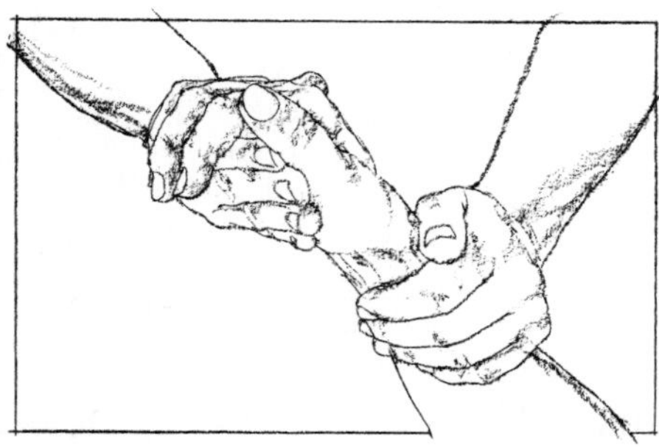

---

1. Move the hand downward. (flexion) ☐

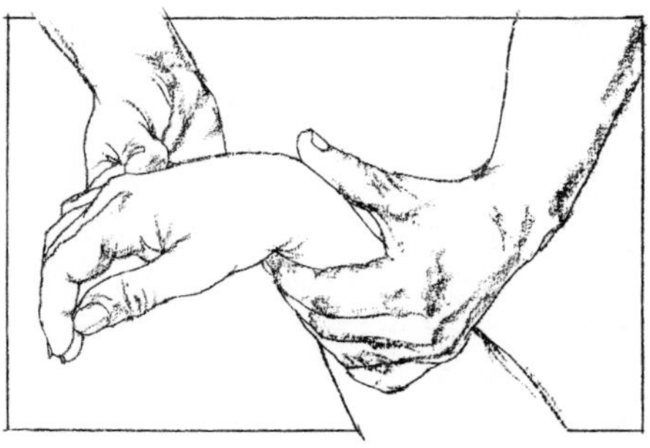

---

2. Straighten the wrist. (extension) ☐

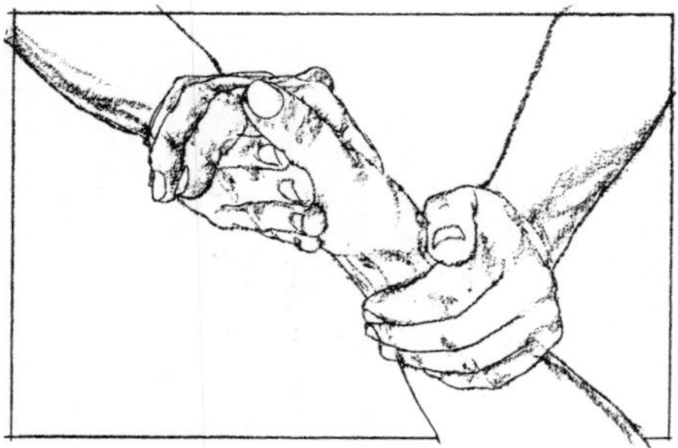

3. Move the hand back. (**hyperextension**) ☐

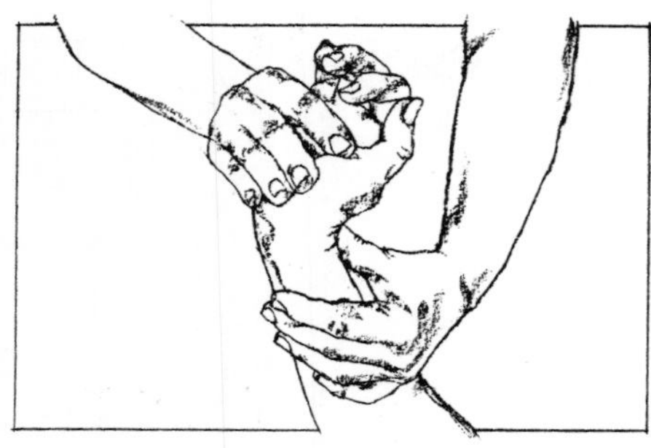

4. Move the wrist from side to side. (adduction and abduction) ☐

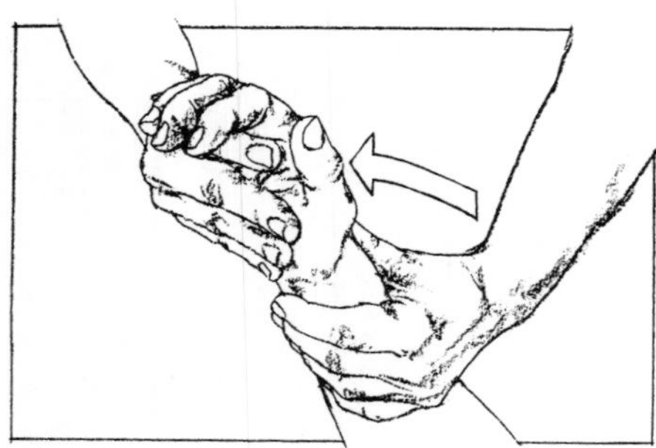

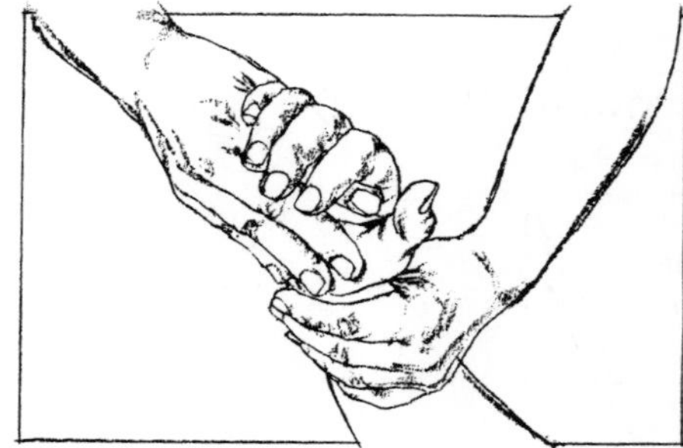

5. Tilt the hand down toward the feet, then bring the thumb up toward the nose. **(ulnar and radial deviation)** ☐

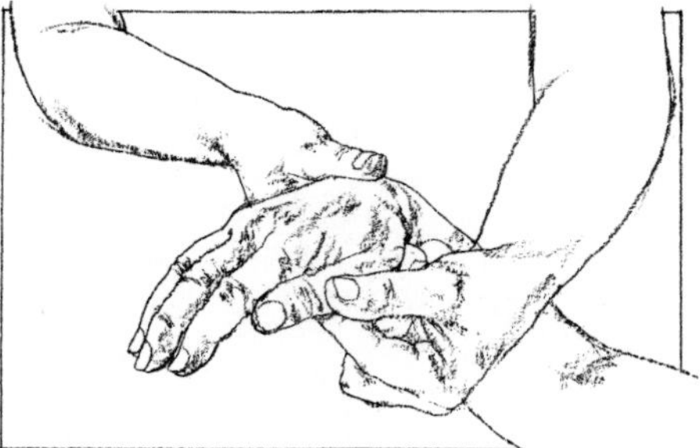

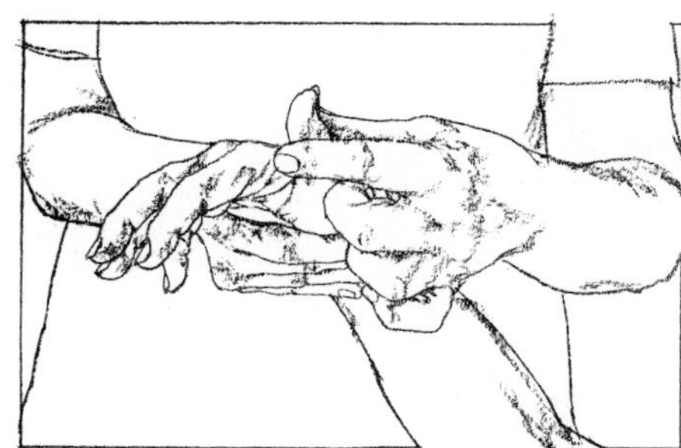

Fingers and Thumb

Hold the resident's hand. ☐

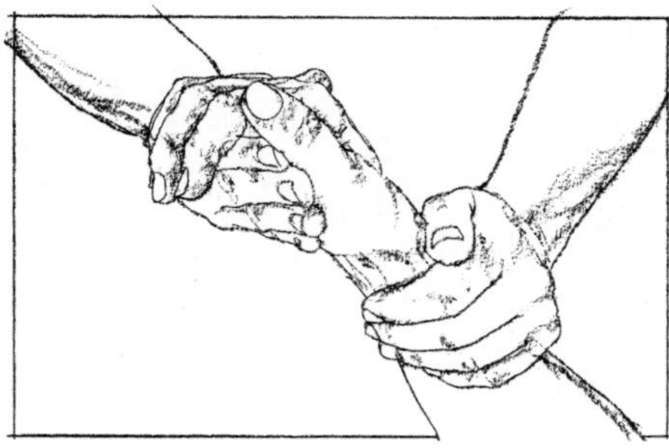

---

1. Make a fist to flex the fingers. ☐

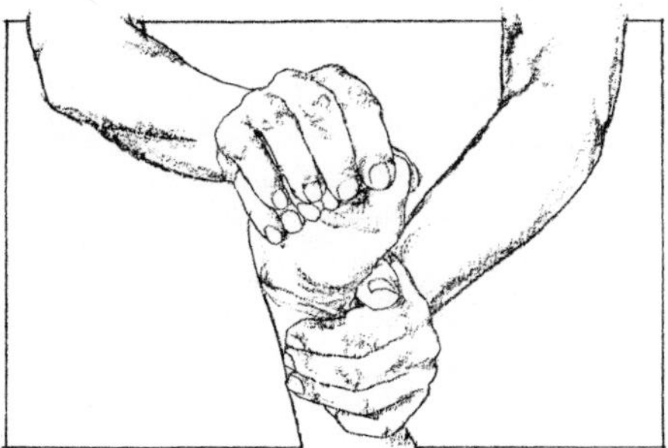

---

2. Straighten the fist by extending the fingers, one at a time. ☐

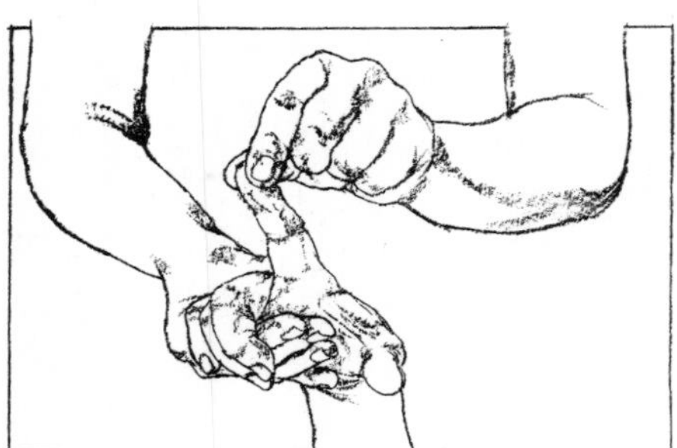

3. Holding two fingers at a time, spread each finger and thumb apart and back. (abduction and adduction) ☐

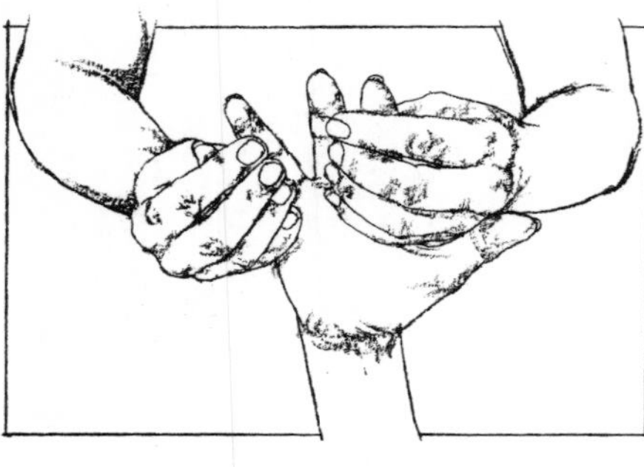

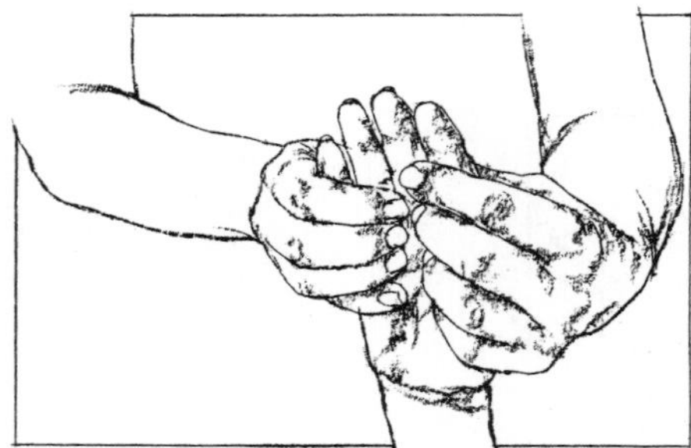

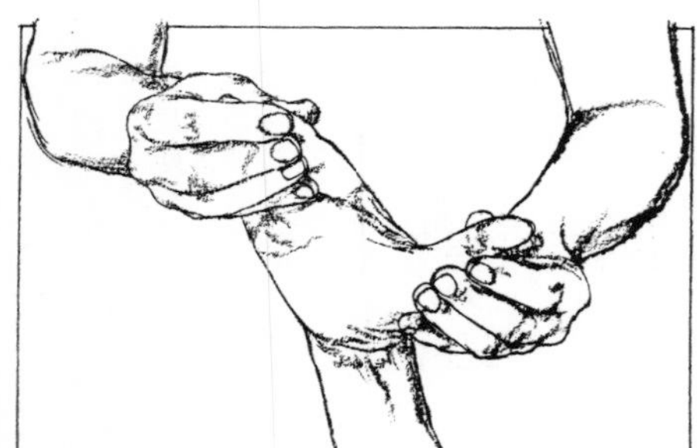

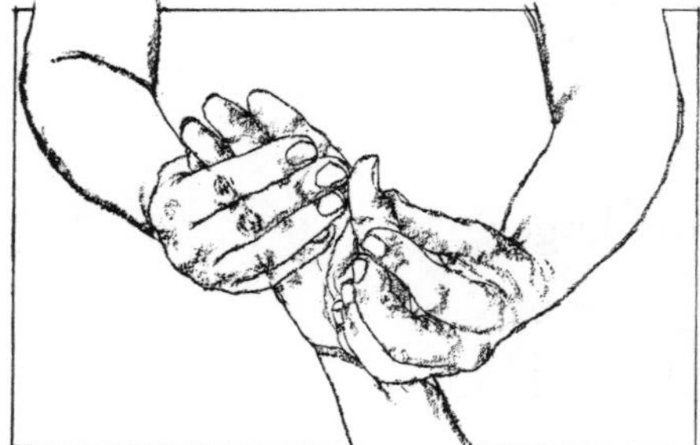

4. Bend the resident's thumb into their palm and move the thumb to the side of the fingers. (adduction and abduction) ☐

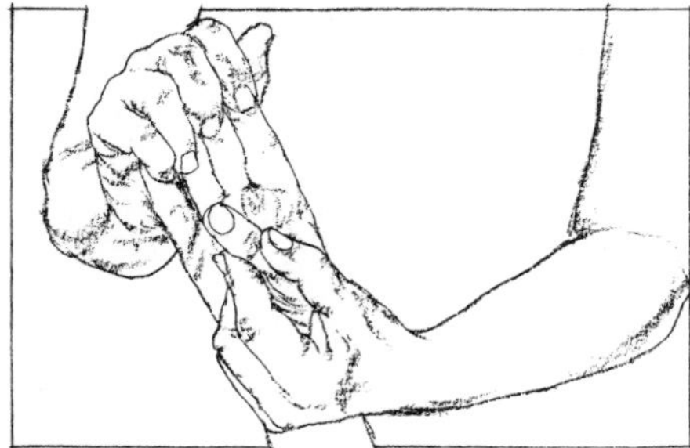

5. Bring the thumb to the tip of each finger. (thumb opposition) ☐

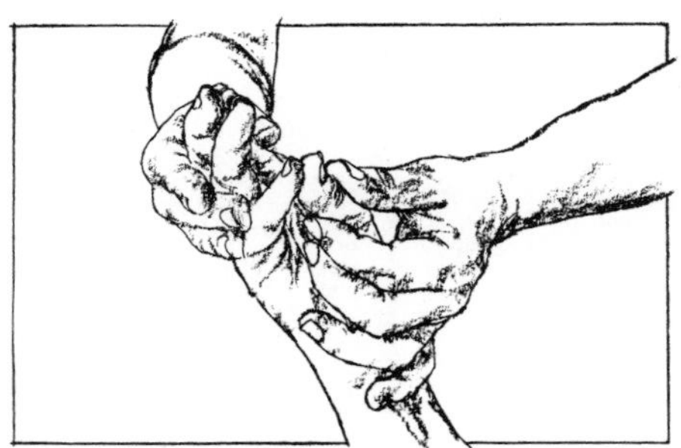

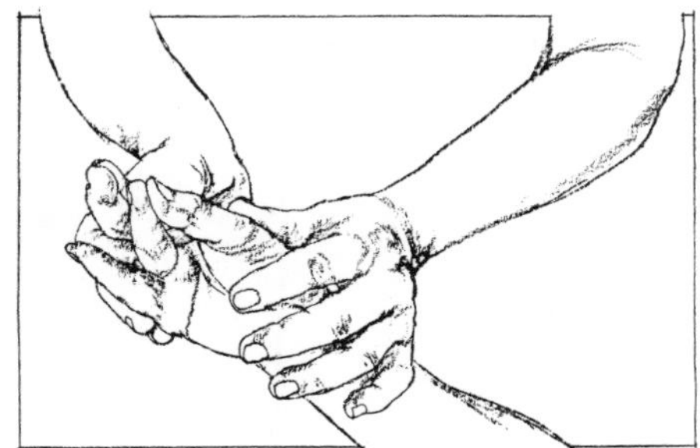

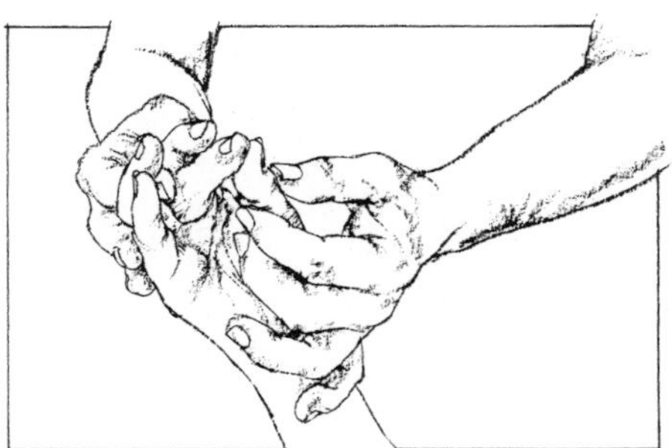

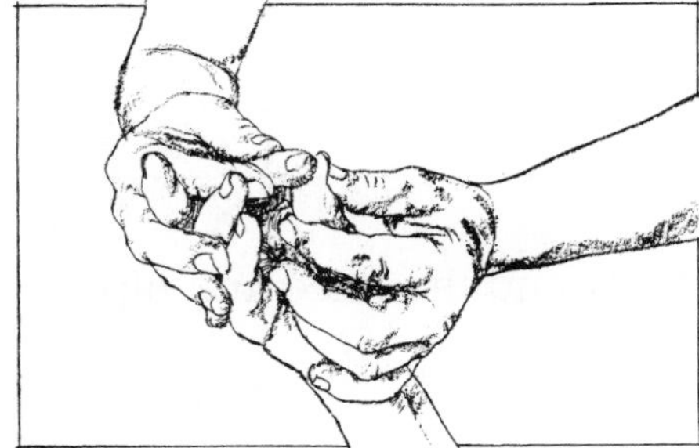

Hip and Knee

Put one hand under the resident's knee and the other under the resident's ankle. ☐

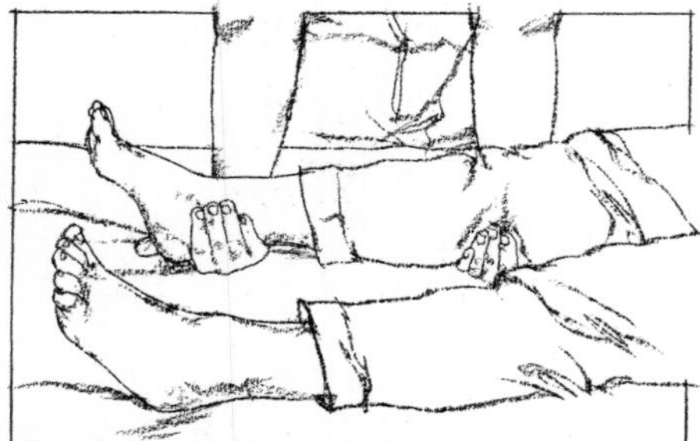

---

1. Bend the resident's knee and move it up toward the resident's head to flex the knee and hip. ☐

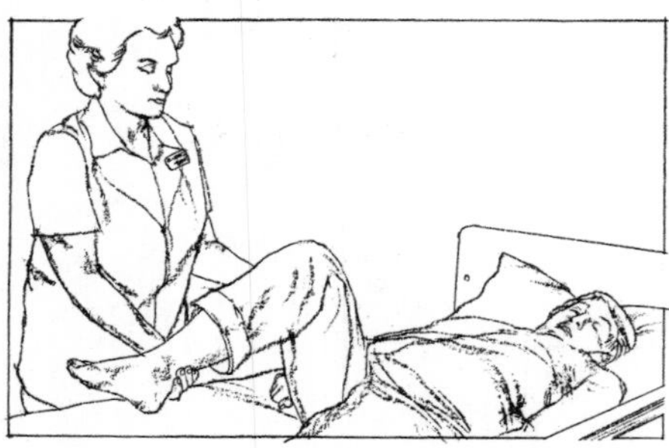

---

2. Straighten the knee to extend the knee and hip, and lower to bed. ☐

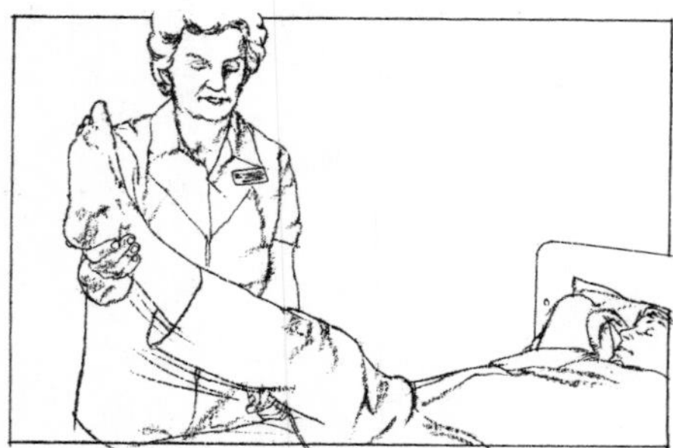

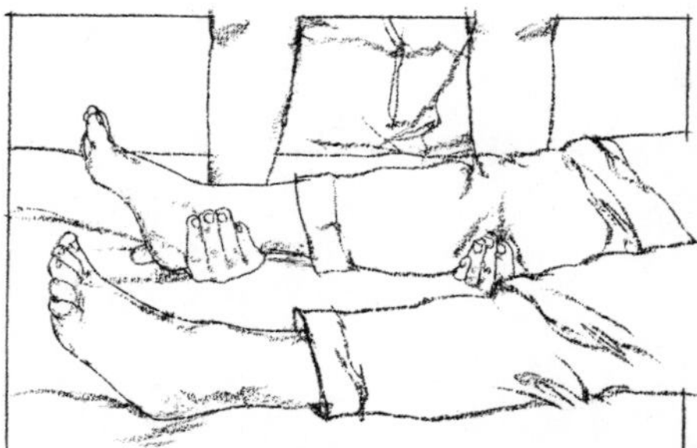

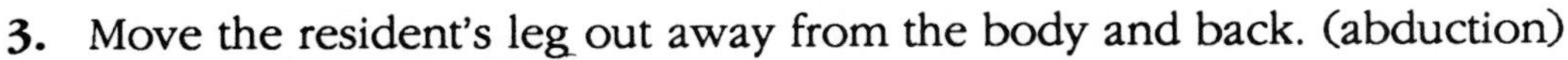

3. Move the resident's leg out away from the body and back. (abduction) ☐

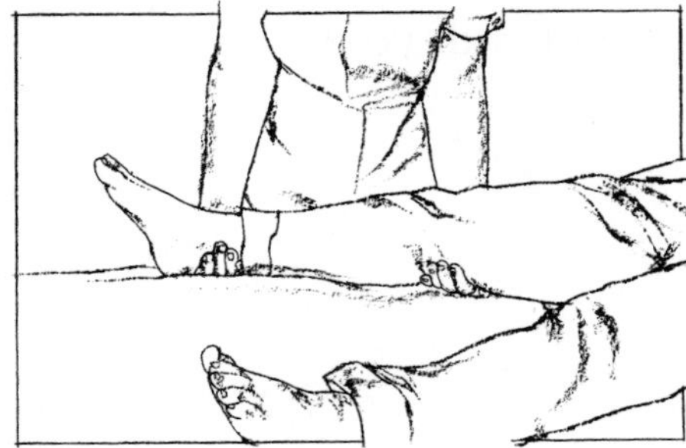

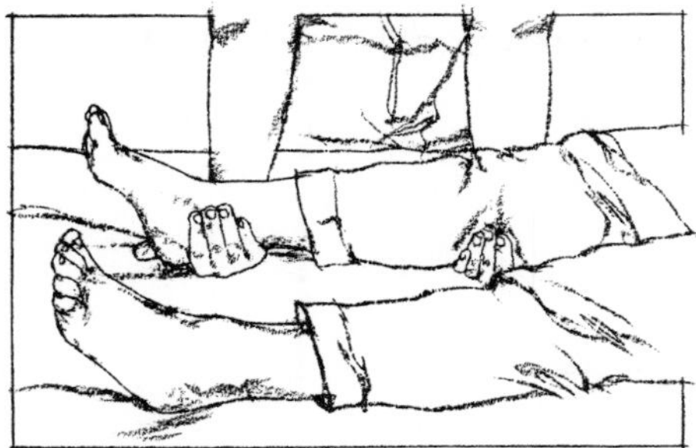

4. Move the leg back to center toward the other leg. (adduction) ☐

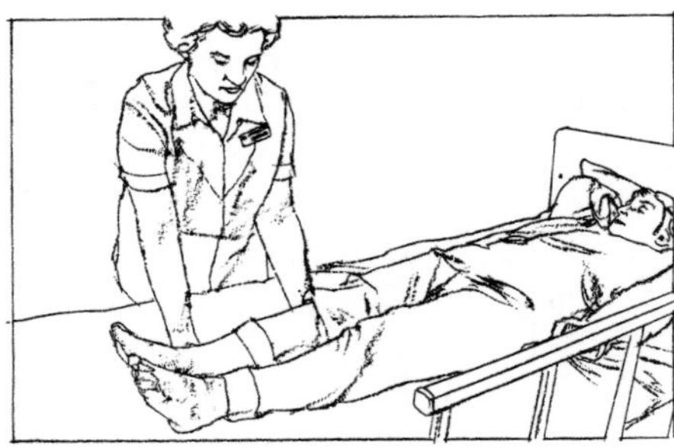

5. Turn the leg inward and outward to rotate the hip. ☐

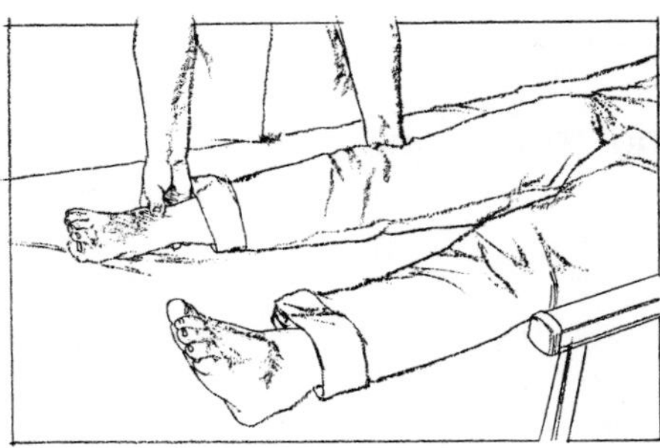

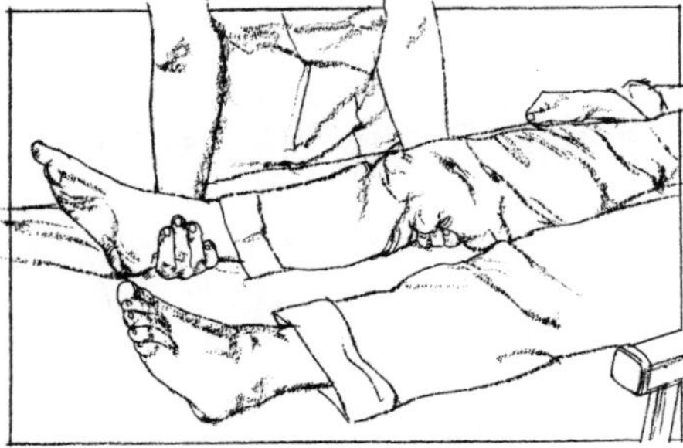

Ankle

1. Put one hand under the resident's ankle and grasp their foot with your other hand. ☐

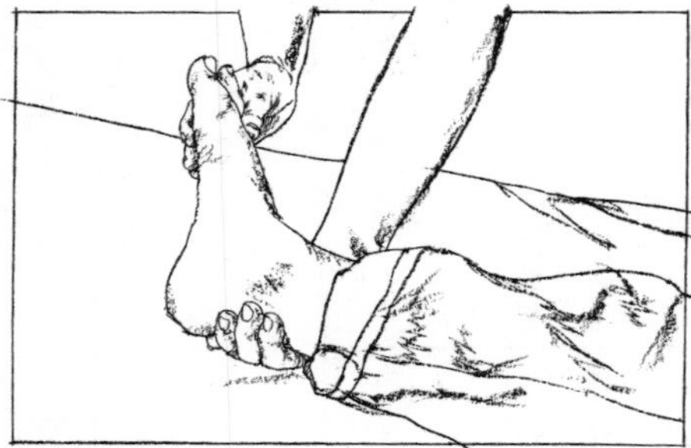

2. Push the foot forward toward resident's head and then downward. (flexion and extension) ☐

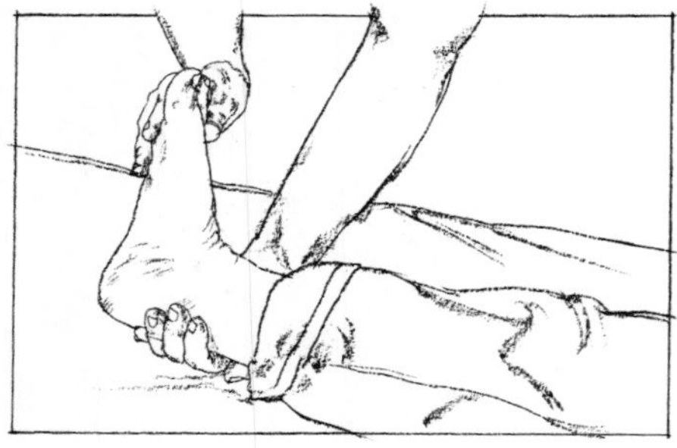

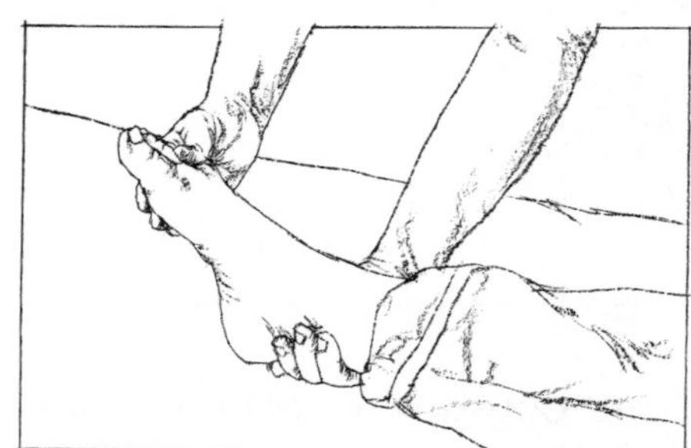

3. Turn the foot inward and then outward. (adduction and abduction). ☐

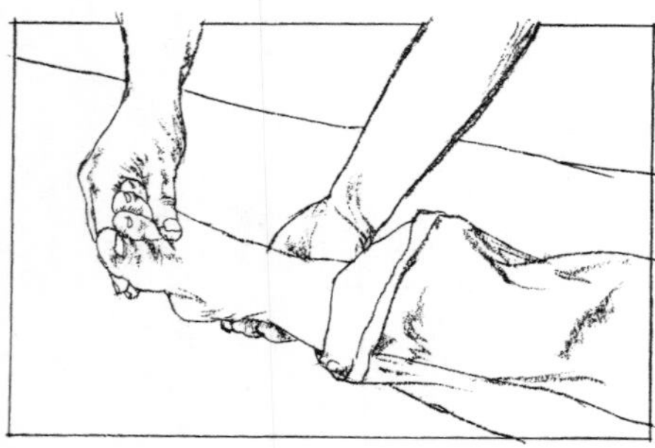

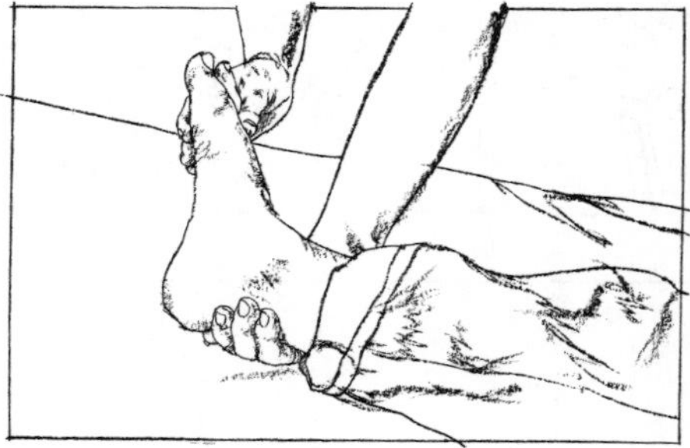

Toes

1. Put one hand under the resident's foot and the other on the top of their foot over the toes and curl the toes downward. (flexion) ☐

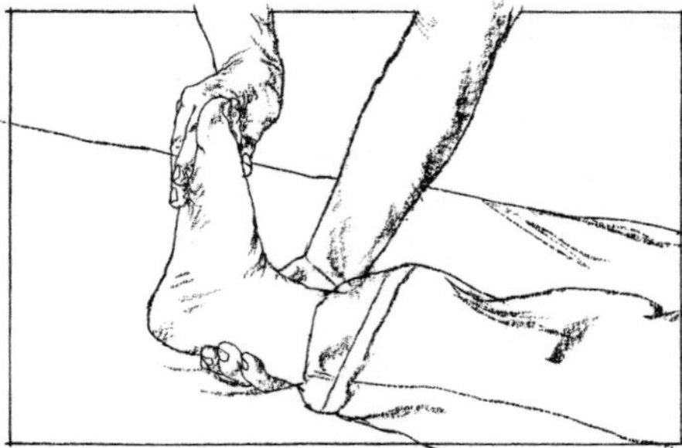

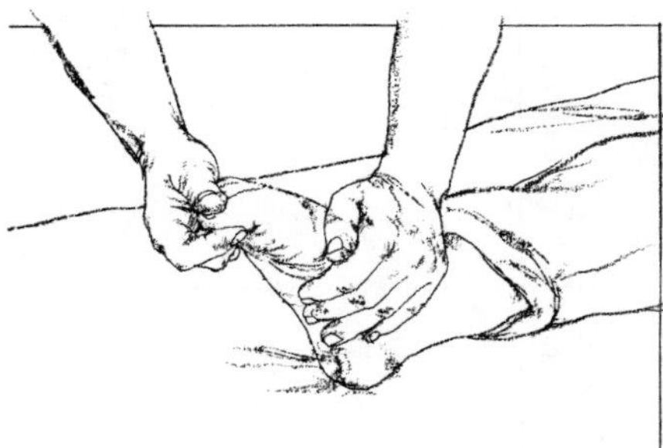

2. Straighten the toes. (extension) ☐

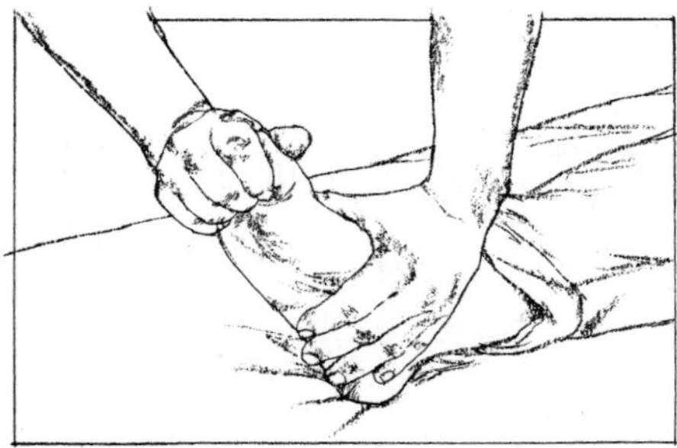

3. Holding two toes, spread each toe. (abduction)

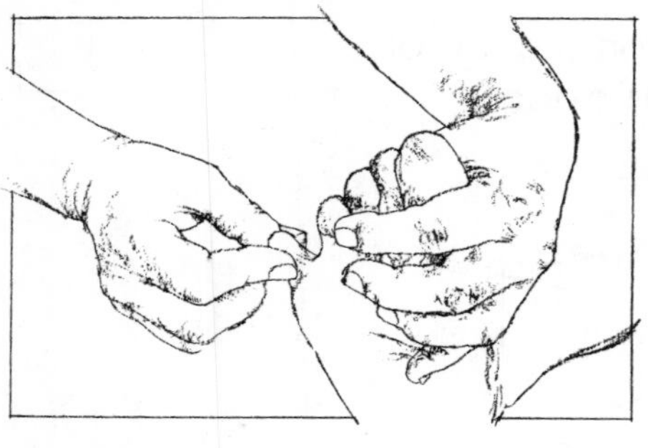
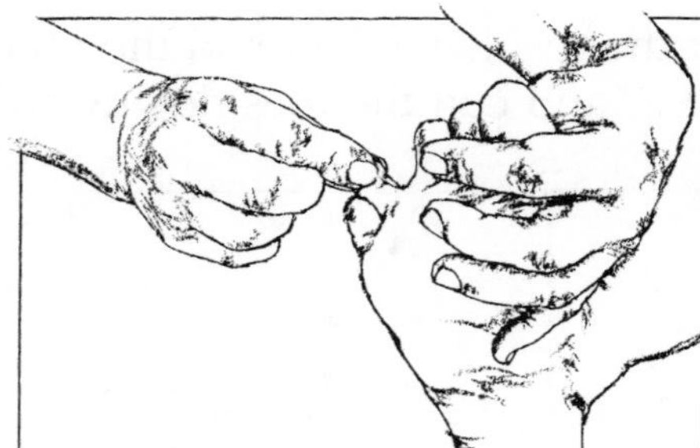
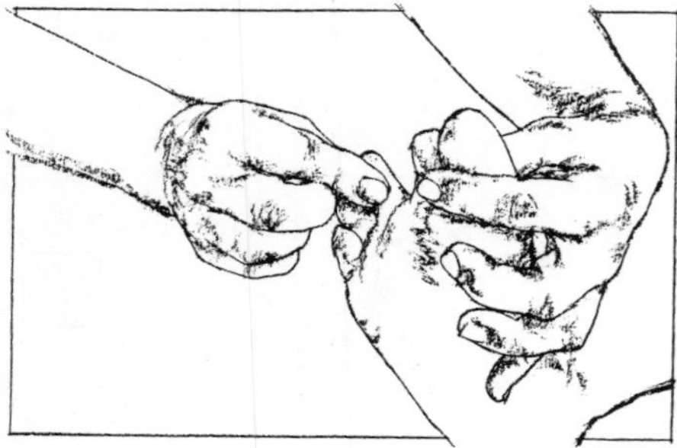
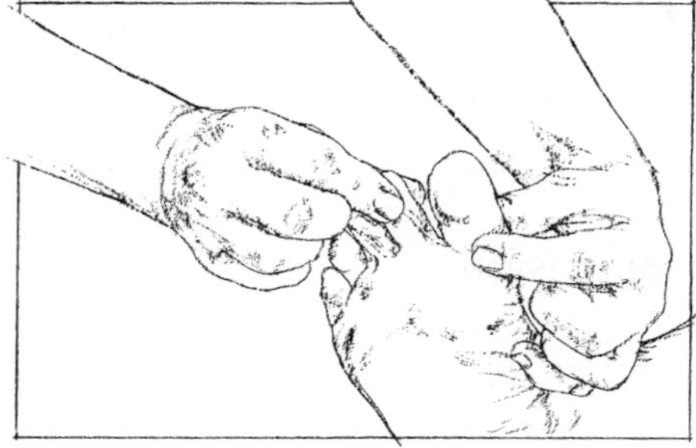

4. Pull up side rail, move to the other side and repeat the sequence on the opposite side of the body.

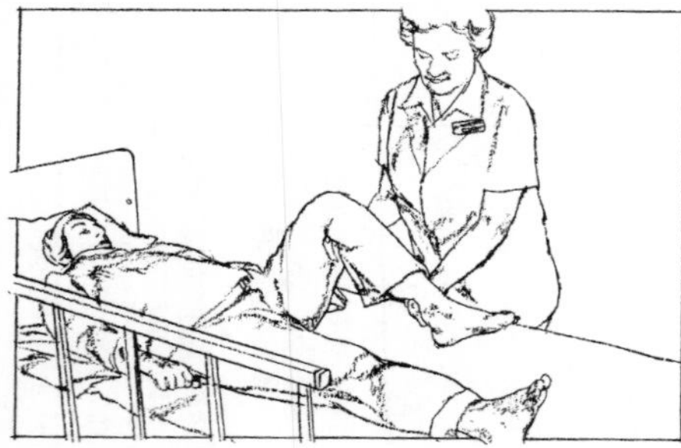

Skill 9: Giving a Complete Bed Bath

Name: ______________________________ Date: ________________

Precautions

- Remember to check water temperature. It should be warm to touch.
- Always wash, rinse, and dry each body part one at a time to prevent chilling and exposure.
- Inspect skin for injuries or changes in condition.
- Use soap sparingly and never leave it in the water.
- Put the towel under each part of the body as you wash it to protect the bedding.
- Always wash the perineal area of a female resident from front to back to prevent infection.
- Be gentle and thorough when cleaning the perineal area.

Procedure

Competency check

1. Lower the resident's head as far as they can tolerate. Lower the side rail on the side where you are working.

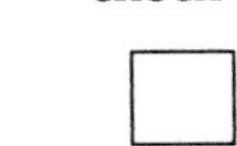

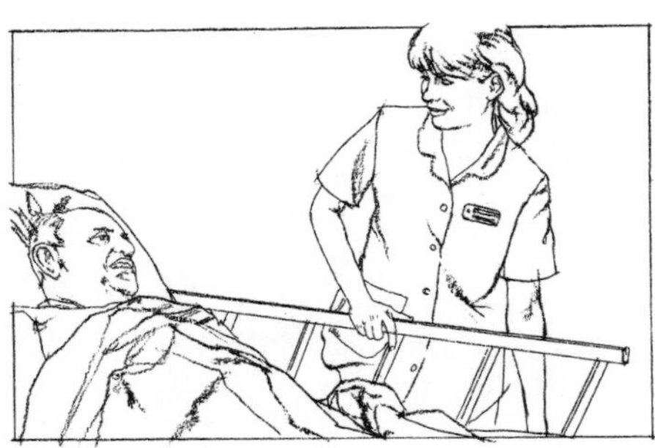

Rationale: Putting the resident in this position will prevent you from injuring your back.

2. Put the bath blanket over the resident. ☐

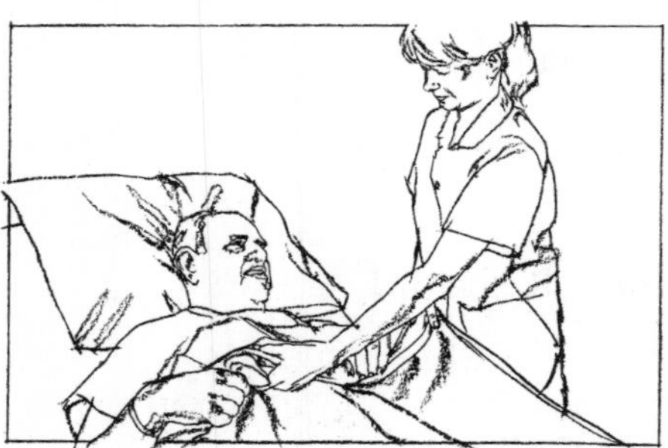

3. Have the resident hold the blanket under their chin and remove the top sheet by placing your hand under the bath blanket and rolling the top sheet to the bottom of the bed. ☐

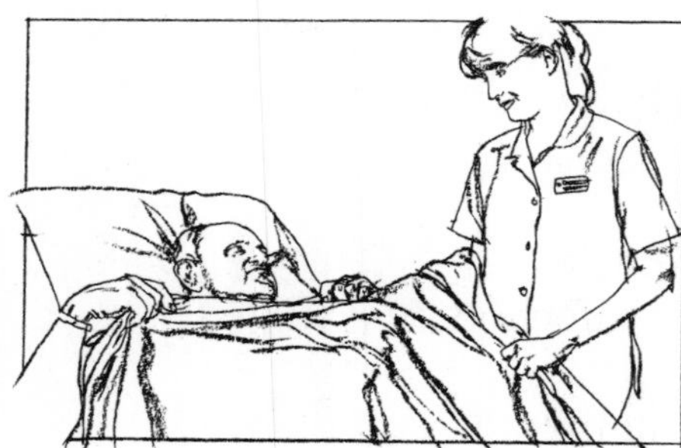

Rationale: These steps protect the resident's privacy and prevent chilling.

4. Take off the sheet and put it at the foot of the bed between the mattress and the footboard. ☐

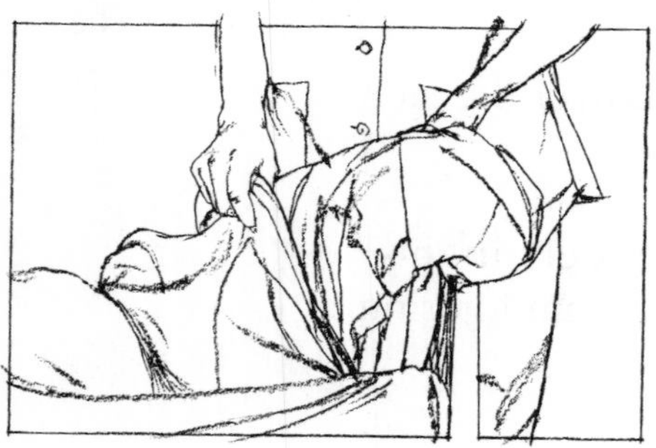

5. Take off the resident's gown by slipping it off each arm and pulling it from under the bath blanket on the side closest to you.

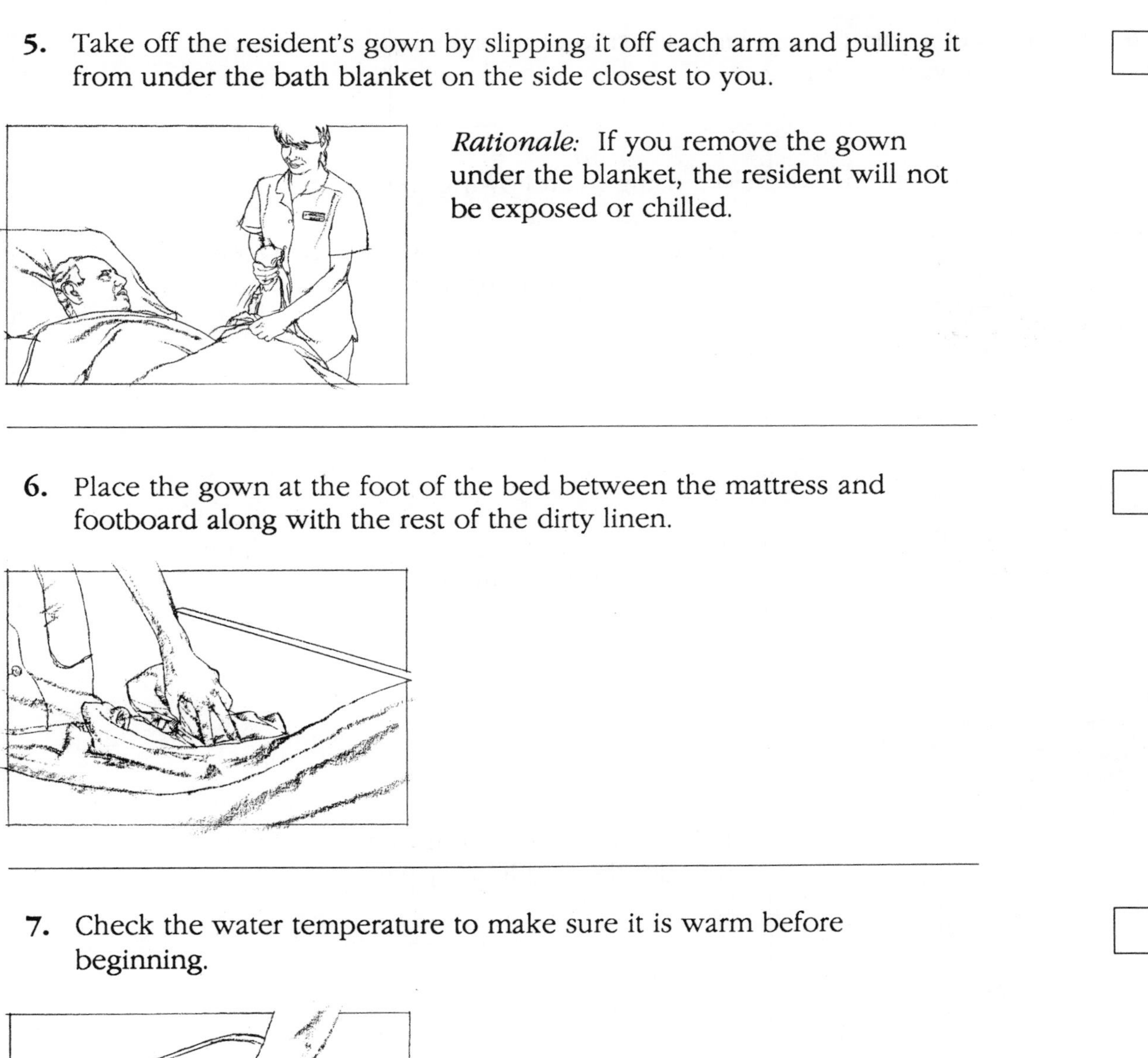

Rationale: If you remove the gown under the blanket, the resident will not be exposed or chilled.

6. Place the gown at the foot of the bed between the mattress and footboard along with the rest of the dirty linen.

7. Check the water temperature to make sure it is warm before beginning.

8. Put a towel across the resident's chest to protect the bath blanket while you wash their face. ☐

---

9. Make a mitt with the washcloth using the following steps: ☐

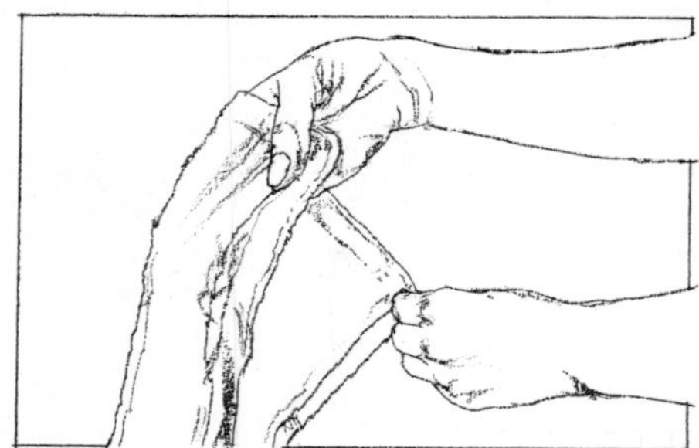

Hold a corner of the washcloth between your thumb and fingers.

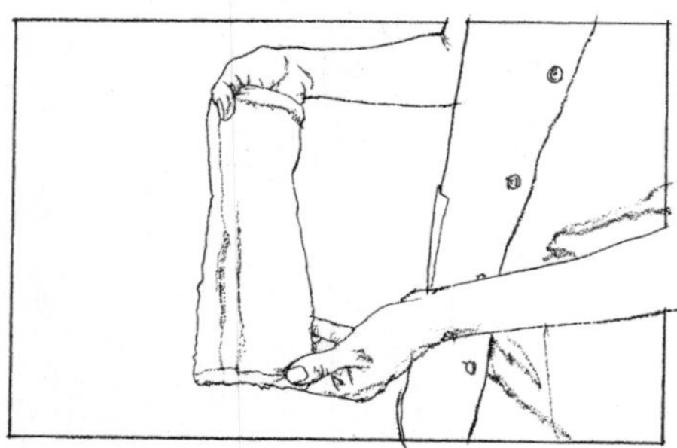

Wrap the rest of it around your hand and hold it with your thumb.

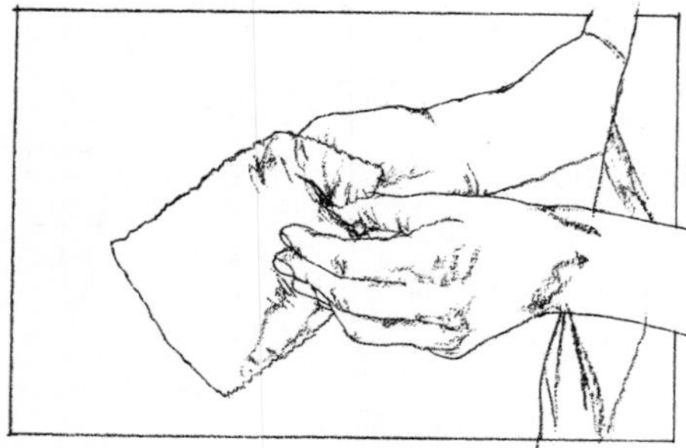

Fold the cloth over your fingers and tuck it under the fold in your palm.

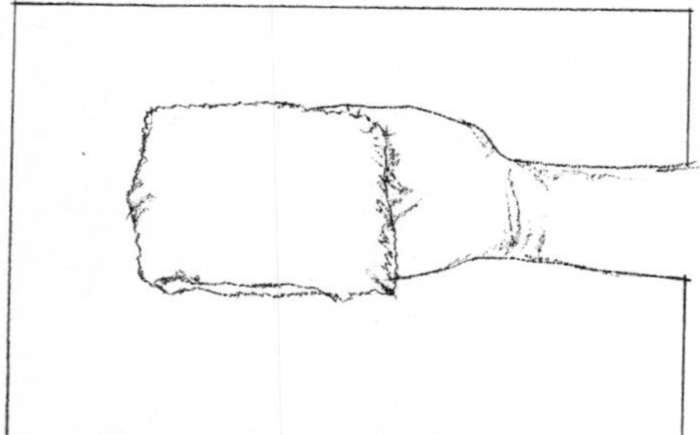

Rationale: Making a mitt prevents the edge of the washcloth from dragging over the resident's skin and causing chilling.

---

10. Without using soap, wash, rinse, and dry each eye, beginning from the inner corner of the eye (near the nose) and moving to the outer corner. ☐

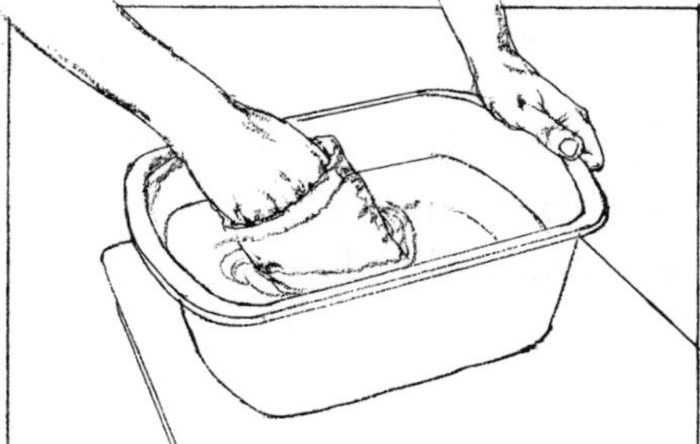

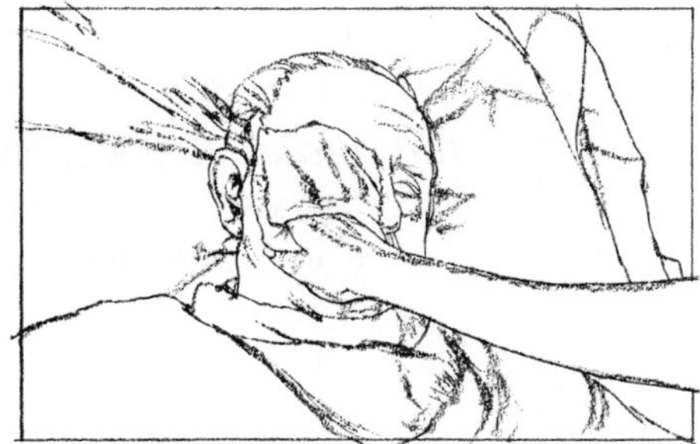

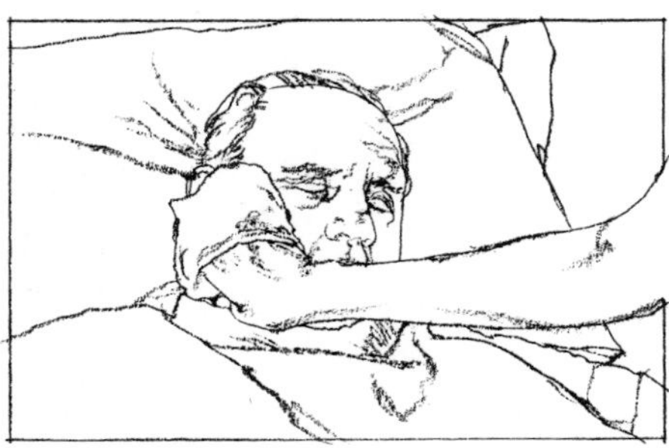

Rationale: Using this procedure prevents the spread of germs from one eye to the other.

Repeat this procedure on the other eye, using the opposite end of the mitt.

---

11. Wash, rinse, and dry the resident's face, neck, and ears. Make sure to wash and dry behind the ears. ☐

Note: Ask the resident if they want soap to be used on their face.

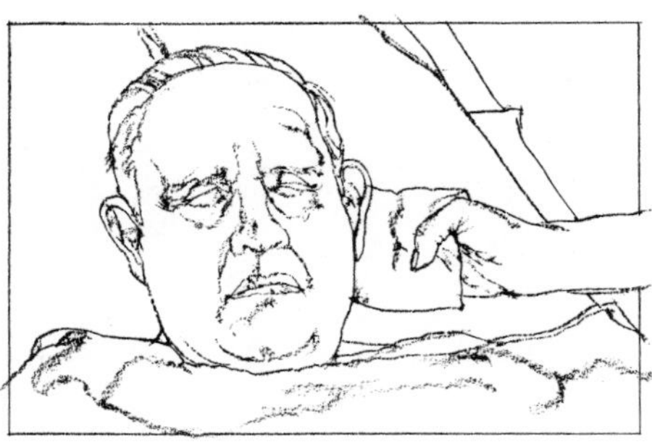

---

12. Put the towel under the arm furthest from you. Wash, rinse, and dry the shoulder, arm, and underarm (axilla). ☐

Note: Remember to work on one side of the resident at a time if the bed is *not* elevated.

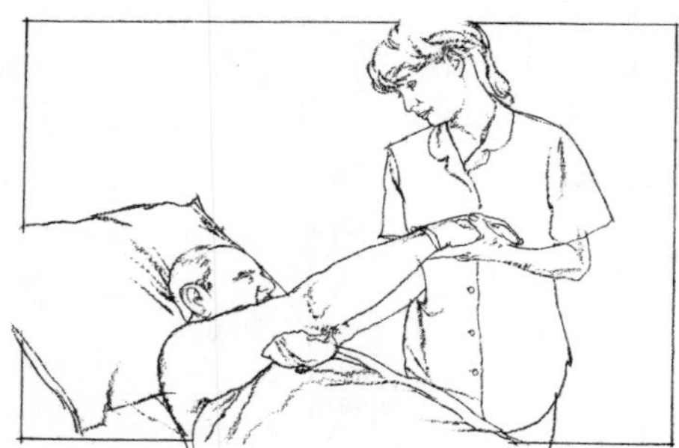

Rationale: If you begin with the arm furthest away, you will not drip on the part you have already cleaned and dried.

---

13. Wash, rinse, and dry the hand. ☐

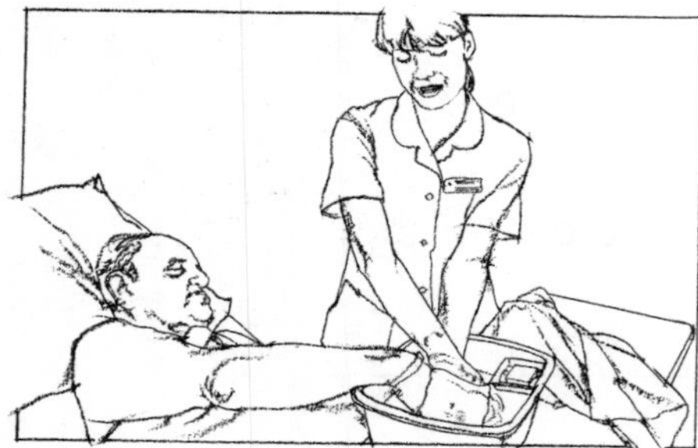

Wash the other arm and hand using the same procedure.

Note: Place the hands in the basin when possible to promote thorough cleaning, and to loosen dirt under the nails.

Nail care may be done at this point

---

14. Put the towel over the resident's chest on top of the bath blanket, then reach under the towel and fold the bath blanket down leaving the towel in place so the resident is not exposed.

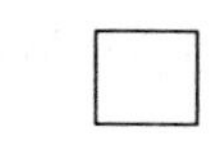

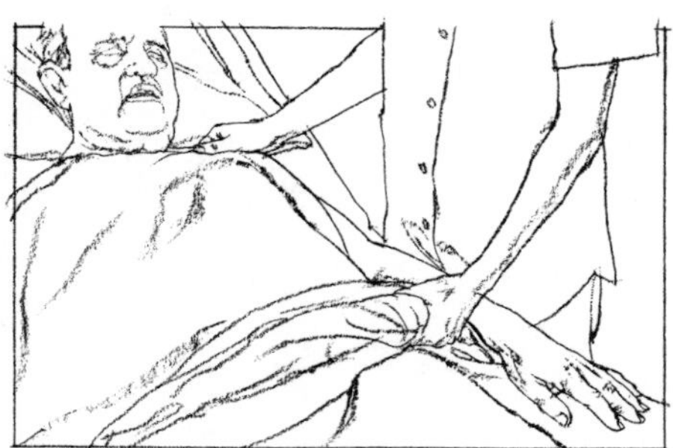

15. Fold back the towel to expose the side of the chest and abdomen furthest from you. Then wash, rinse, and dry the area. Inspect under the breast and skinfolds as you work. Re-cover the chest with the towel.

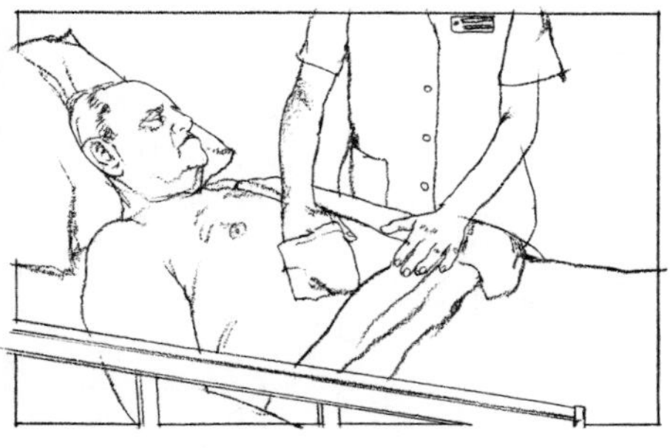

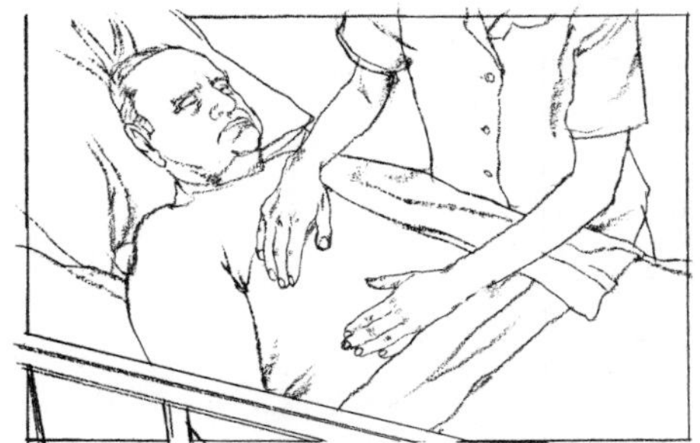

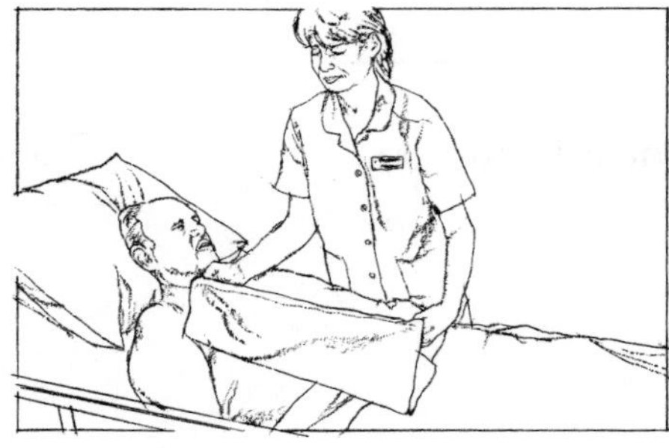

Wash the other side of the chest using the same procedure. ☐

Note: Make sure the skin is completely dry. Moisture in skin folds can result in skin cracking, and later, skin breakdown.

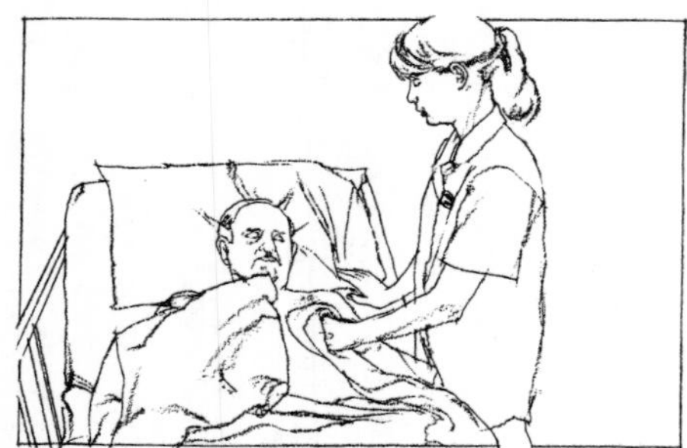

16. Check to make sure the water temperature is still warm and that the water has not become too soapy. Change the water if necessary. ☐

Note: Remember to raise the side rail if you leave the bedside.

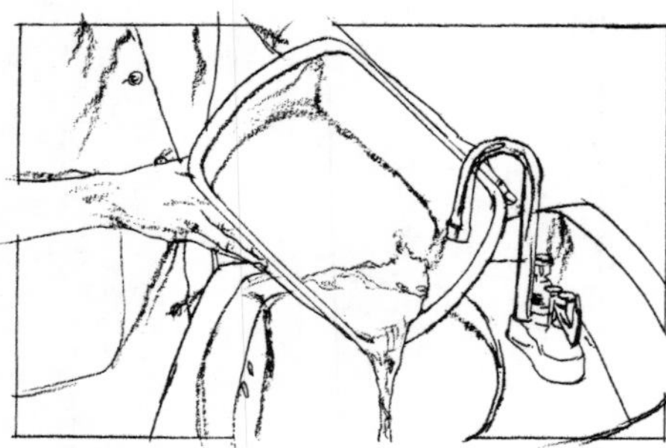

17. Fold the bath blanket away from the resident's leg furthest from you, and place a towel under the leg. ☐

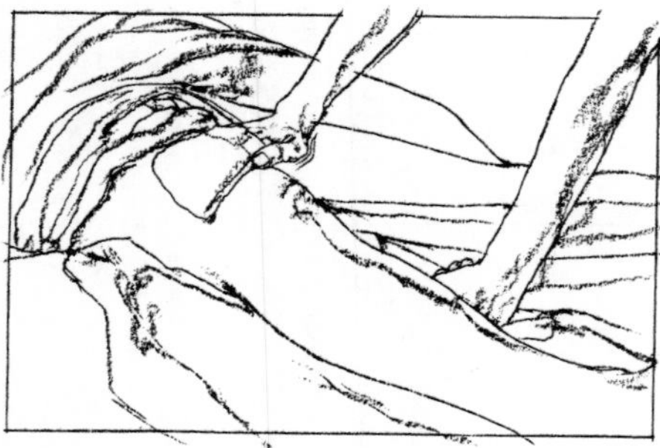

18. Wash, rinse, and dry the resident's leg. ☐

---

19. Wash, rinse, and dry the resident's foot. ☐

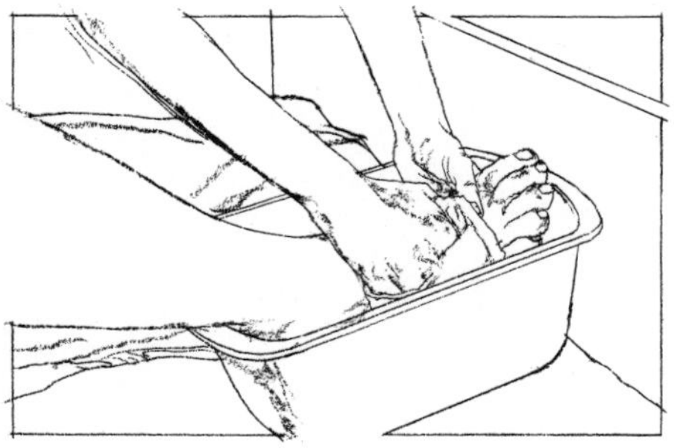

Wash the other leg and foot using the same procedure.

Note: Place the feet in the basin when possible to promote thorough cleaning, and to loosen dirt under the nails.

Foot care may be done at this point

---

20. Help the resident turn onto one side using the procedure learned in Skill 2. ☐

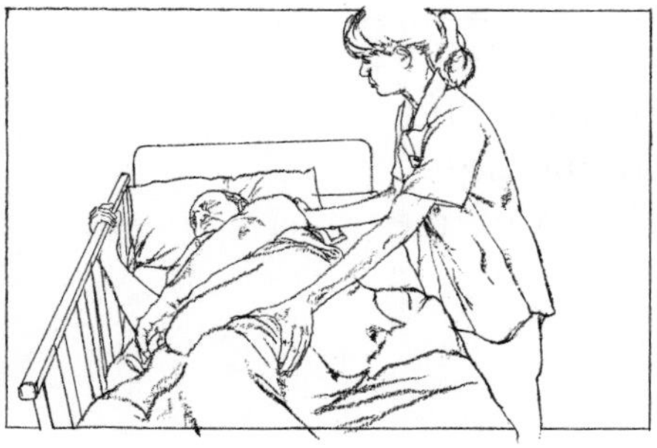

---

21. Protect the sheet with a towel. Wash, rinse, and dry the resident's neck, back, and buttocks. Inspect the skin as you work.

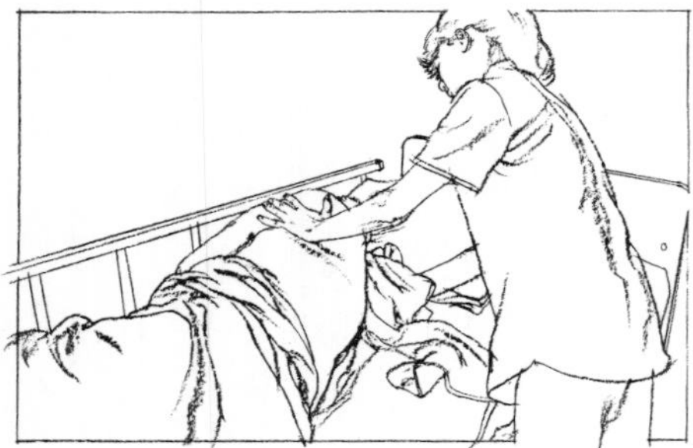

Back Rub

1. Squeeze some lotion onto the palm of your hand and warm it by rubbing your hands together.

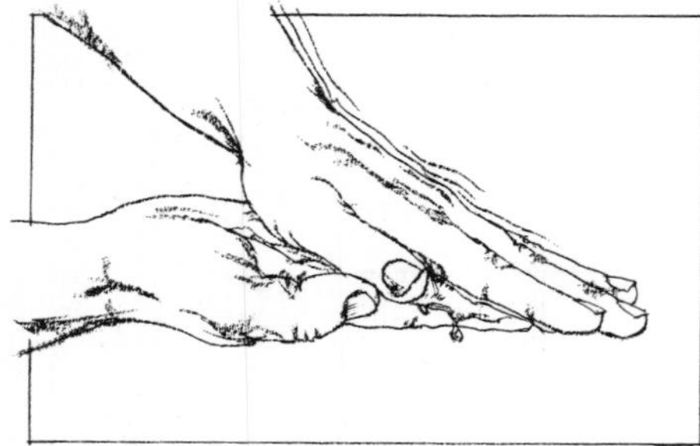

2. Gently rub the resident's back, starting at the base of the back and moving upward toward the shoulders. Without interrupting the motion or taking your hands away, rub down their back. Continue the back rub for 3 to 5 minutes.

   Note: Remember to use good body mechanics.

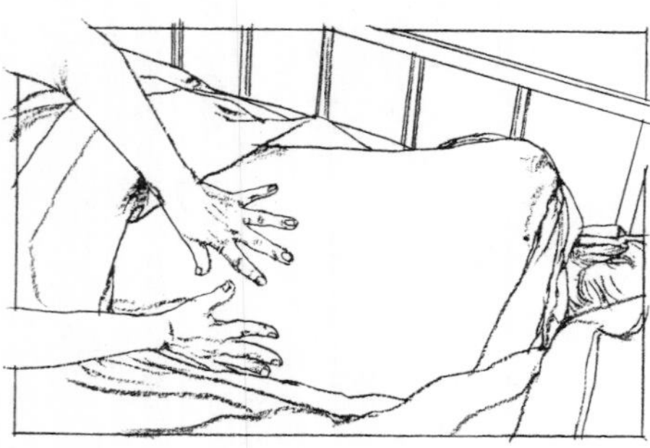

Rationale: Moving your hands in this direction promotes comfort and stimulates circulation toward the heart. Maintaining even, continuous strokes will relax and comfort the resident.

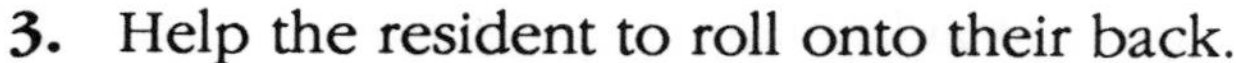

3. Help the resident to roll onto their back.

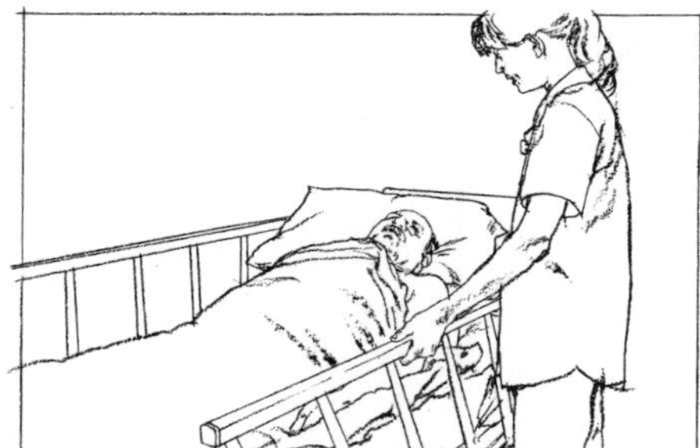

4. Pull up the side rail for the resident's safety.

Perineal Care

1. Change the water.

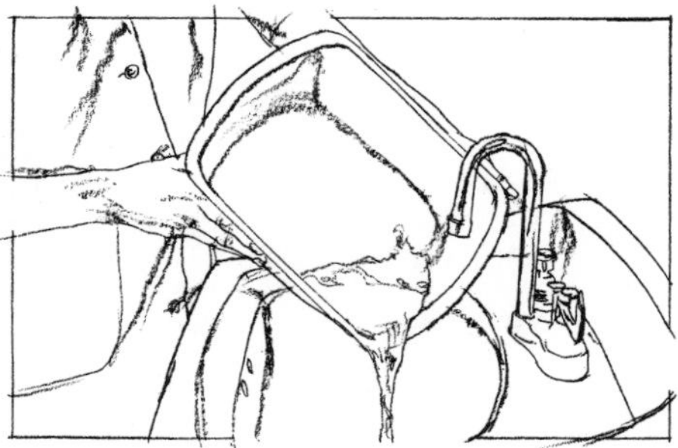

---

2. Put a disposable bed protector under the resident's buttocks to protect the bedding.

   Note: If the resident is able to do their own perineal care, offer them a washcloth, soap, and clean water. Allow the person a few minutes alone to bathe themselves.

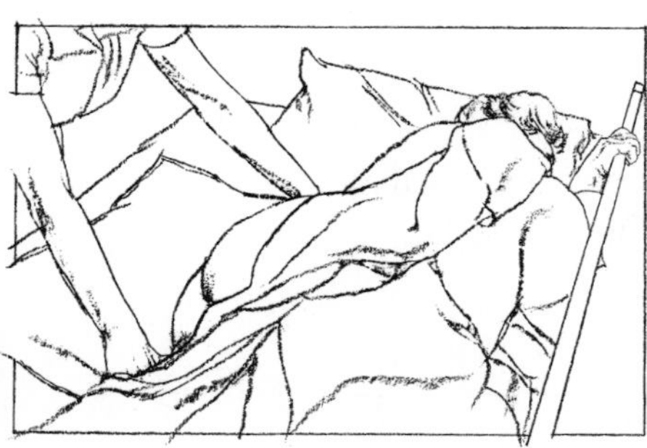

---

3. Drape the resident's perineal area using the following steps:

   Help the resident to bend their knees and spread their legs.

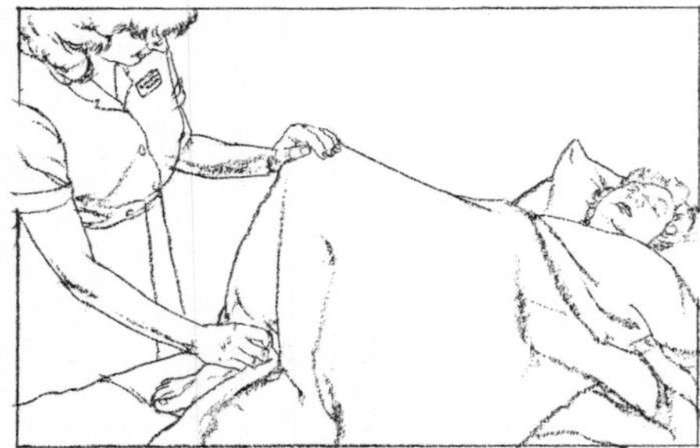

Place the bath blanket over the resident like a diamond with one corner at the neck, a corner at each side, and one corner between the legs.

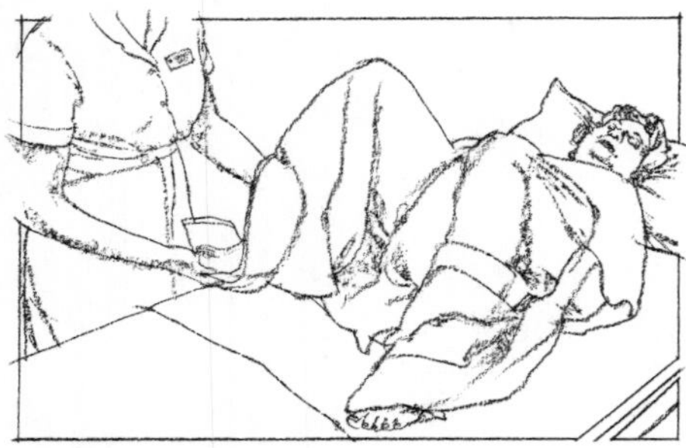

Wrap each side corner around the resident's feet by bringing the corner under and around the foot to secure the blanket.

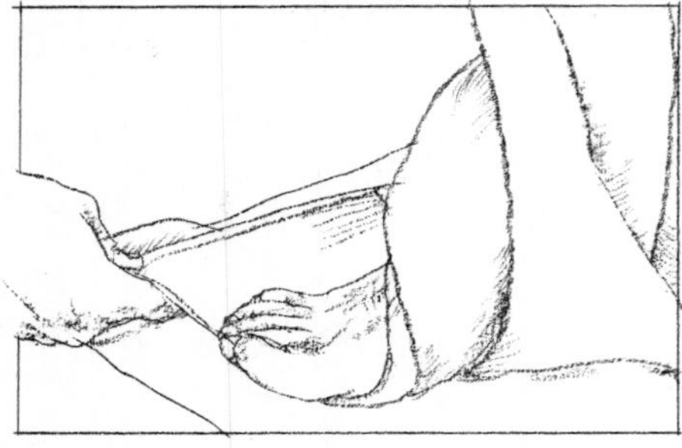

Rationale: This method exposes only the part of the resident that must be exposed.

For female resident

1. Elevate the pelvis using one of the following methods: ☐

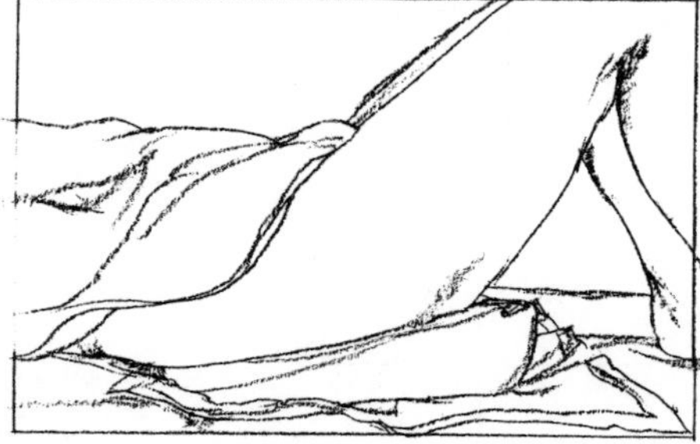

A folded towel or bath blanket under the buttocks.

A warm bedpan

Rationale: This position elevates the pelvis so you can get a better view of the perineal area. The bedpan will also collect excess water during care.

---

2. Put on disposable gloves for infection control. ☐

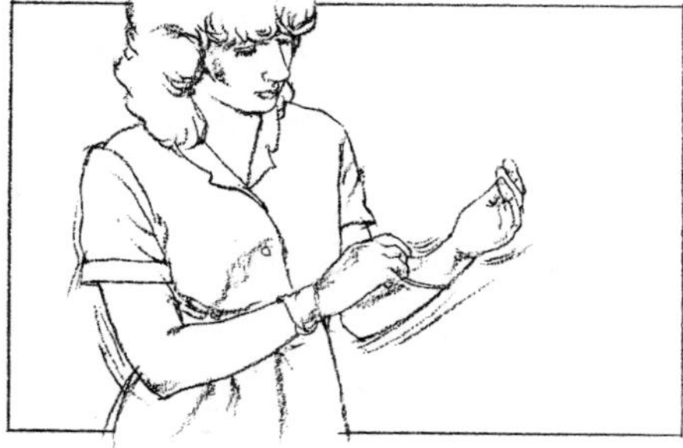

---

3. Make the washcloth into a mitt. ☐

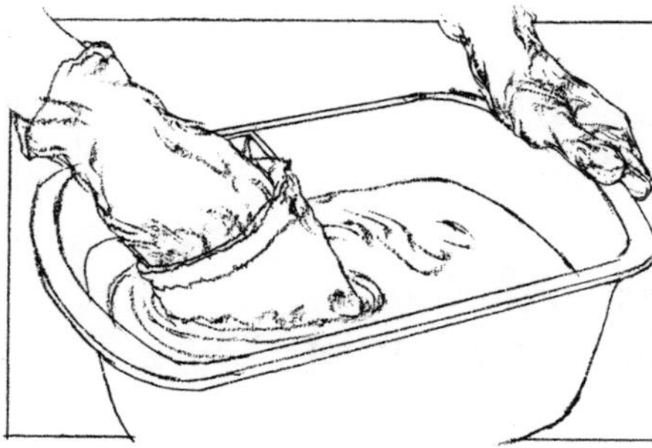

---

4. Lift the drape to expose the resident's perineal area. ☐

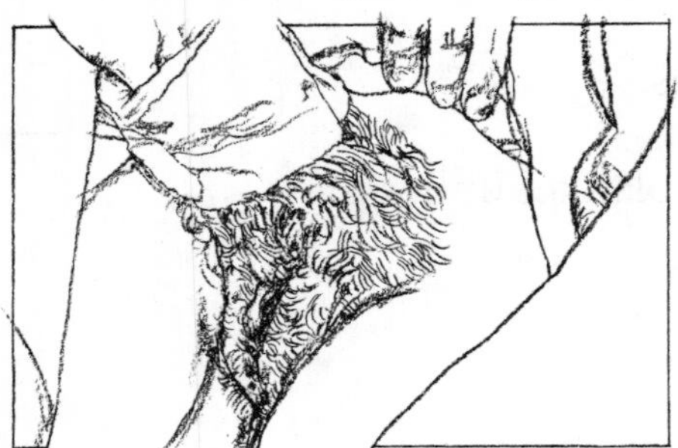

---

5. Separate the labia. In one even stroke wash the sides of the labia. Then wash down the middle, using a different area of the washcloth for each stroke to prevent the spread of germs. ☐

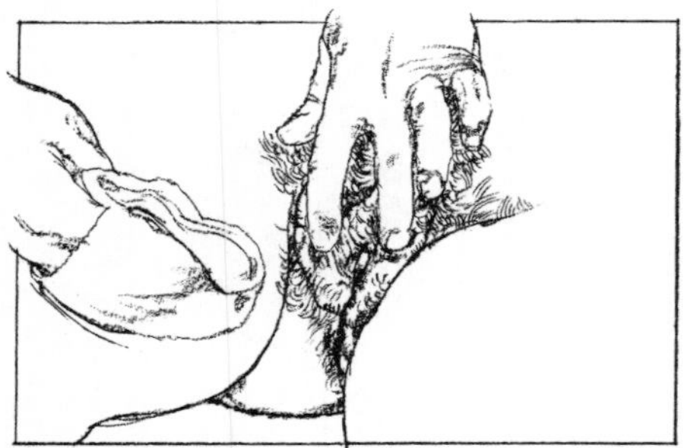

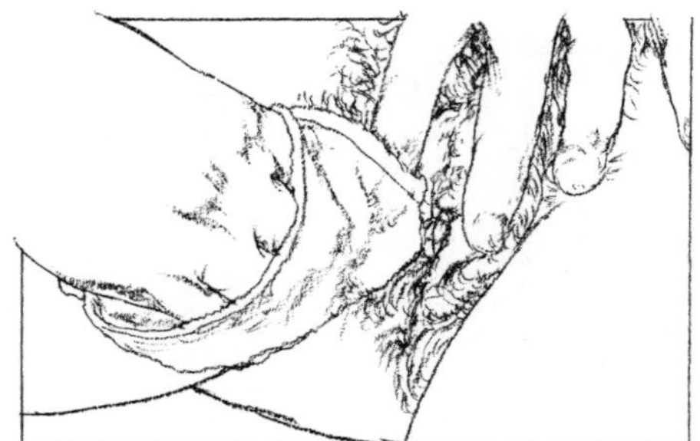

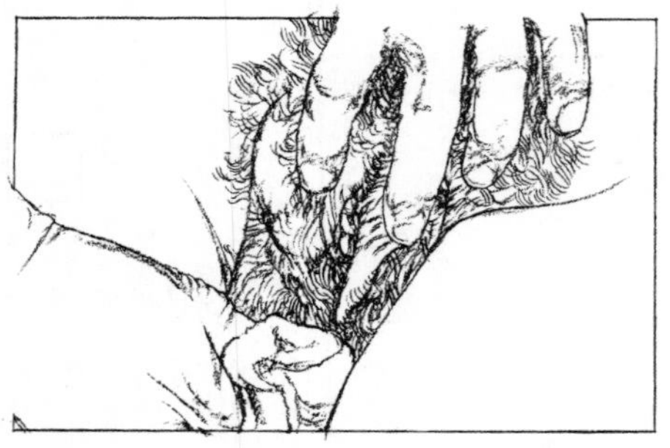

Note: Always wash from the pubic area to the anal area to prevent contaminating the clean area (the urethral opening) with bacteria from the anal area.

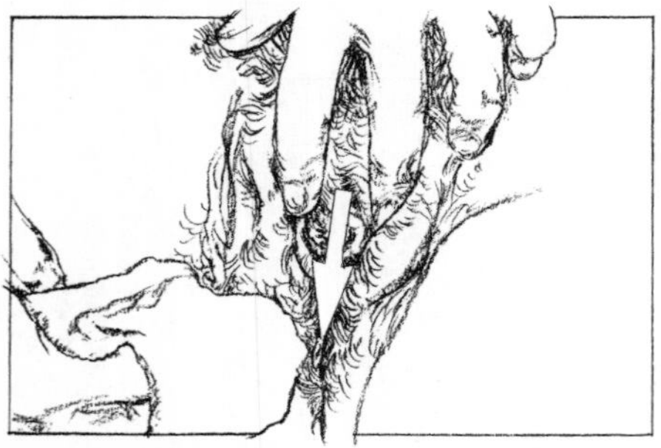

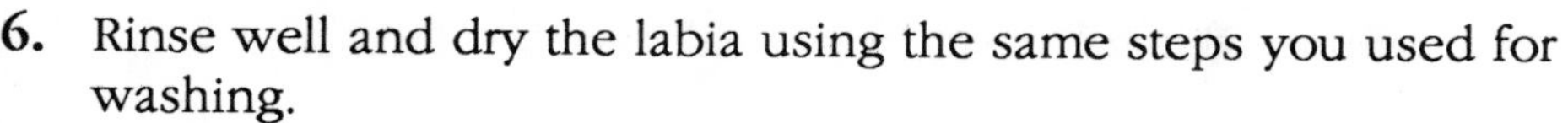

6. Rinse well and dry the labia using the same steps you used for washing. ☐

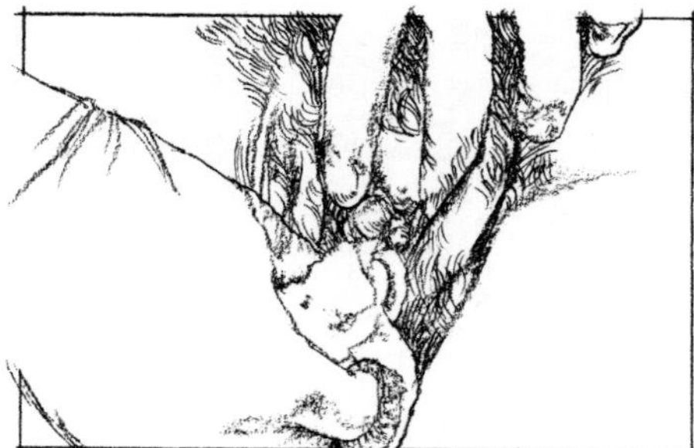

---

7. Remove the towel, blanket or bedpan and turn the resident on her side to wash the anal area using the procedure in Skill 2. ☐

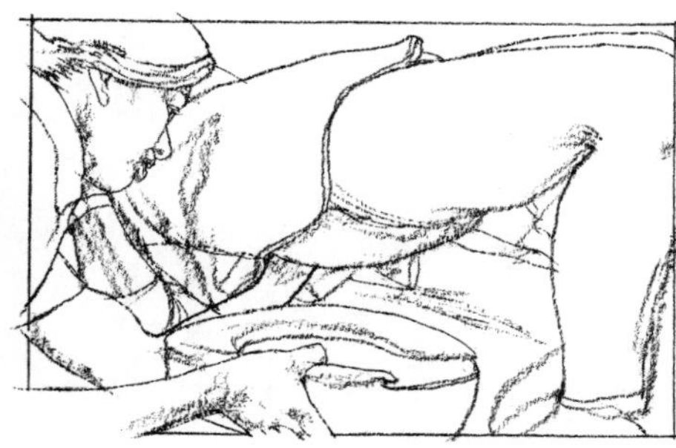

---

8. Wash, rinse, and dry the anal area going in the direction away from the genital area using a different area of the washcloth for each stroke. ☐

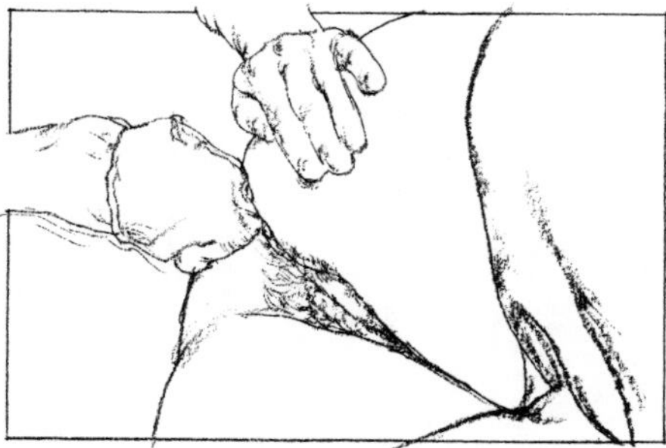

For male resident

1. Put on disposable gloves for infection control. ☐

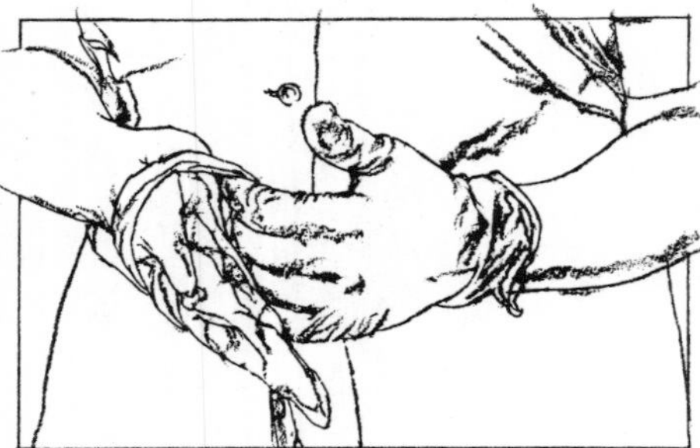

2. Make the washcloth into a mitt. ☐

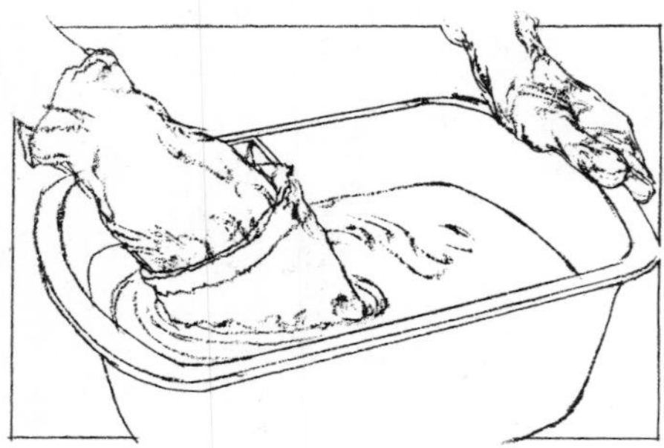

3. Lift the drape to expose the resident's perineal area. ☐

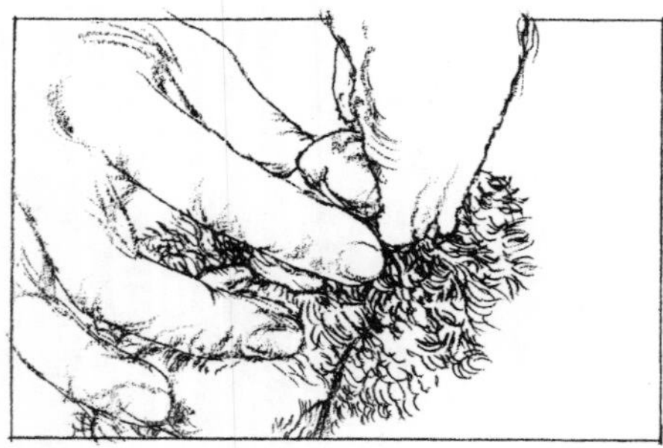

4. Hold the penis and wash, rinse, and dry the tip. ☐

Note: Always wash from the urethral opening outward, using a different area of the washcloth for each stroke, to prevent contaminating the clean area of the urethral opening.

5. Wash the shaft of the penis in the same way working in the direction of the pubic area.

   Note: If resident is not circumcised, carefully pull back foreskin and wash, rinse, and dry the penis.

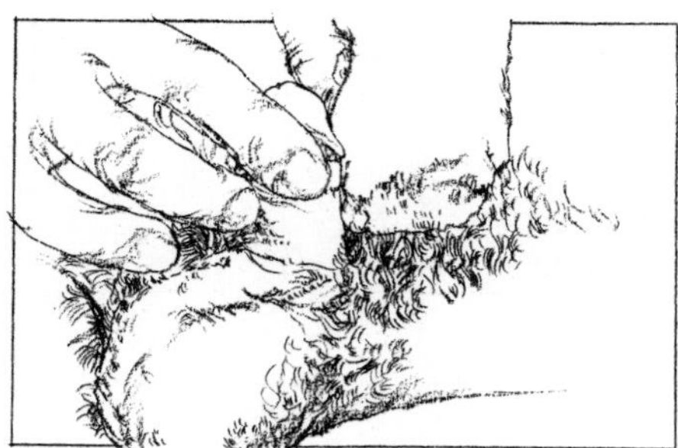

---

6. Help the resident to spread his legs and wash, rinse, and dry the scrotum. Clean between the skin folds in this area and under the scrotom thoroughly.

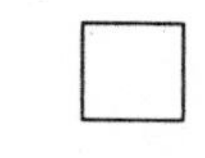

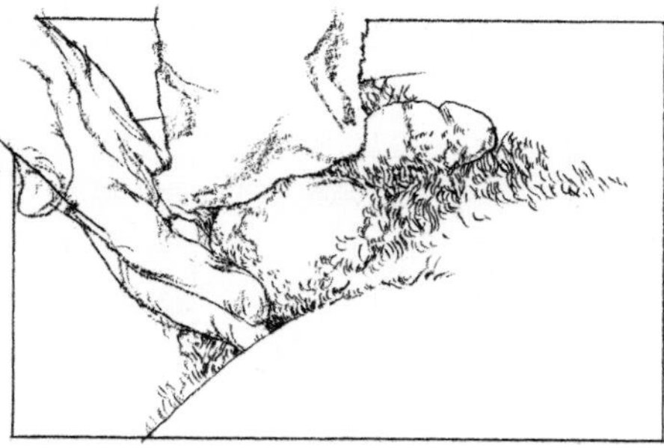

---

7. Help the resident to roll onto his side using the procedure described in Skill 5.

---

8. Wash, rinse, and dry the anal area. ☐

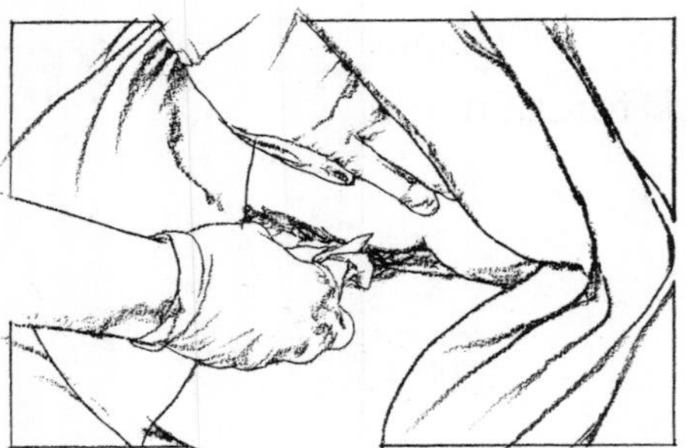

Rationale: Moisture between the skin folds may cause skin breakdown.

Skill 9: Brushing and Flossing

Name: ______________________________ Date: ______________

Precautions

- Never insert floss into the gumline. Gums are sensitive and easily cut.
- Never use full-strength mouthwash. It may harm delicate gums.

Procedure

Competency check

1. Help the resident to turn their head toward you so you can see better. ☐

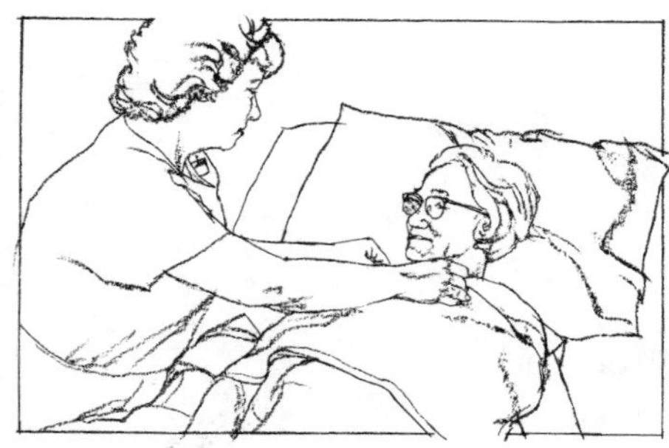

Rationale: Turning the resident's head while brushing teeth prevents aspiration of fluid.

2. Unfold the towel and place it across the resident's chest to protect the resident's bedding and clothing. ☐

3. Place the emesis basin on the towel and have the resident hold it, if possible. ☐

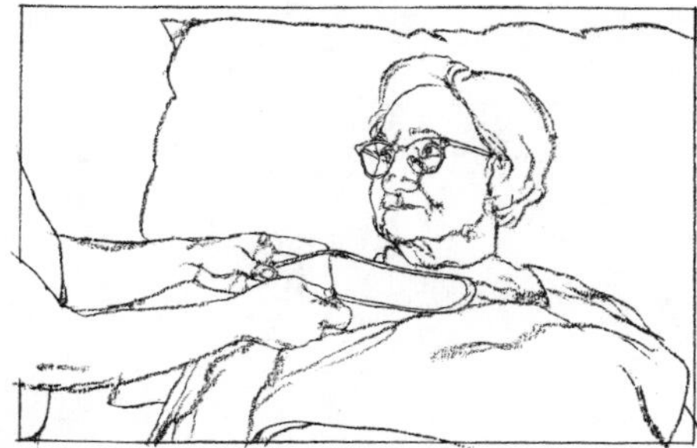

Rationale: The emesis basin will catch the solution.

4. Put toothpaste on a wet toothbrush.

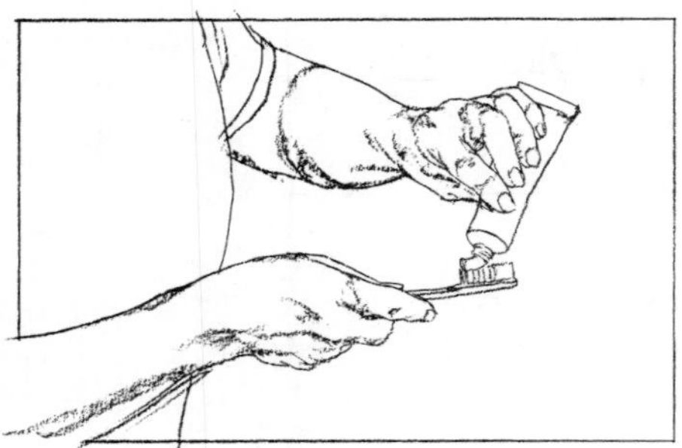

Rationale: Toothpaste will spread more easily on a moist brush.

5. Put on disposable gloves.

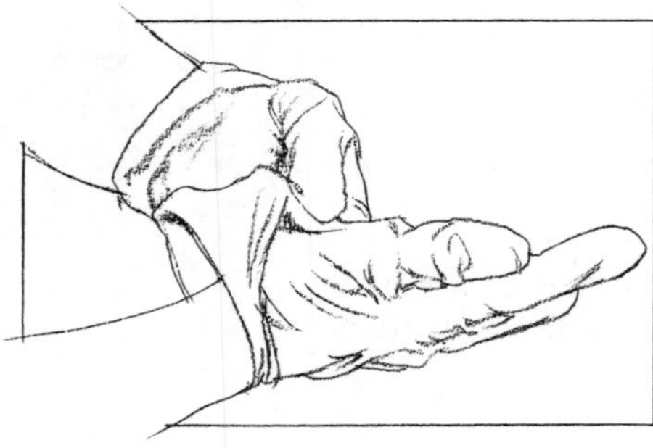

Rationale: Wearing disposable gloves protects the nurse assistant if the resident's gums are bleeding.

6. Give the resident a mouthful of the solution to rinse their mouth. Hold the emesis basin under the chin to catch the solution.

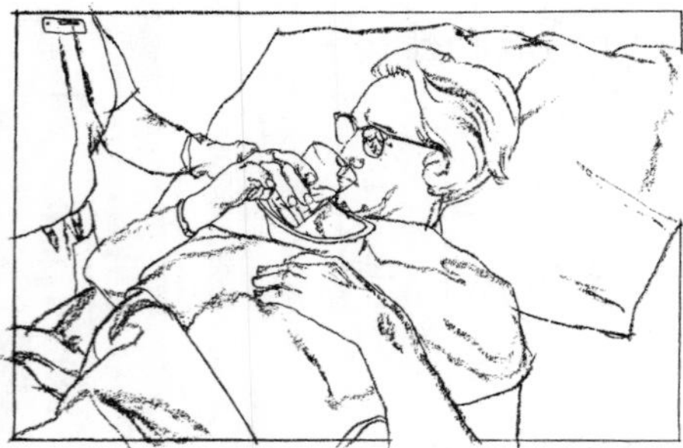

7. Brush the upper teeth and gums first, then lower teeth and gums. Be sure to brush the resident's tongue gently.

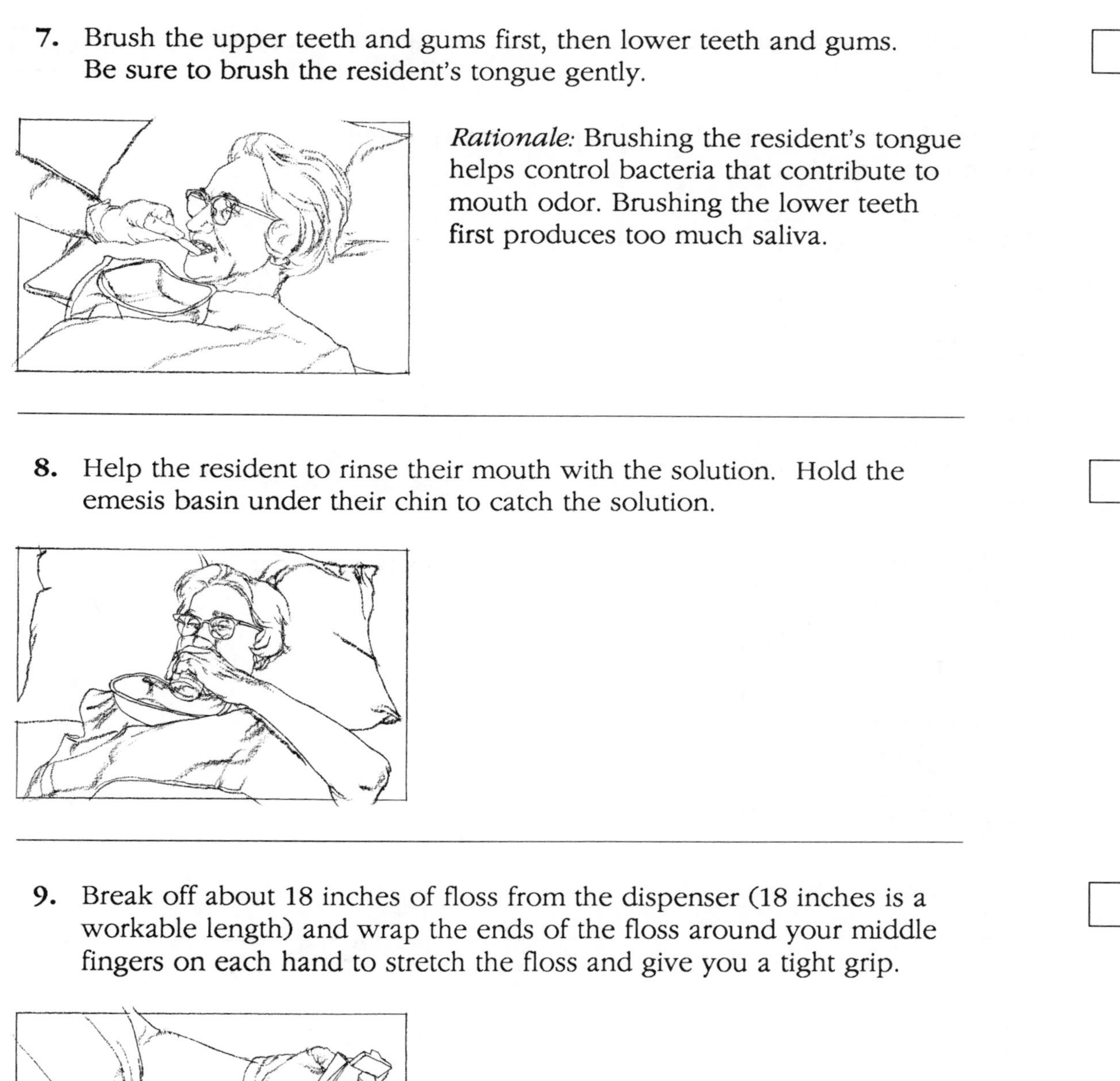

Rationale: Brushing the resident's tongue helps control bacteria that contribute to mouth odor. Brushing the lower teeth first produces too much saliva.

---

8. Help the resident to rinse their mouth with the solution. Hold the emesis basin under their chin to catch the solution.

---

9. Break off about 18 inches of floss from the dispenser (18 inches is a workable length) and wrap the ends of the floss around your middle fingers on each hand to stretch the floss and give you a tight grip.

---

10. Gently insert floss between teeth, but not into the gumline. Continue until all teeth are flossed. ☐

Note: Avoid inserting the floss into the gumline to prevent cutting gums and causing bleeding.

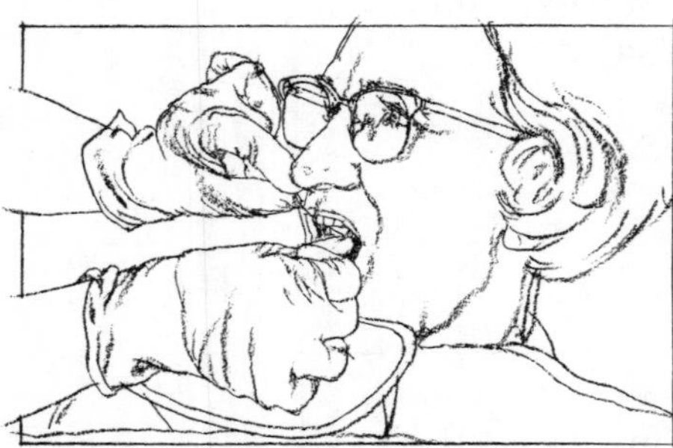

---

11. Help the resident rinse their mouth. Hold the emesis basin under their chin to catch the solution. ☐

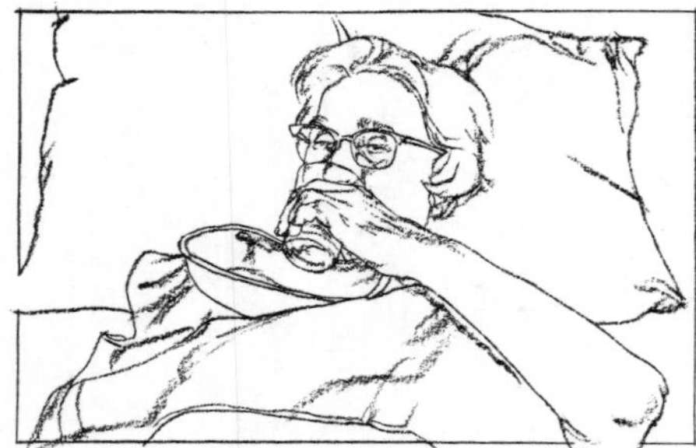

Skill 10: Denture Care

Name: ______________________________ Date: ______________

Procedure

Competency check

1. Open disposable trash bag. ☐

2. Open toothettes or lemon glycerine swabs. ☐

3. Put on disposable gloves. ☐

Note: Putting on disposable gloves is optional for this procedure.

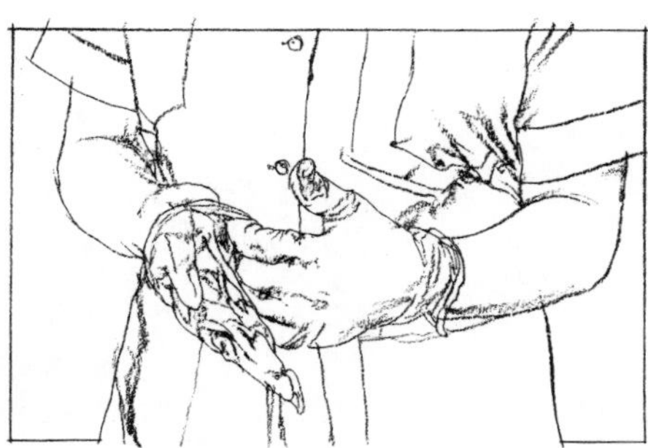

4. Ask the resident to remove their dentures and put them in the emesis basin. If the resident needs help, hold teeth firmly with a tissue, and with a rocking motion gently remove the teeth and put them in emesis basin. ☐

Note: Using a rocking motion to remove dentures breaks the seal holding the dentures in place.

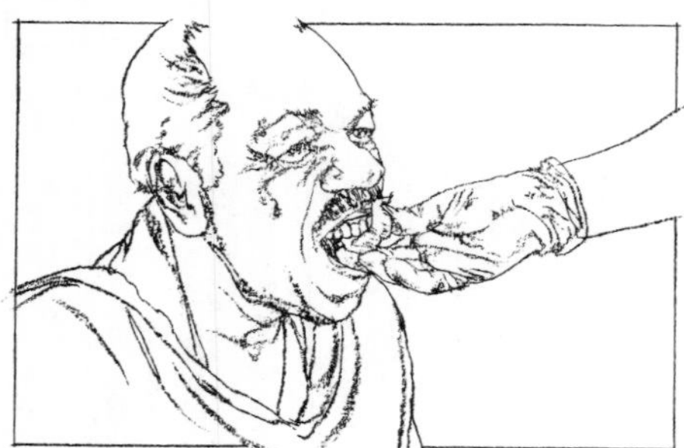

---

5. Clean the dentures in the sink by brushing all surfaces to assure proper oral hygiene. ☐

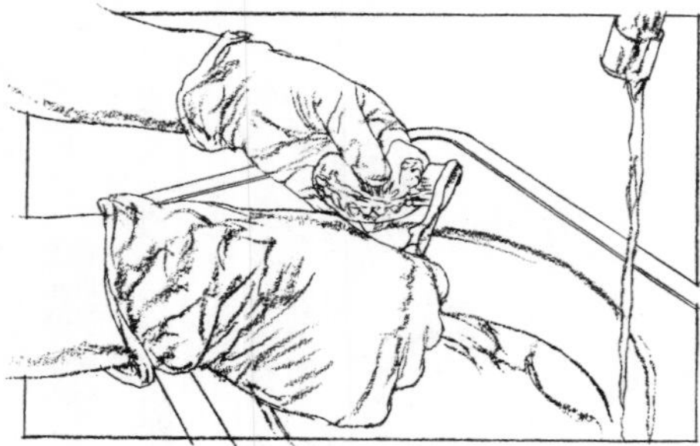

---

6. Rinse dentures under cool running water. ☐

Note: Hot water may change the shape or warp the dentures.

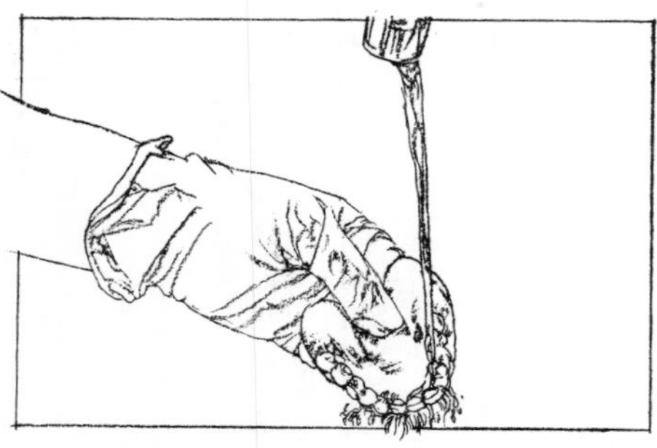

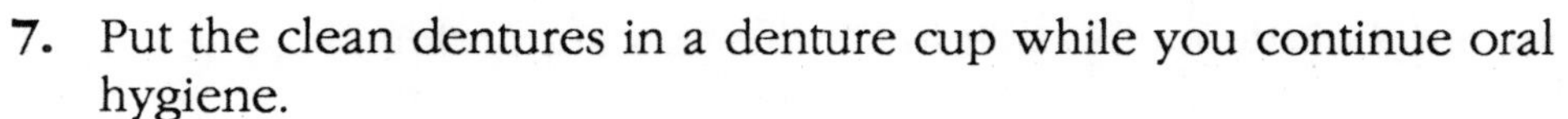

7. Put the clean dentures in a denture cup while you continue oral hygiene.

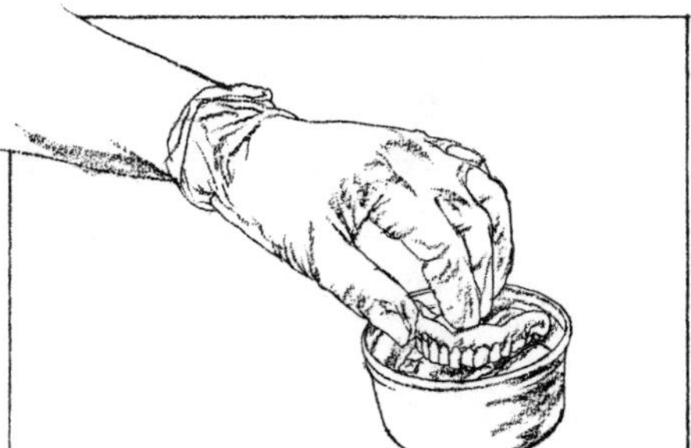

---

8. Help the resident clean their gums with toothettes dipped in mouthwash solution or with lemon and glycerine swabs.

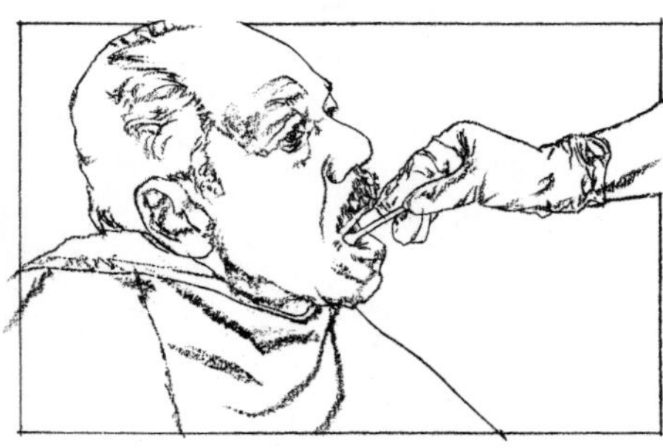

---

9. Help the resident rinse their mouth with mouthwash solution. Hold the emesis basin under the chin to catch the solution.

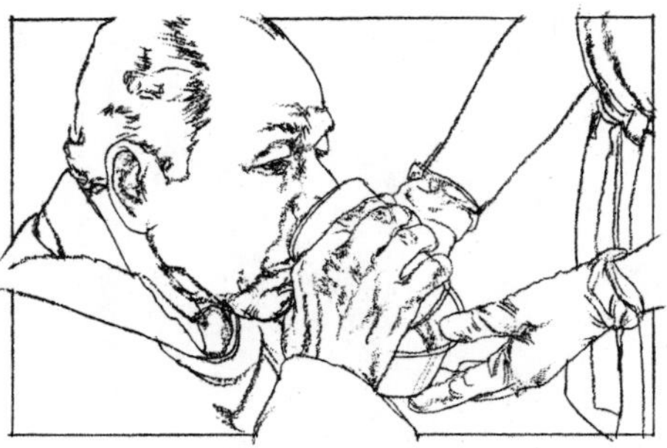

---

10. Help the resident put their dentures back in. If the resident prefers, put the clean dentures in a denture cup with enough water to cover them. ☐

Note: If dentures are stored in a cup, they should never be allowed to dry because they might warp.

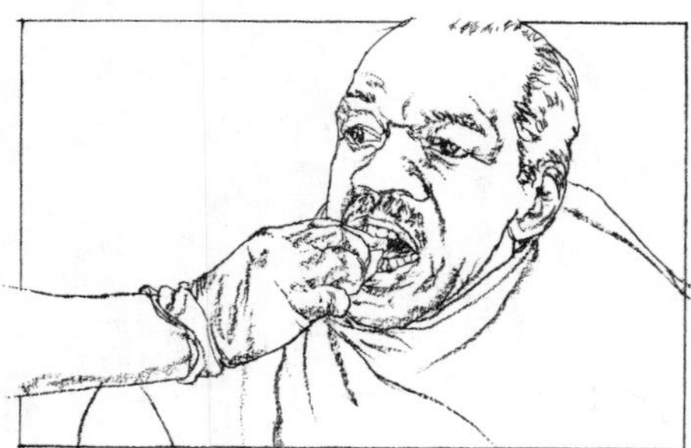

Skill 11: Mouth Care for the Unconscious Resident

Name: ______________________________ Date: ______________

Precautions

- When working on an unconscious resident, never use force to open the mouth.
- Always position the person's head to the side to prevent aspiration, because unconscious residents cannot swallow fluids.

Procedure

Competency check

1. Turn the resident's head toward you so you can see better. ☐

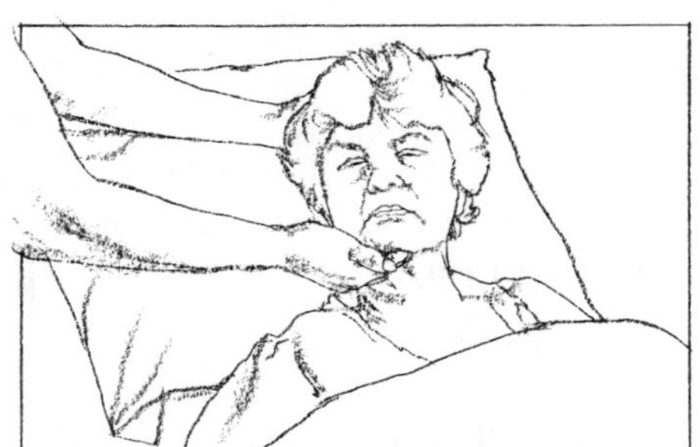

Rationale: Turning the resident's head while cleaning teeth prevents aspiration of fluid.

2. Spread a towel under the resident's head and put a towel across their chest to protect the resident's bedding and clothing. Put the emesis basin under their chin to catch the solution. ☐

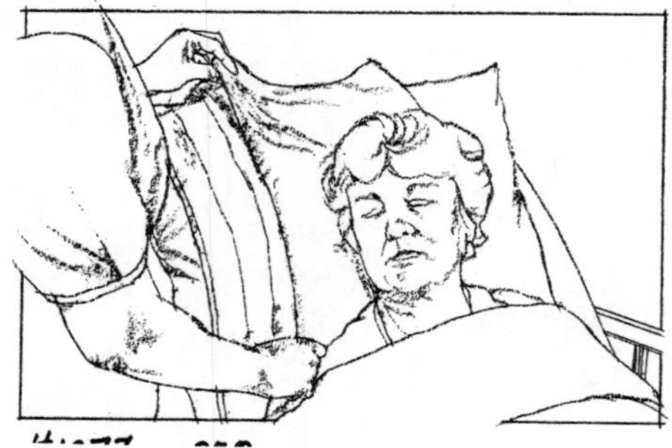

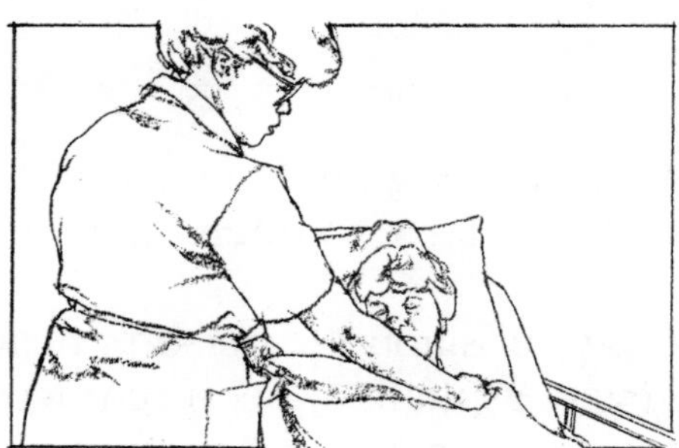

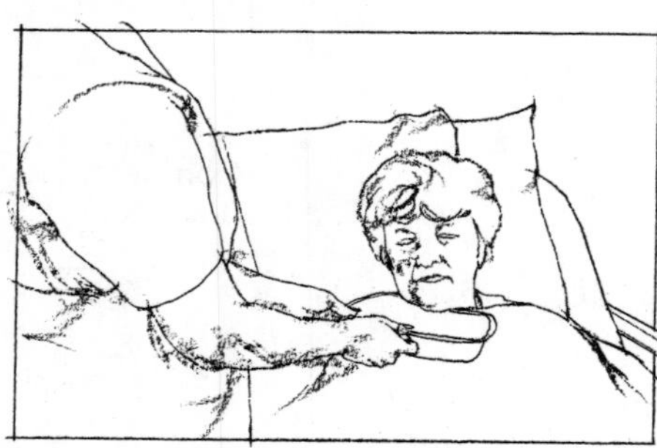

---

3. Prepare equipment for use (equipment should be ready to use before putting on gloves): ☐

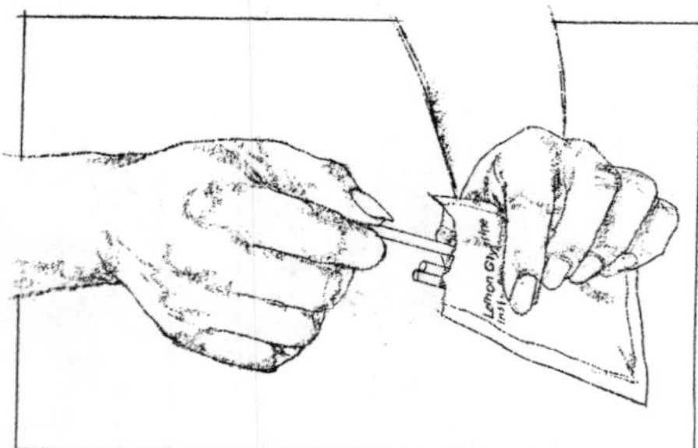

Mix half-mouthwash, half-water solution. Open packages of toothettes or swabs.

---

4. Put on gloves.

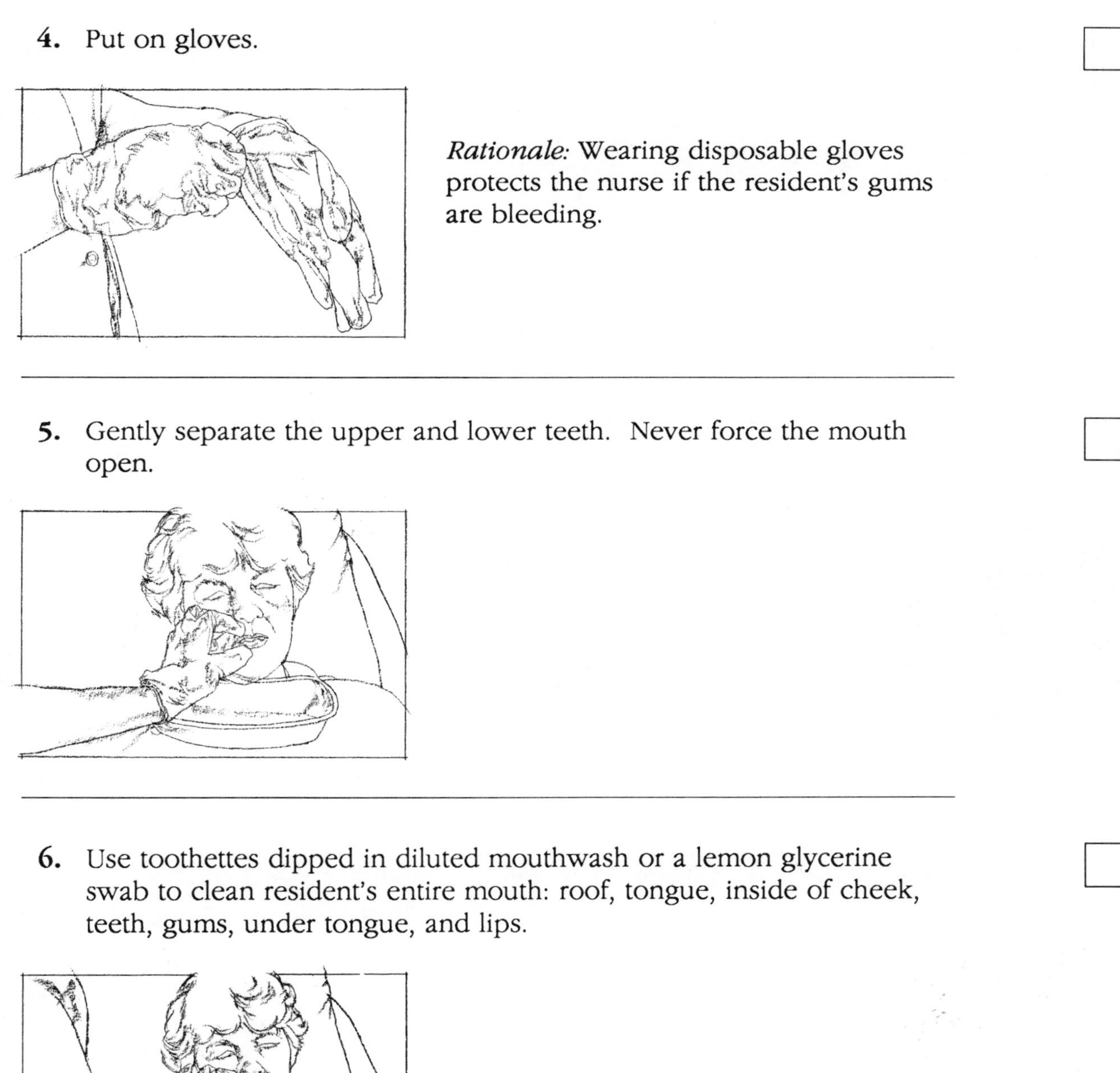

Rationale: Wearing disposable gloves protects the nurse if the resident's gums are bleeding.

5. Gently separate the upper and lower teeth. Never force the mouth open.

6. Use toothettes dipped in diluted mouthwash or a lemon glycerine swab to clean resident's entire mouth: roof, tongue, inside of cheek, teeth, gums, under tongue, and lips.

Skill 12: Brushing and Combing Hair

Name: ______________________ Date: ______________

Precautions

- Always brush hair gently so as not to pull out any hair.
- Never use a comb with sharp teeth that may hurt the scalp.

Procedure

Competency check

1. Brush hair gently and slowly. Start at the ends of the hair and work your way up to the scalp ☐

   Note: If hair is tangled, use a wide-tooth comb. Forcing and pulling on a tangled mass breaks many hairs. Sometimes alcohol will loosen a tangle.

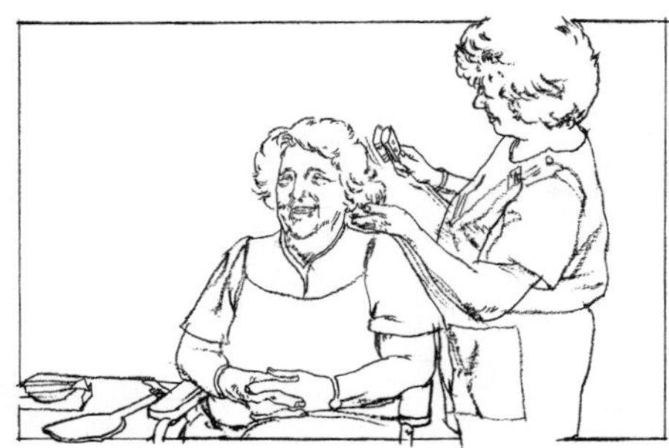

Rationale: Brushing hair gently will avoid damaging it and will stimulate circulation.

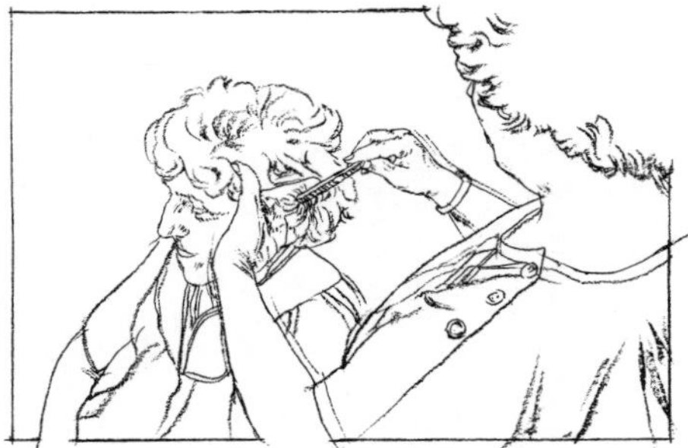

2. Style the resident's hair the way they like it. ☐

Note: Remember, the resident should decide how their hair is styled.

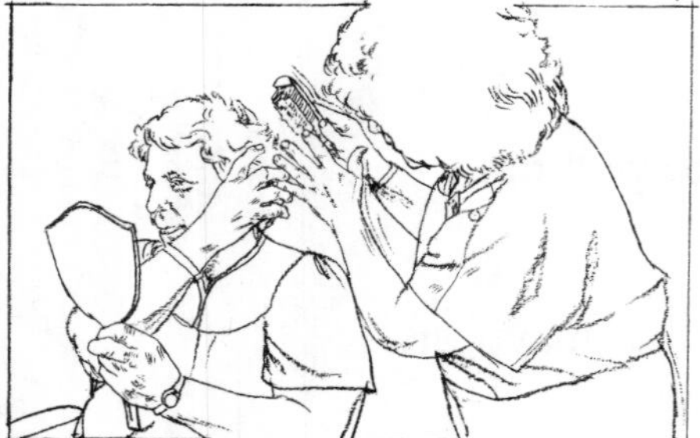

Skill 13: Shaving

Name: ______________________________ Date: ______________

Precautions

- Never use an electric razor in a room if anyone is receiving oxygen.
- Never share razors among residents.

Procedure

Competency check

1. Assist the resident to a sitting position and put the towel over the chest to protect clothing. ☐

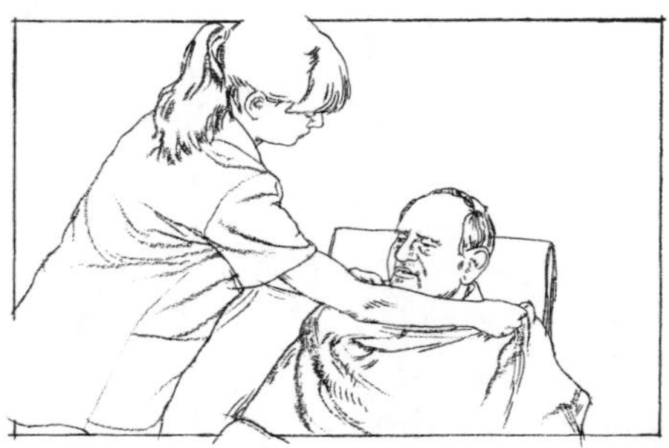

2. Prepare equipment for use: ☐

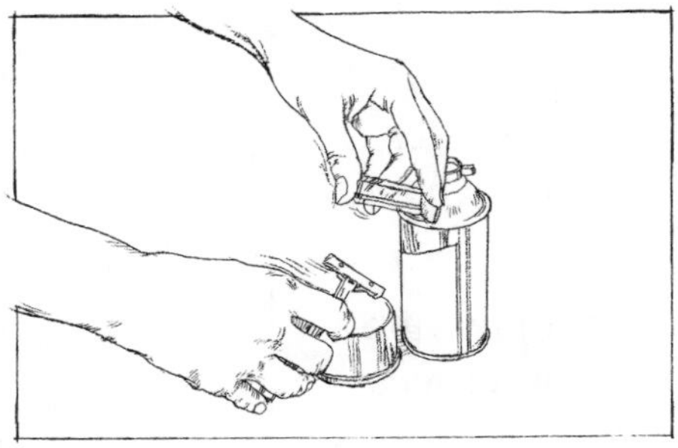

Open shaving cream
Remove cap on razor

3. Inspect the resident's skin for moles, birthmarks, or lesions.

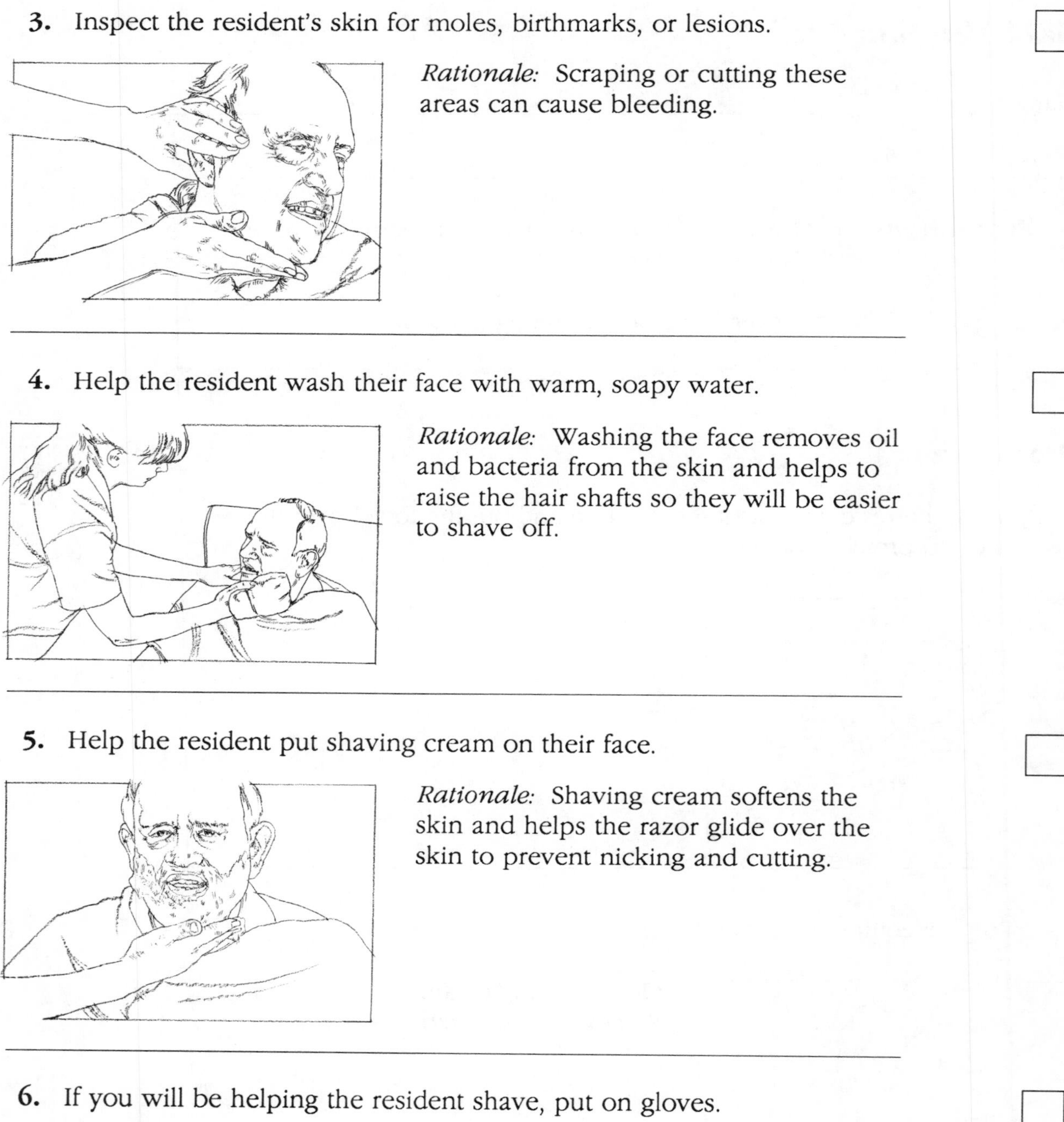

Rationale: Scraping or cutting these areas can cause bleeding.

4. Help the resident wash their face with warm, soapy water.

Rationale: Washing the face removes oil and bacteria from the skin and helps to raise the hair shafts so they will be easier to shave off.

5. Help the resident put shaving cream on their face.

Rationale: Shaving cream softens the skin and helps the razor glide over the skin to prevent nicking and cutting.

6. If you will be helping the resident shave, put on gloves.

Rationale: If any bleeding occurs while you are shaving the resident, the gloves will protect you from possible infection.

7. With the fingers of one hand hold the skin tight as you shave downward in the direction that the hair grows. ☐

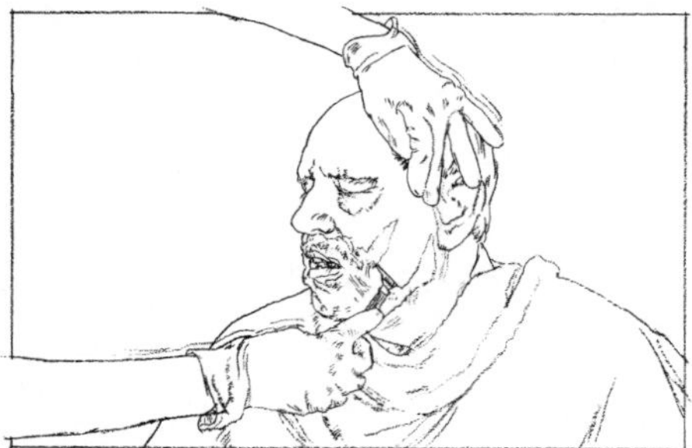

Rationale: Shaving in the direction the hair grows will produce a smoother shave without irritating the skin.

---

8. Rinse the razor often to remove hair so the cutting edge remains clean. ☐

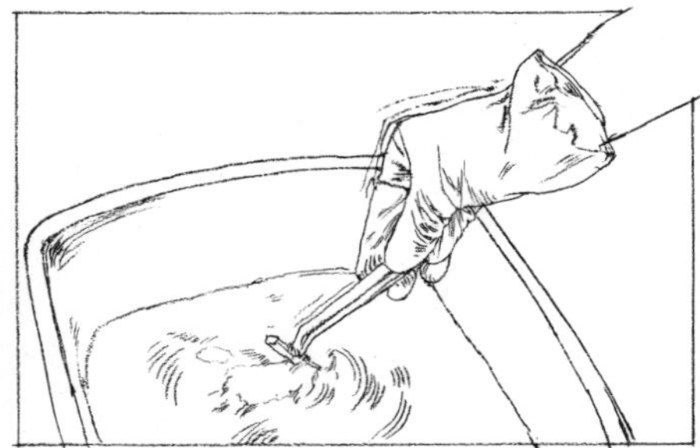

---

9. Use shorter strokes around chin and lips. Work downward on the neck under the chin. ☐

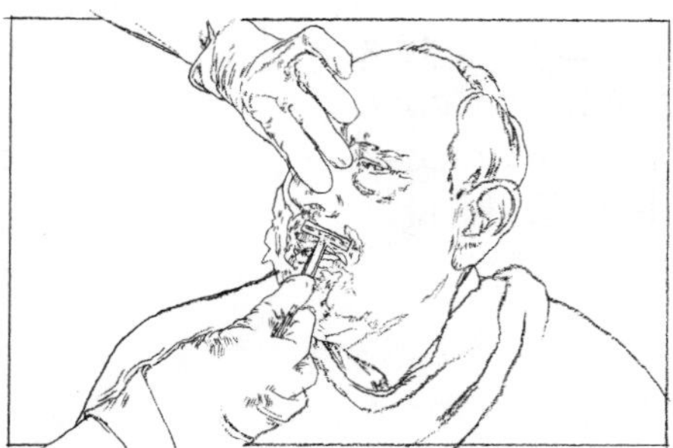

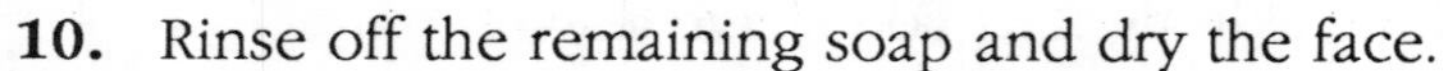

10. Rinse off the remaining soap and dry the face.

Note: Soap may irritate the skin if not rinsed thoroughly.

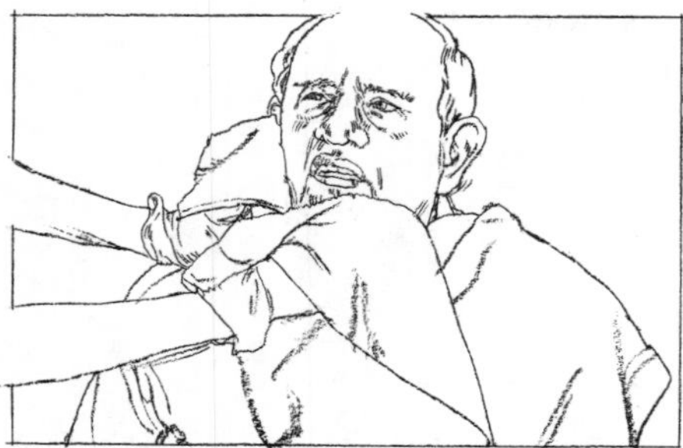

11. Give the resident a mirror so he can inspect shaved area.

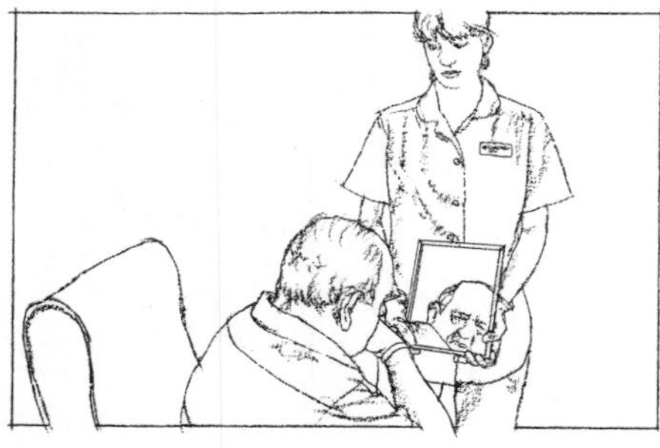

12. Apply after-shave lotion if resident desires.

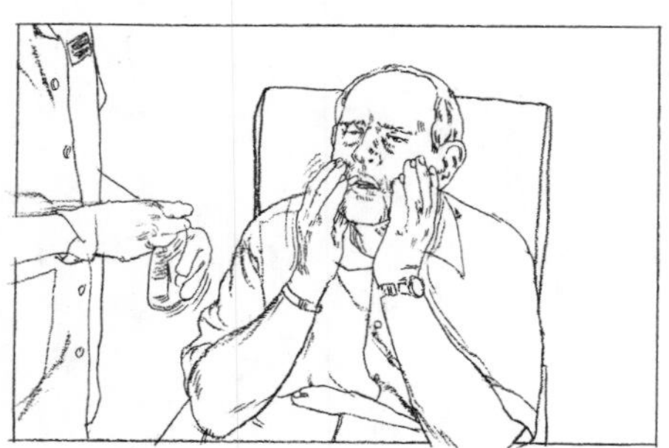

Rationale: Alcohol in after-shave acts as antiseptic for any tiny abrasions or cuts. When after-shave evaporates, it causes a cooling sensation that feels refreshing.

Skill 14: Cleaning and Trimming Fingernails

Name: ______________________________ Date: ______________

Precaution

- Nails should always be kept trimmed and smooth to prevent injury to the skin.

Procedure

Competency check

1. Soak the resident's hands in warm water for 5 minutes and then wash them. ☐

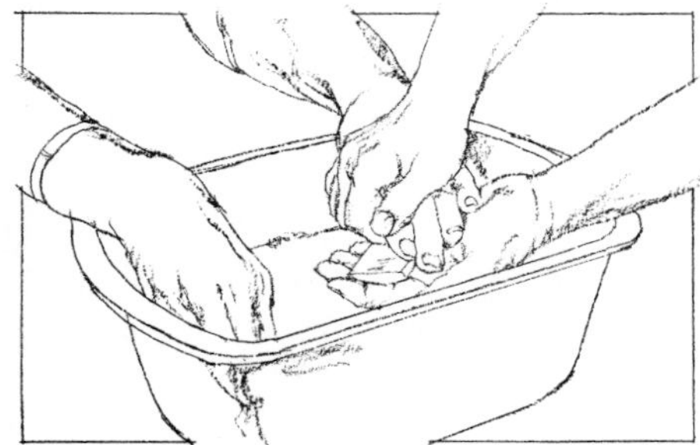

Rationale: Soaking will soften the nails and make them easier to trim.

---

2. Push cuticle back gently with a washcloth to prevent hangnails. ☐

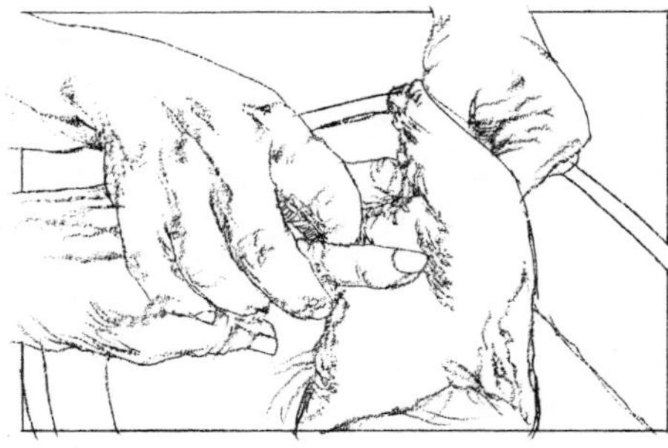

---

3. Clean under the nails with the orange stick to prevent injury to skin tissue. ☐

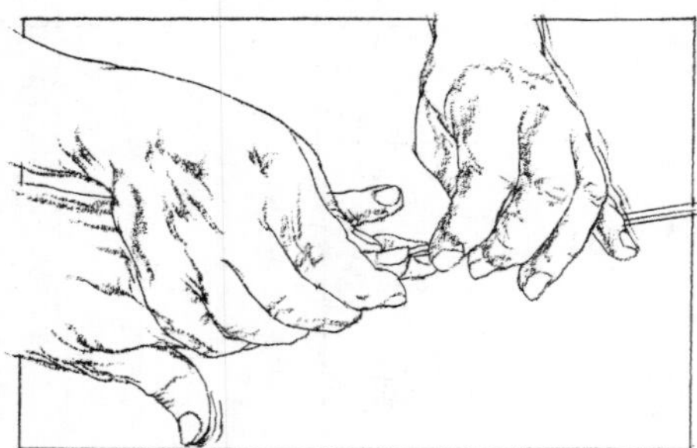

4. Change the water and rinse the resident's hands. ☐

Note: Do not rinse in soapy water. It will be irritating and drying.

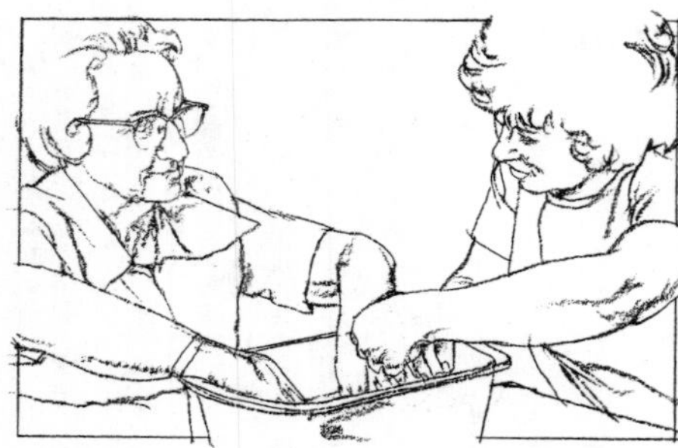

5. Dry the resident's hands. ☐

Note: Make sure the hands are dry to prevent chapping.

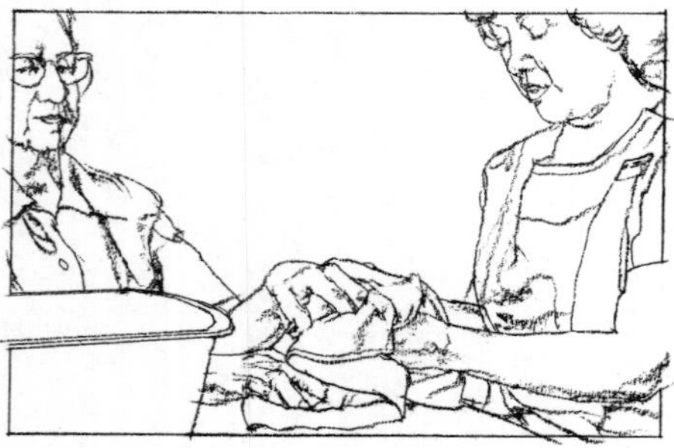

6. Use clippers to cut fingernails straight across and a nail file to shape, trim, and smooth them. ☐

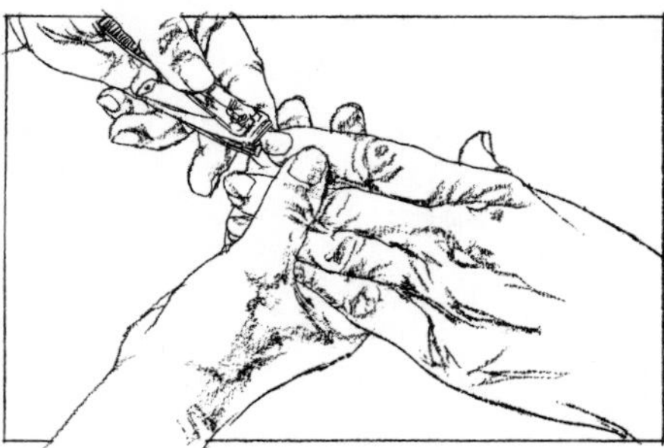

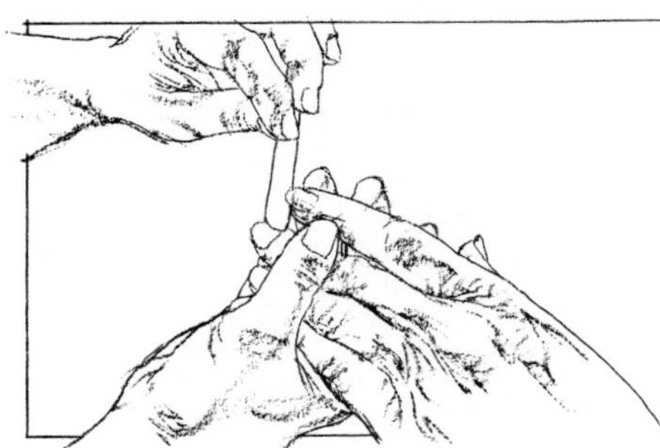

7. Put on lotion and gently massage the resident's hands from the fingertips toward the wrist. ☐

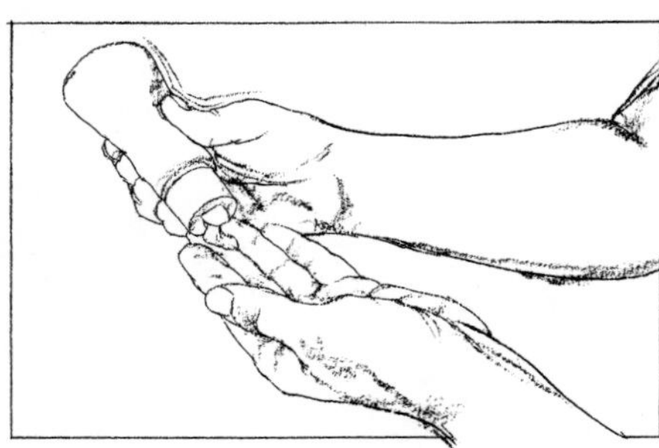

Rationale: Working in this direction helps blood circulation.

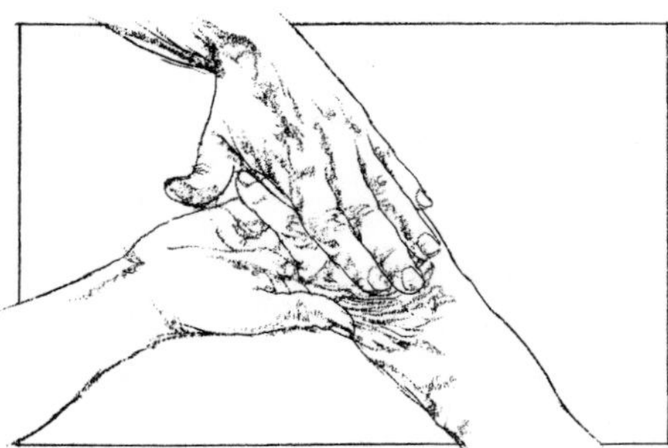

Skill 15: Giving Foot Care and Cleaning Toenails

Name: ______________________________ Date: ______________

Precaution • Never cut the resident's toenails.

Procedure

Competency check

1. Soak the resident's feet for at least 5 minutes and then wash them. ☐

Rationale: Soaking will loosen dirt under the nails and make them easier to clean.

2. Clean under toenails with an orange stick to prevent injury to skin tissue. ☐

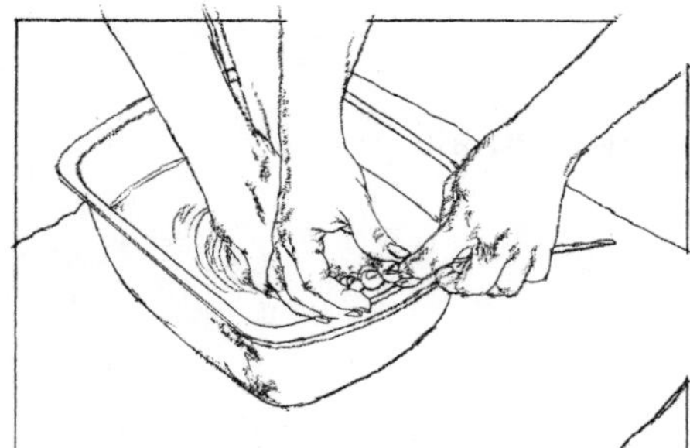

3. Change the water and rinse the resident's feet. ☐

Note: Do not rinse in soapy water. It will be irritating and drying.

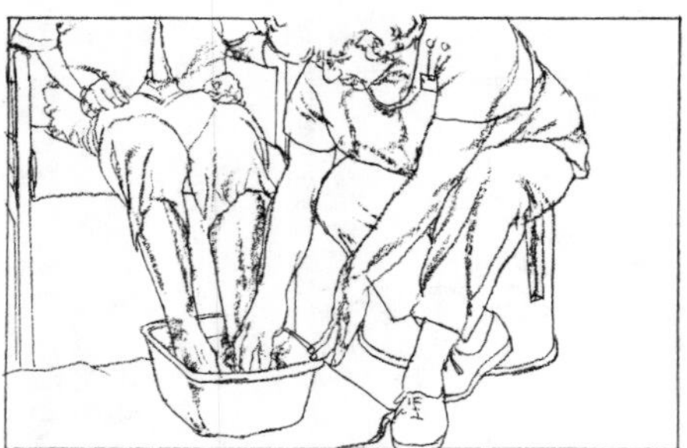

---

4. Dry the feet thoroughly. ☐

Note: Make sure the area between the toes is dry. Any moisture between toes can cause skin breakdown.

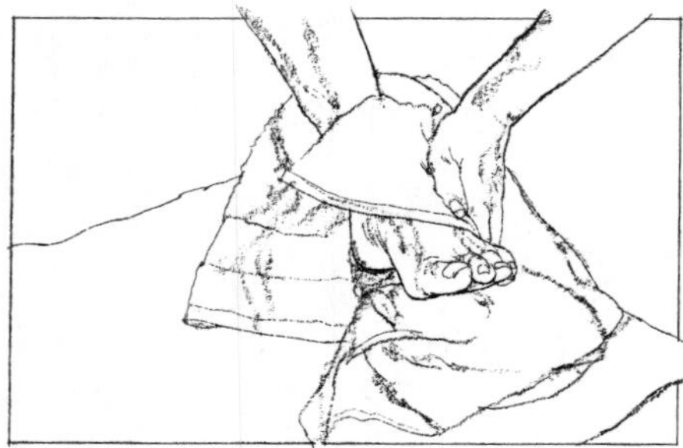

---

5. Inspect the condition of the skin on the feet, including between all toes. ☐

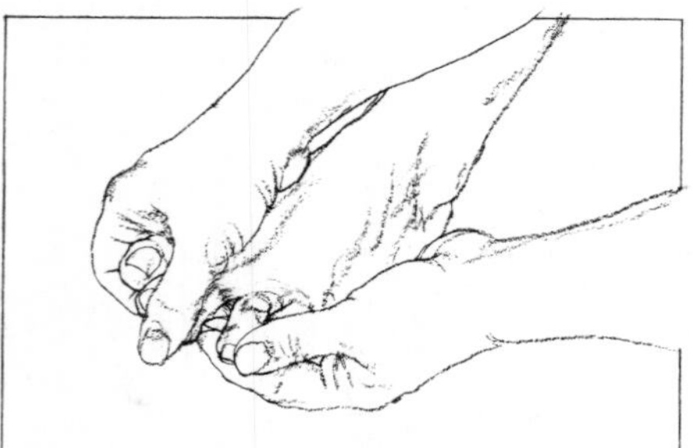

---

6. Gently massage the feet with lotion. Begin with toes and move upward. ☐

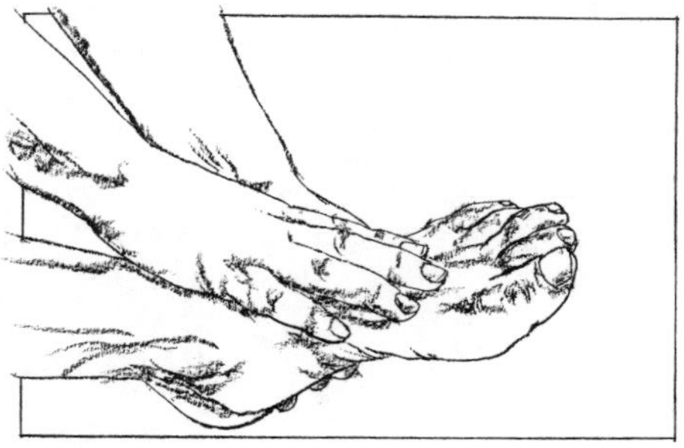

Rationale: This motion helps blood circulation.

---

7. Help the resident put on clean socks and shoes. ☐

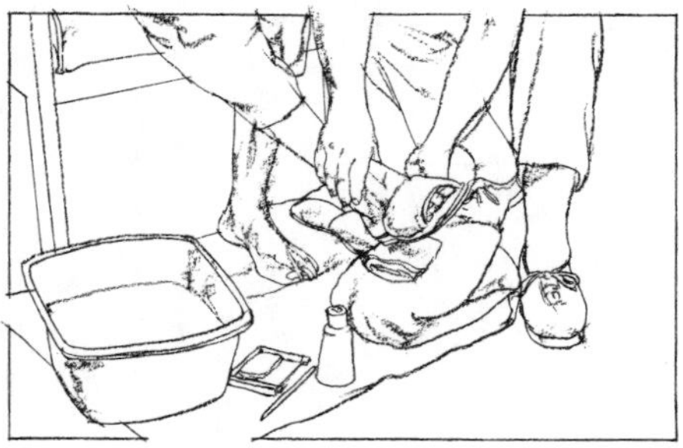

Skill 16: Dressing the Resident

Name: ______________________________ Date: ______________

Procedure

Competency check

1. Assist the resident to put on socks or stockings and help them to sit on the side of the bed. ☐

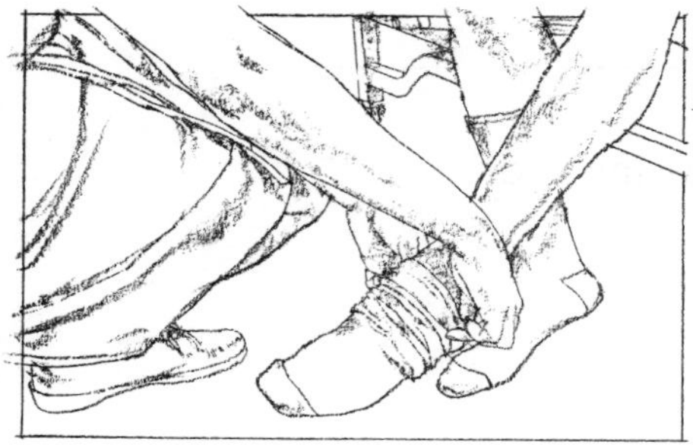

Rationale: This position will make dressing easier.

2. Help the resident put on underwear and pants. (To do this, have the resident put both legs in the legs of underpants and legs of pants while sitting.) ☐

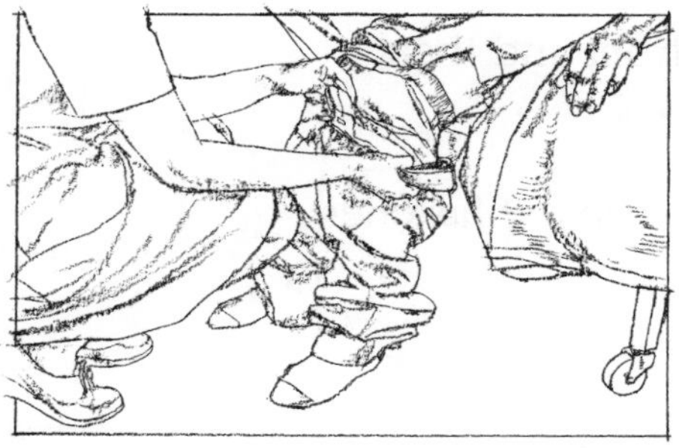

3. Put on resident's shoes and assist to a standing position. ☐

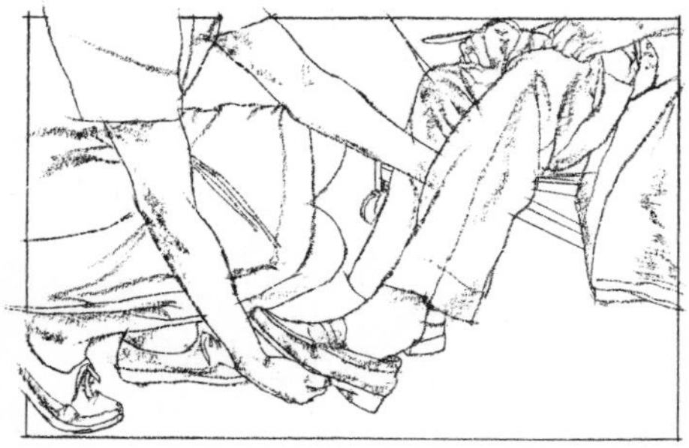

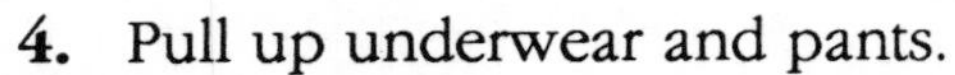

4. Pull up underwear and pants.

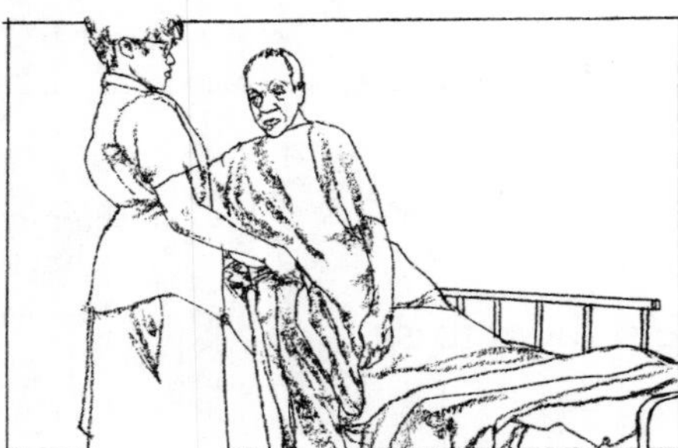

5. Assist resident to sit back down so you can finish dressing them.

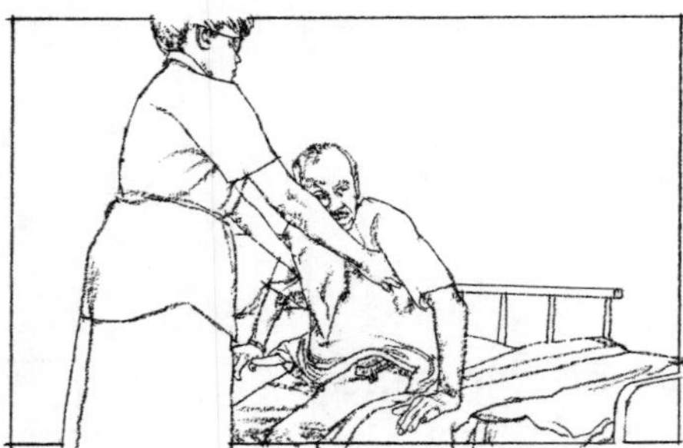

6. If the resident is female, help her to hook the bra in front and then turn it around so hooks are in back.

Rationale: It is easier to see the fastener this way.

7. Help the resident put her arms through the shoulder straps.

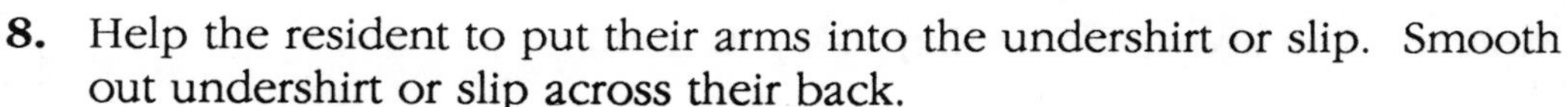

8. Help the resident to put their arms into the undershirt or slip. Smooth out undershirt or slip across their back. ☐

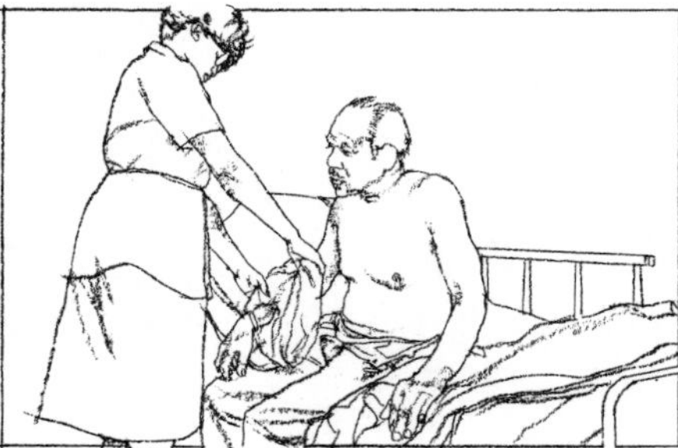

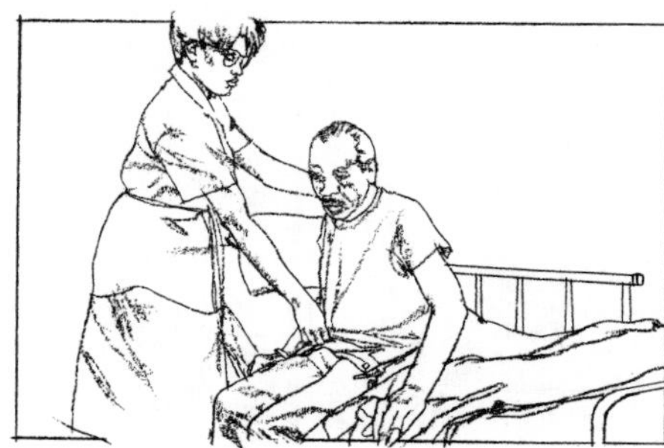

---

9. Help the resident to put on the dress or shirt by putting arms into sleeves, then smoothing out the back of the dress or shirt and fastening it. ☐

Note: Put weaker arm in sleeve first.

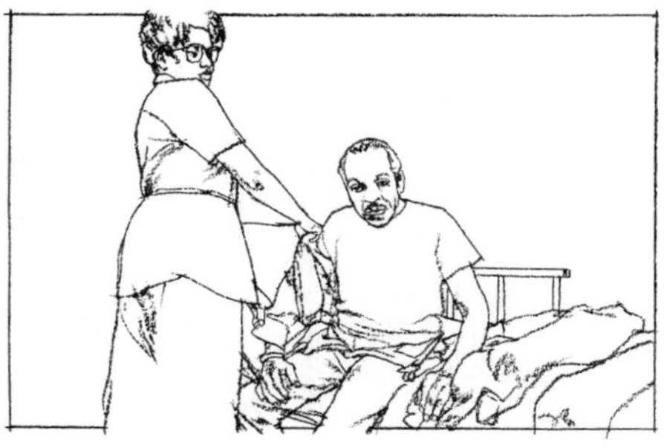

---

10. Have the resident stand again and tuck in the shirt and fasten or zip pants. ☐

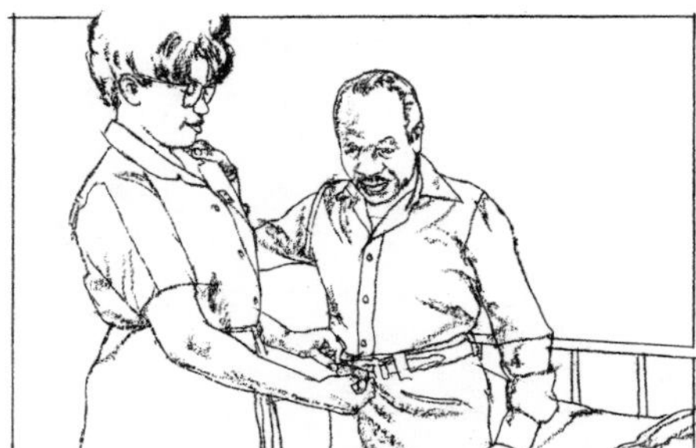

---

11. Help the resident with accessories if they ask you to do so. ☐

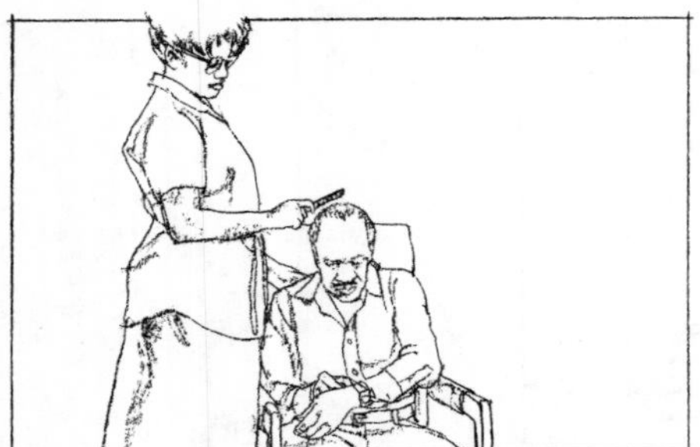

Skill 17: Undressing the Resident

Name: ______________________ Date: ______________

Procedure

Competency check

1. Help the resident to take off their shirt or dress. ☐

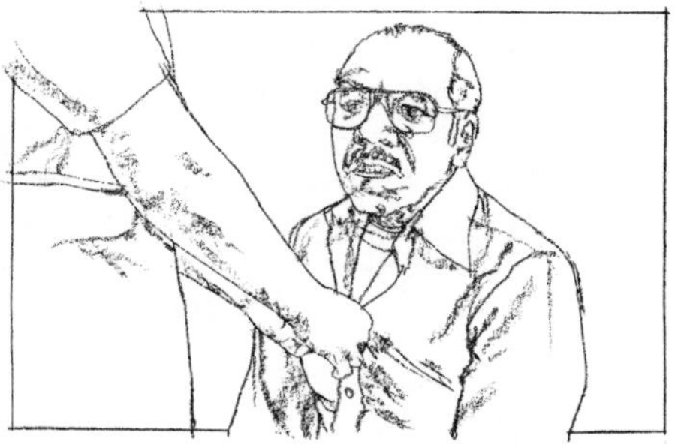

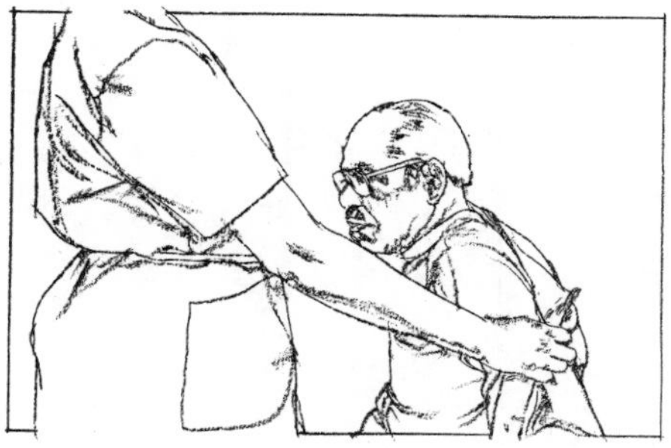

2. Help the resident to take off their undershirt or bra. ☐

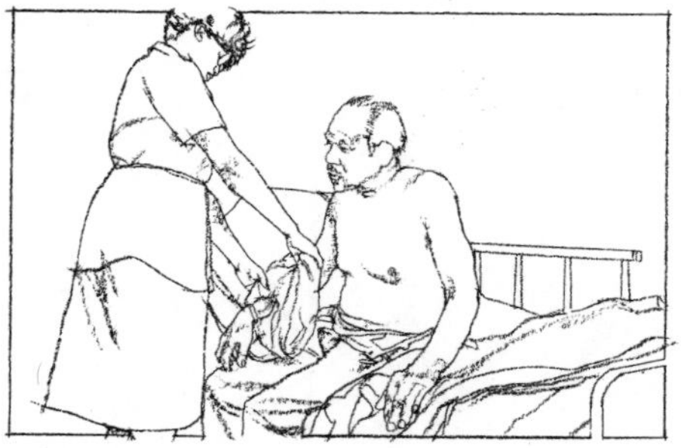

3. Help the resident put on their nightgown or pajama top. ☐

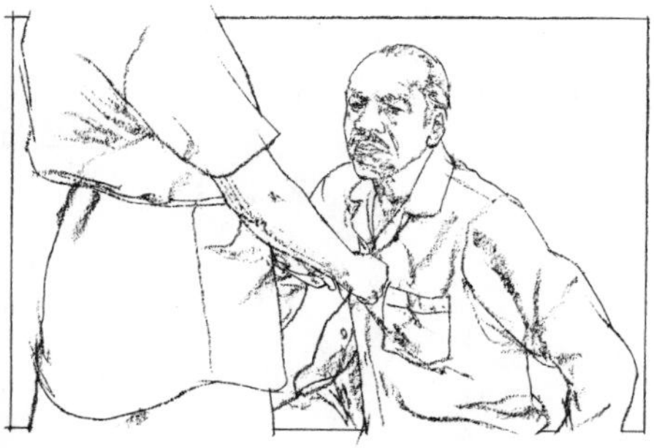

4. Help the resident to take off their shoes and socks. ☐

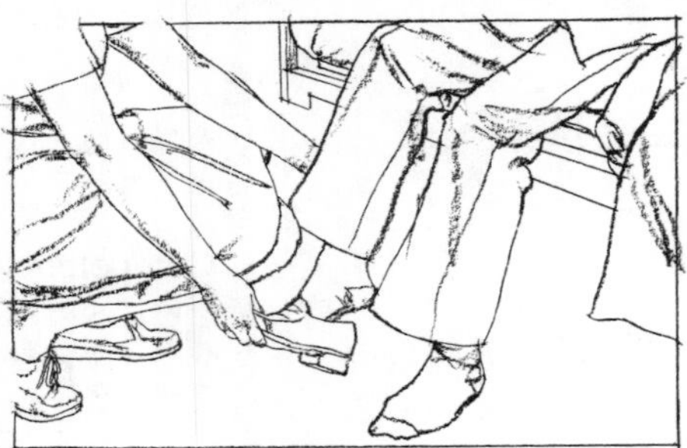

5. Help the resident to lie down in bed. ☐

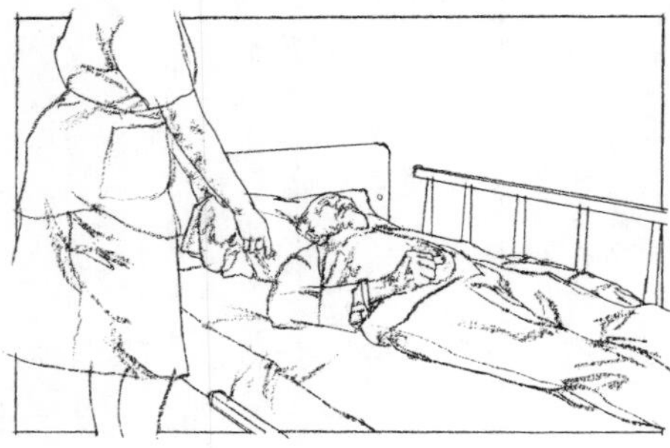

6. Help the resident to remove their pants. Ask them to raise their hips so you can slip the pants over their hips. ☐

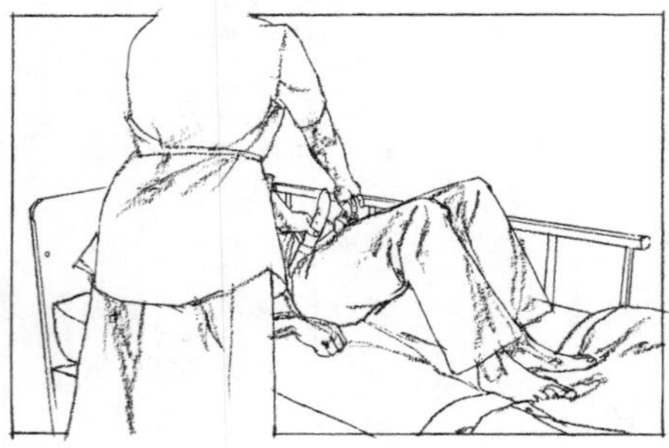

7. Help the resident to put on their pajama pants. Ask them to raise their hips so you can slip the pants over their hips. ☐

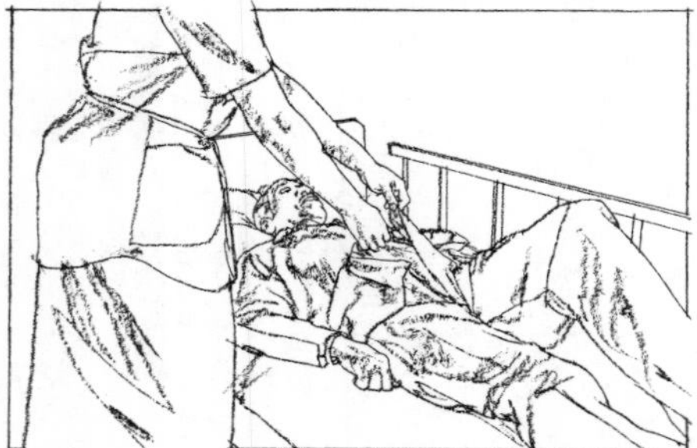

Skill 18: Assisting With a Bedpan or Urinal

Name: ______________________ Date: ____________

Precaution	• Never leave a resident on a bedpan or urinal for more than 5 minutes without checking on them. Pressure sores can develop if they are left longer.

Procedure

Competency check

1. Make sure bedpan is warm and dry. Put powder on the rim to make it easier to put it under the resident. ☐

2. Lower the side rail. ☐

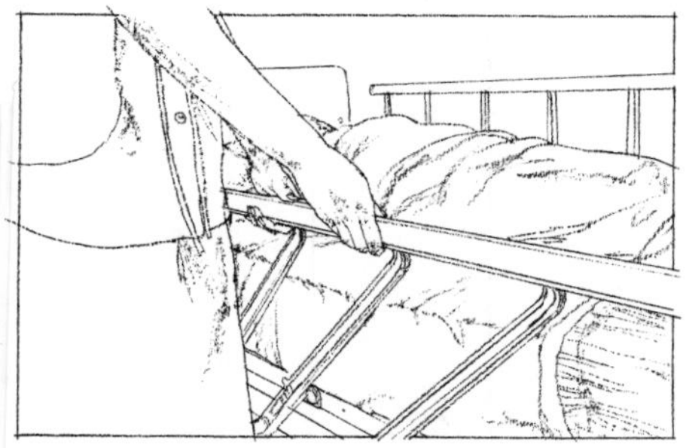

3. Fold top linens out of the way, keeping the resident's lower body covered. Be sure resident's clothing is out of the way. ☐

4. Help the resident onto the bedpan. Ask the resident to bend their knees and raise their buttocks by pushing against the mattress with their feet. Help as necessary by slipping your hand under their lower back and lifting slightly. Note: If the resident is unable to help, turn them onto their side away from you and place the bedpan firmly against the buttocks. Gently turn the resident back on the bedpan. ☐

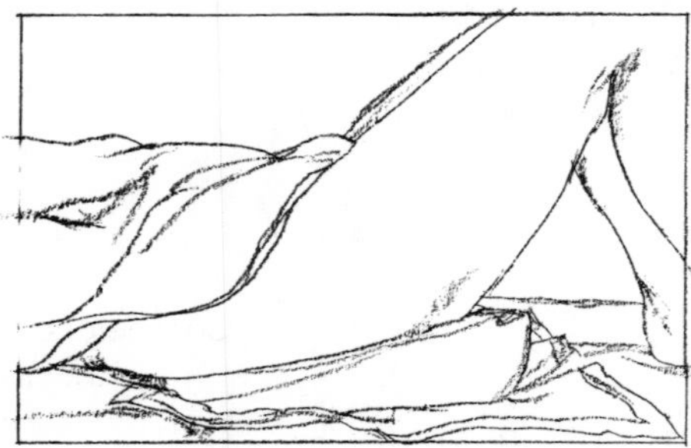

---

5. Give a urinal to a male resident. If they need assistance, put the urinal between their legs and gently put their penis into the urinal opening. ☐

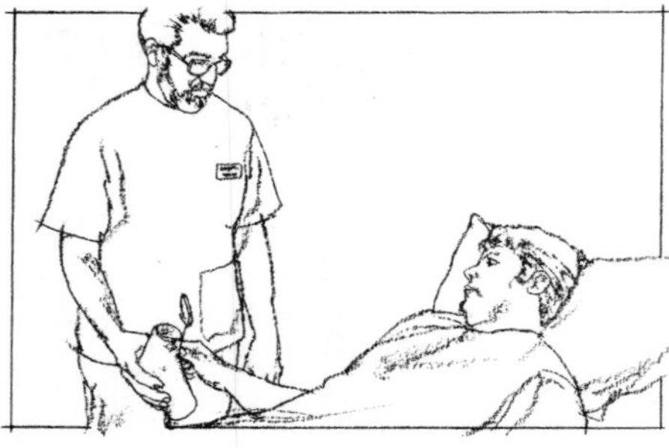

---

6. Put the top linens back over the resident. ☐

---

7. Raise the head of the resident's bed so the resident is in a comfortable sitting position. ☐

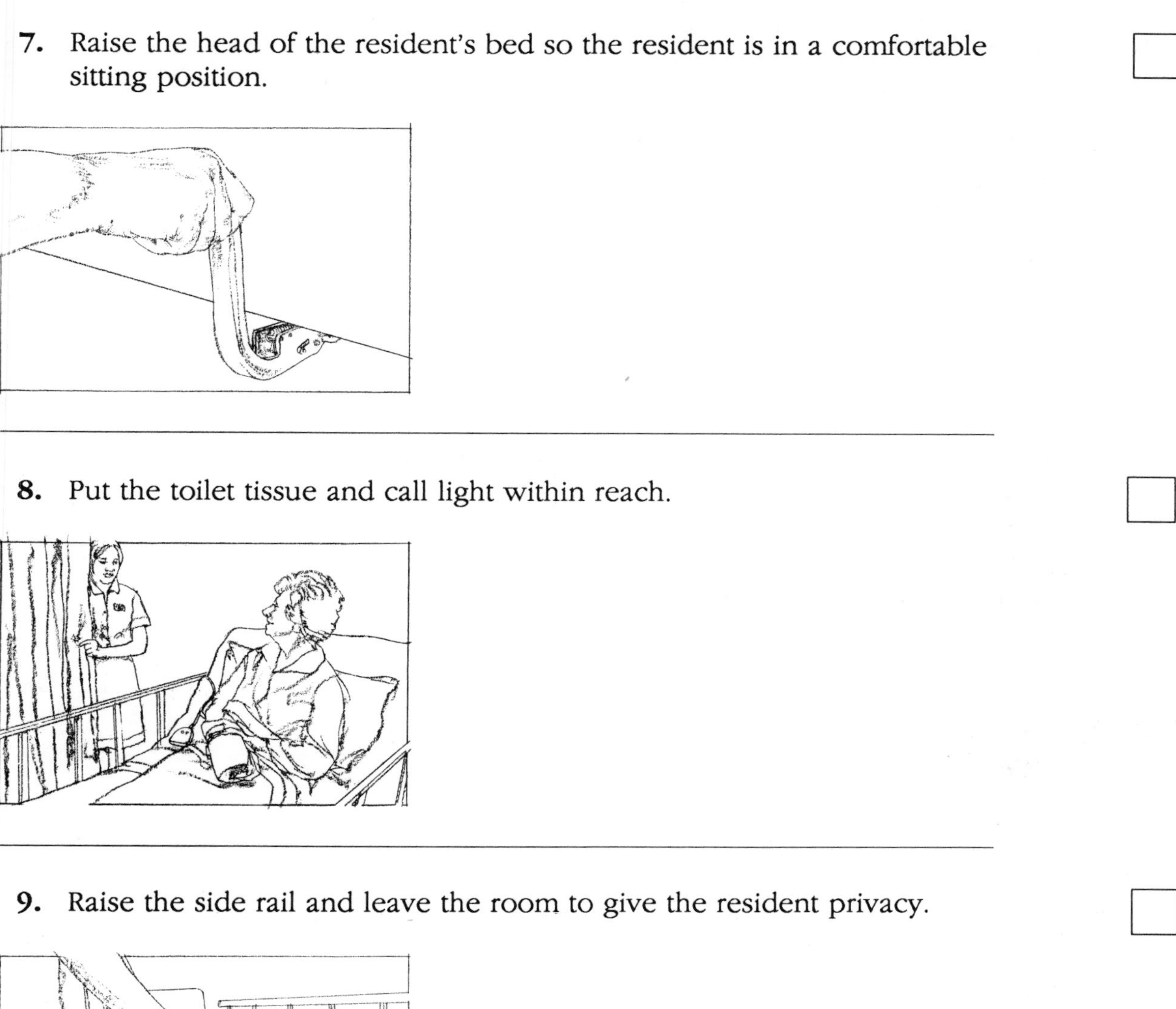

8. Put the toilet tissue and call light within reach. ☐

9. Raise the side rail and leave the room to give the resident privacy. ☐

10. Wash your hands.

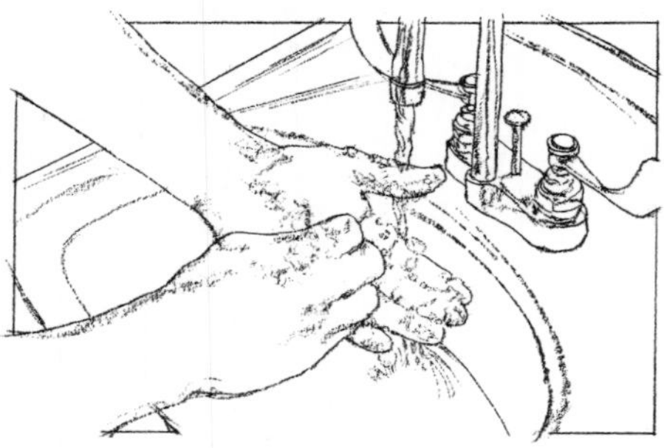

11. Return to the room when resident signals. If the resident cannot signal, check on them, at least every 5 minutes.

12. Put on disposable gloves.

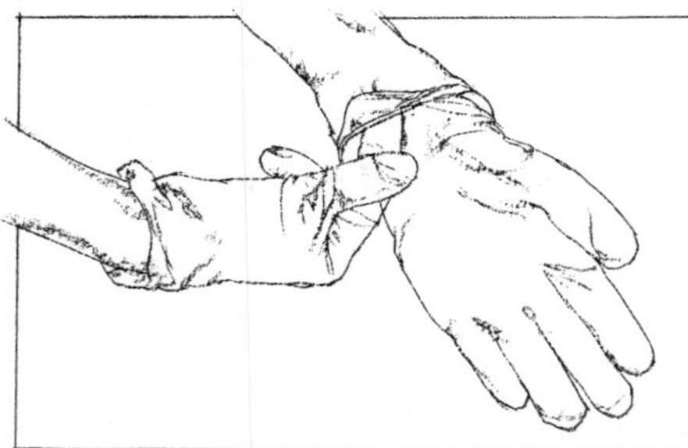

13. Help the resident off the bedpan. Have them raise their hips so you can remove the bedpan, or help them turn onto their side while you remove the bedpan.

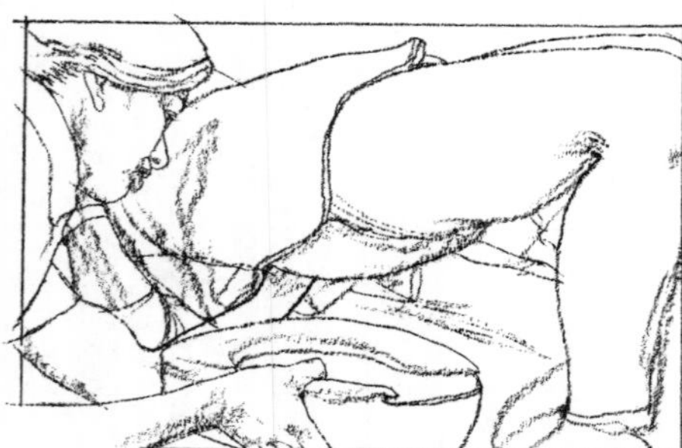

14. Help the resident clean and wipe themself as necessary. Always clean from front to back. Provide perineal care as necessary. ☐

15. Take off gloves and throw them away in the plastic trash bag. ☐

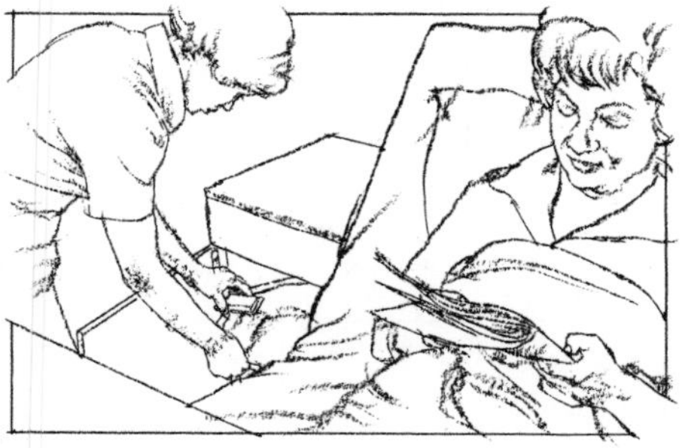

16. Cover the bedpan or urinal. ☐

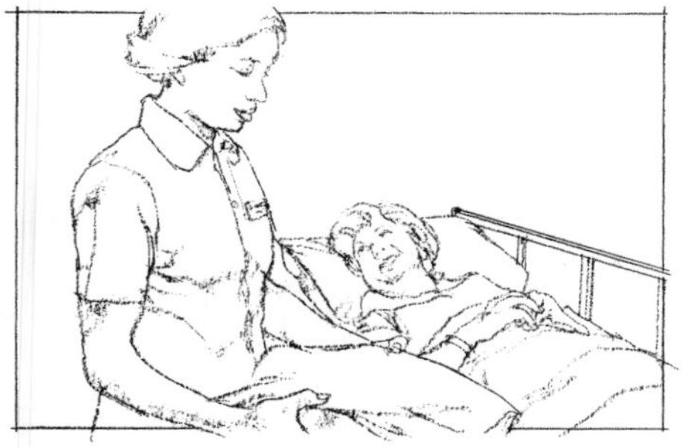

17. Pull the side rail up. ☐

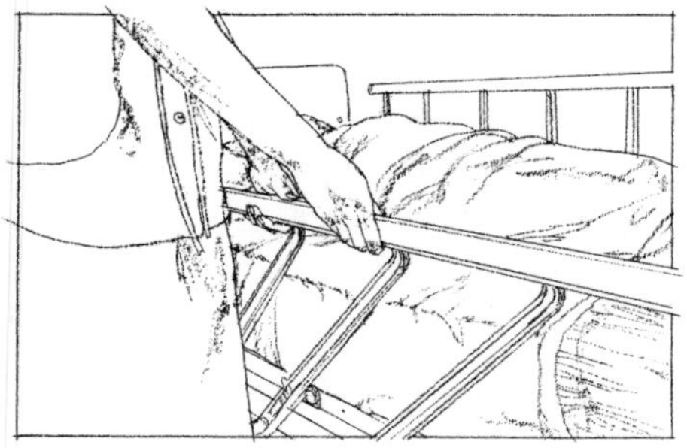

18. Take the bedpan or urinal to the soiled utility room or to the resident's bathroom. ☐

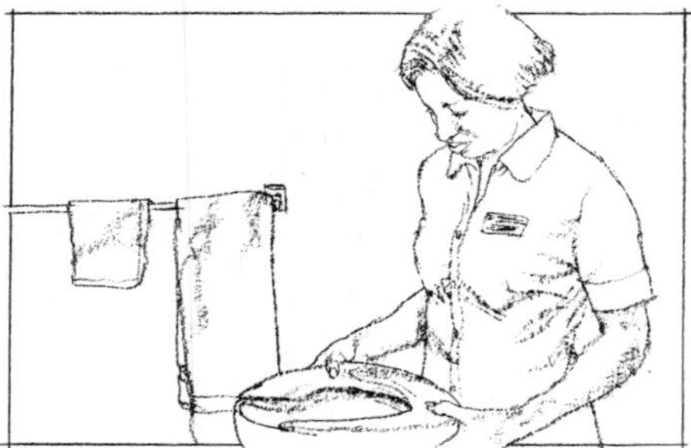

19. Empty the bedpan or urinal. Note: If you see blood in the urine or stool, put on a new pair of gloves before emptying the bedpan/urinal. ☐

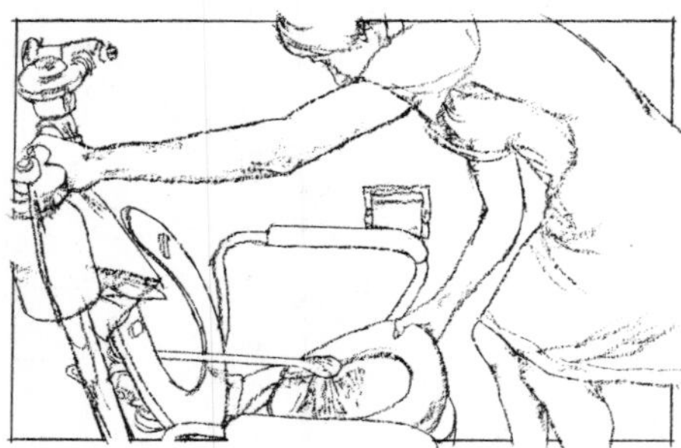

20. Clean and dry the bedpan, and put it away. ☐

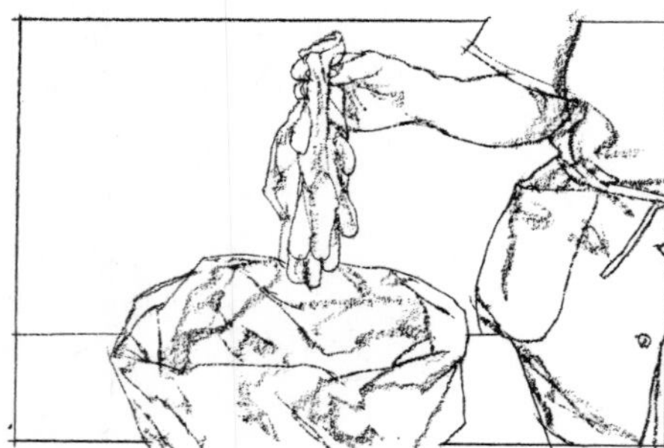

Skill 19:Taking an Oral Temperature With a Glass Thermometer

Name: ______________________ Date: ______________

Precautions

- Never take an oral temperature if a resident :

  Has had recent mouth surgery or has mouth disease
  Is getting oxygen
  Is short of breath or having trouble breathing
  Is confused or unconscious
  Is paralyzed on one side of the body/face
  Can only breathe through their mouth

Procedure

Competency check

1. Put on the thermometer sheath, if used. ☐

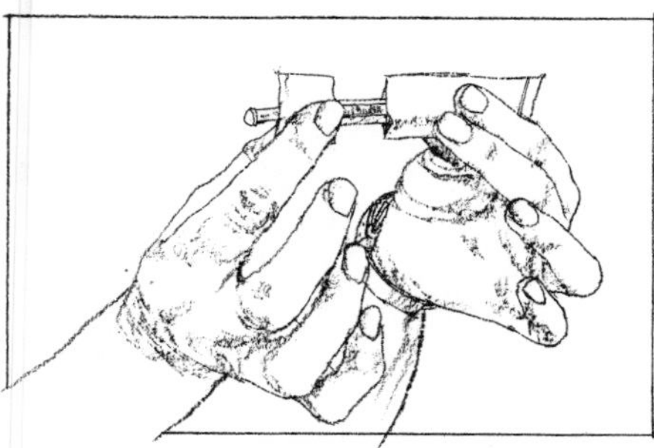

Rationale: Infection control measure

2. Put the thermometer under the resident's tongue and slightly to one side. ☐

Note: The bulk of the thermometer should be touching the mucous membrane under the tongue.

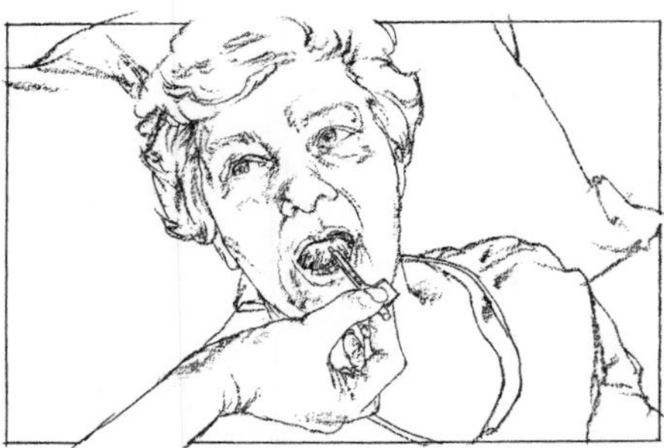

3. Keep the thermometer in the resident's mouth for at least 5 minutes. ☐

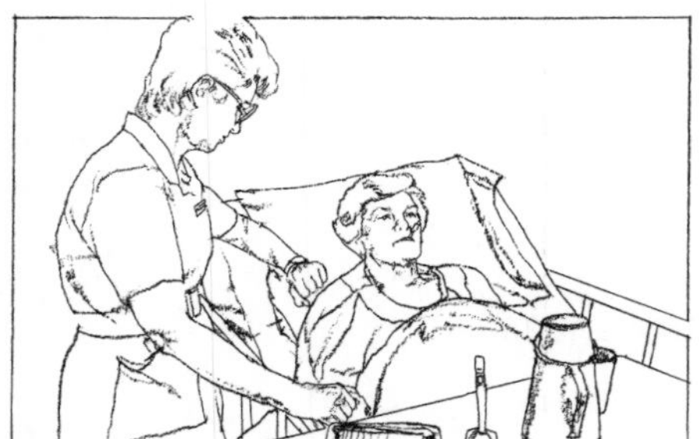

Rationale: Five minutes is needed to measure temperature accurately.

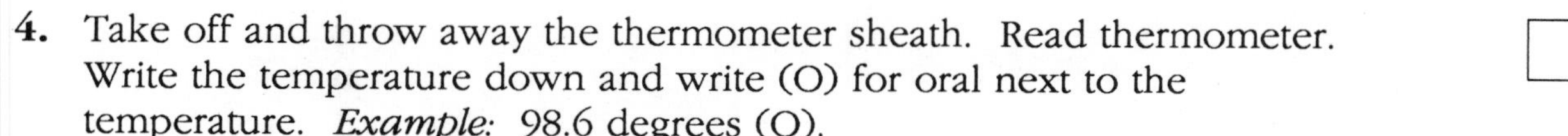

4. Take off and throw away the thermometer sheath. Read thermometer. Write the temperature down and write (O) for oral next to the temperature. *Example:* 98.6 degrees (O).

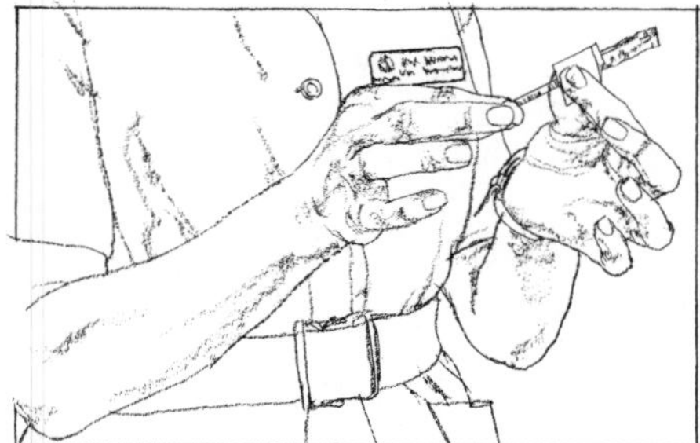

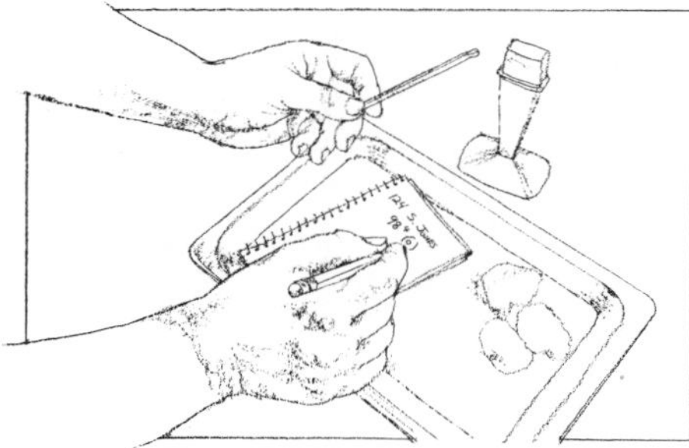

Rationale: Sometimes the nurse assistant may be distracted and forget the temperature.

---

5. Clean the thermometer.

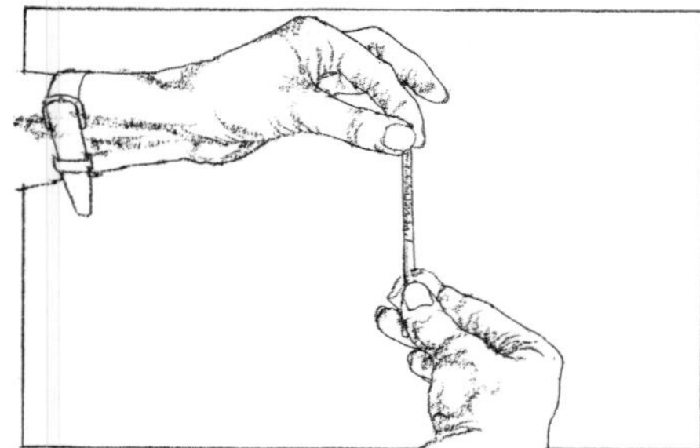

Rationale: Infection control measure

Skill 20:Taking a Rectal Temperature With a Glass Thermometer

Name: ______________________ Date: ______________

Precautions

- Never take a rectal temperature if the resident has:

  Diarrhea
  A blocked rectum
  Had a recent heart attack
  Had recent rectal surgery or injury
  Hemorrhoids

- Never put the rectal thermometer in more than 1 inch.

- Never leave a resident alone or let go of the thermometer when taking a rectal temperature.

Procedure

Competency check

1. Put on the thermometer sheath, if used. ☐

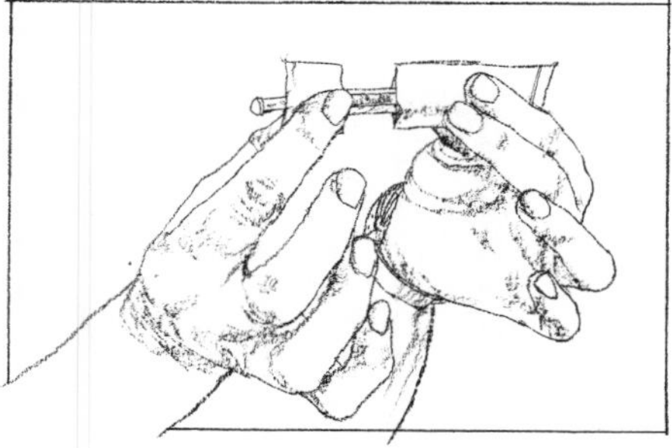

Rationale: Infection control measure

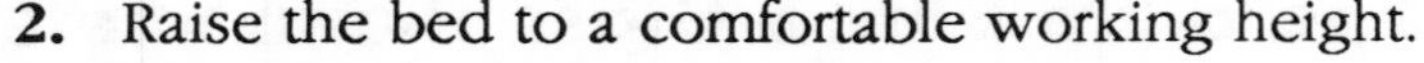

2. Raise the bed to a comfortable working height.

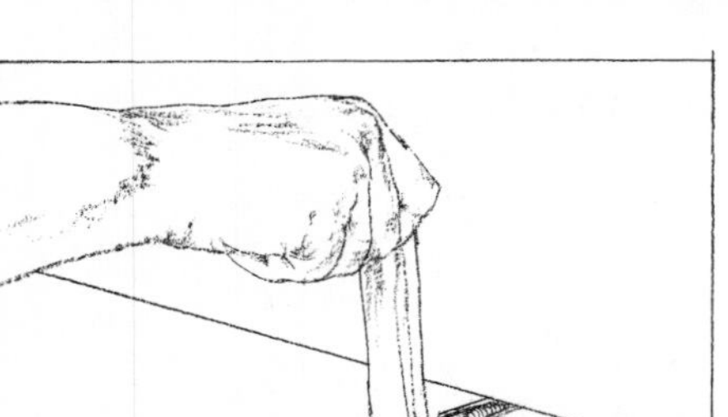

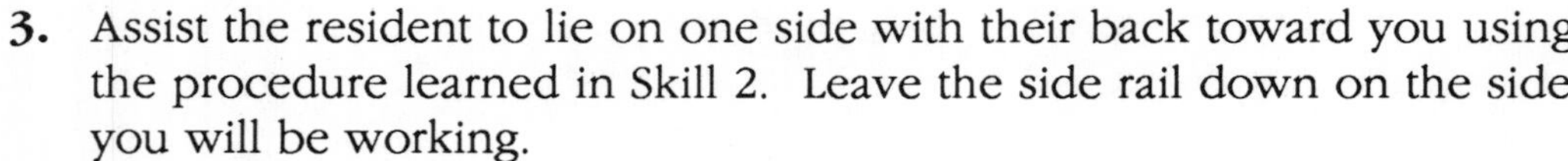

3. Assist the resident to lie on one side with their back toward you using the procedure learned in Skill 2. Leave the side rail down on the side you will be working.

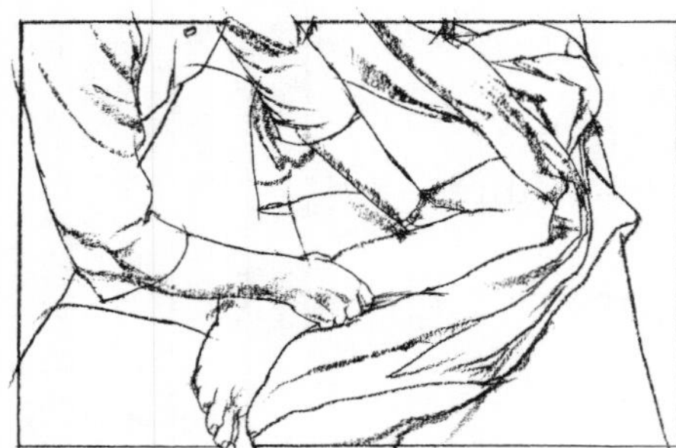

Rationale: Proper position for taking a rectal temperature.

---

4. Cover the resident with the bed sheet so that only the anal area shows.

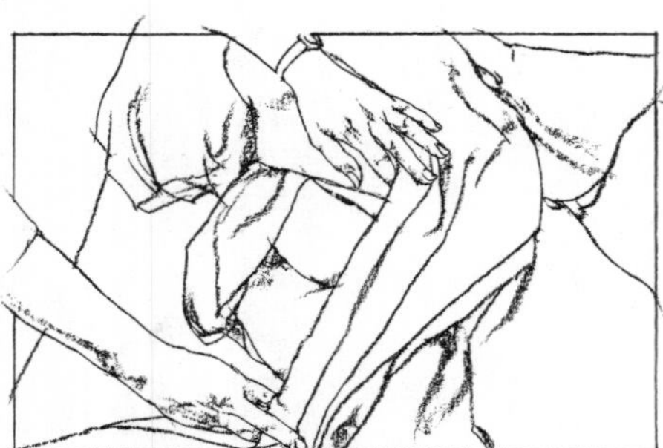

Rationale: Maintains privacy

---

5. Put on disposable gloves (if to be used). ☐

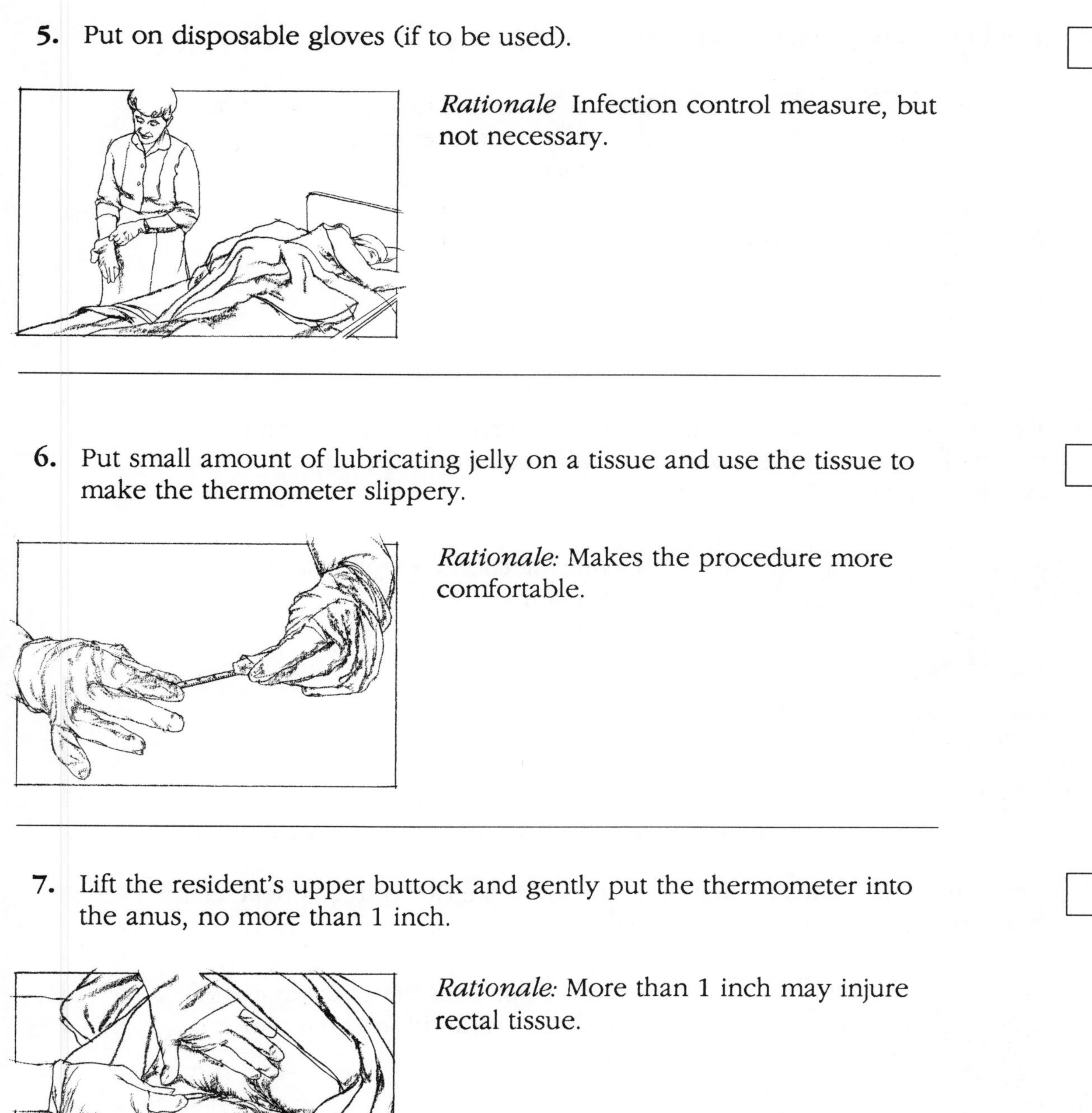

Rationale Infection control measure, but not necessary.

---

6. Put small amount of lubricating jelly on a tissue and use the tissue to make the thermometer slippery. ☐

Rationale: Makes the procedure more comfortable.

---

7. Lift the resident's upper buttock and gently put the thermometer into the anus, no more than 1 inch. ☐

Rationale: More than 1 inch may injure rectal tissue.

---

8. Hold the thermometer in place for at least 3 minutes. ☐

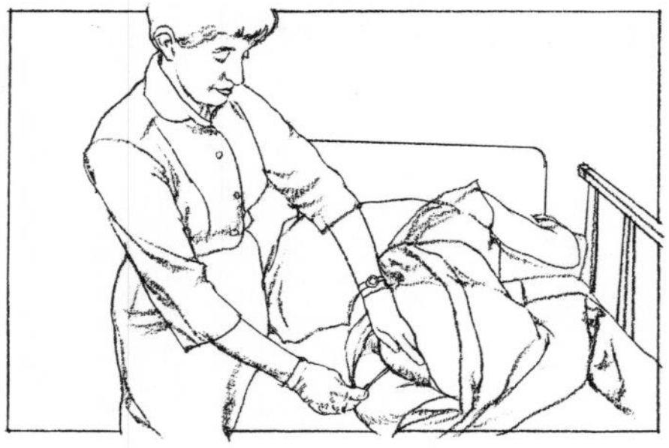

Rationale: Three minutes is the amount of time for accurate temperature measurement.

---

9. Gently take out the thermometer; clean anal area with tissue and take off and throw away thermometer sheath; then throw them away in a plastic trash bag. ☐

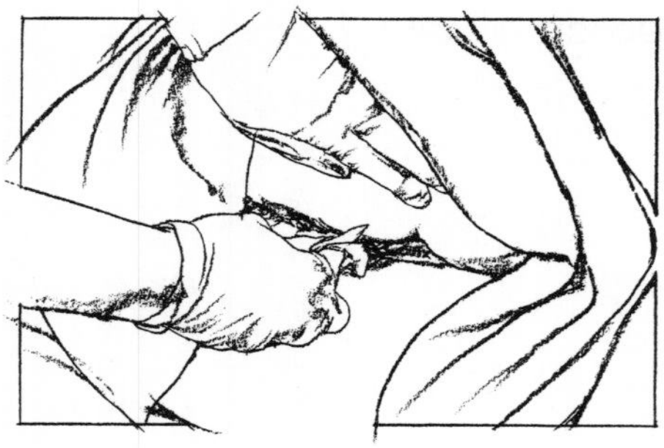

Rationale: Infection control measure and resident's comfort.

---

10. Read and write down the temperature and write (R) for rectal next to the temperature. *Example*: 99.6 degrees (R) ☐

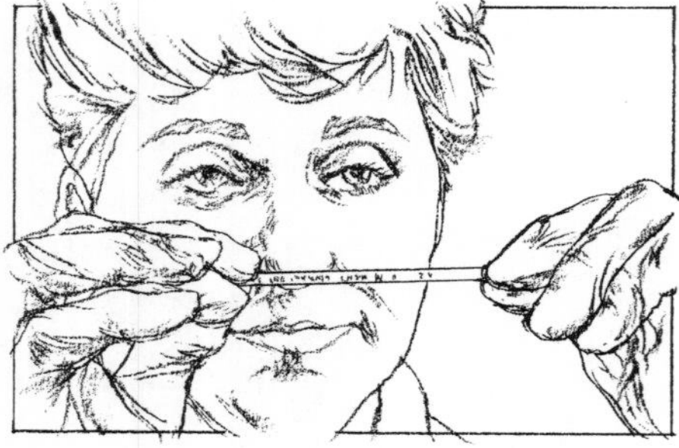

Rationale Sometimes the nurse assistant may be distracted and forget the temperature.

---

11. Clean the thermometer. ☐

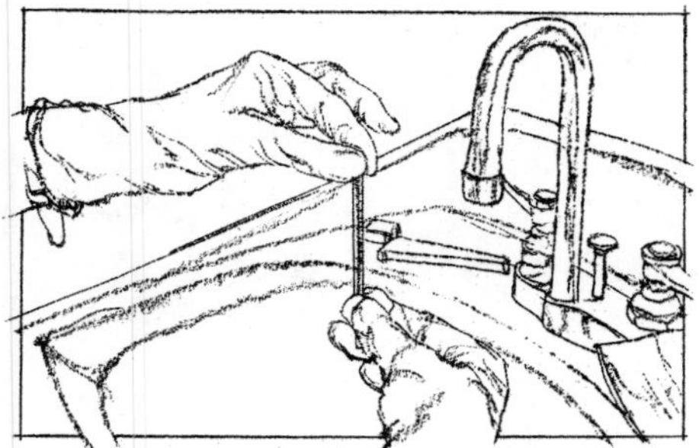

---

12. Remove gloves and throw them away in a disposable bag. ☐

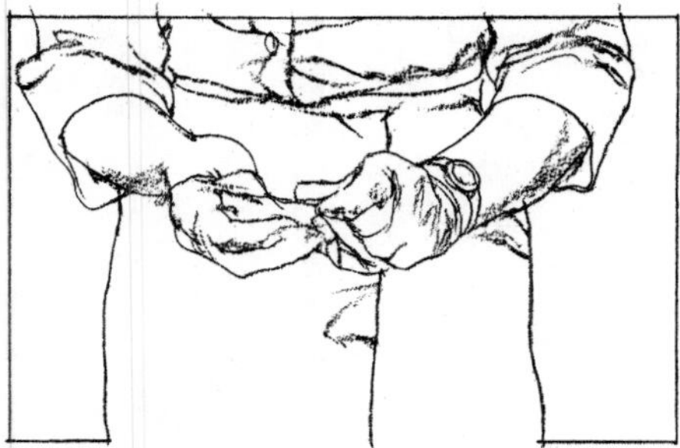

Skill 21: Counting a Radial Pulse

Name: ______________________________ Date: ______________

Precaution	• Never take a resident's pulse with your thumb. The thumb has its own pulse and you may count your pulse rate instead of the resident's.

Procedure

Competency check

1. Make sure the resident is in a comfortable, relaxed position. ☐

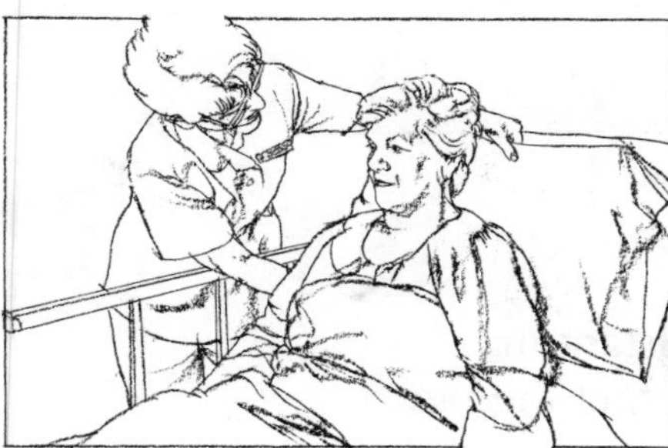

Rationale: If resident is comfortable and relaxed, reading will be more accurate.

2. Gently press your first, second, and third fingers over the radial pulse. ☐

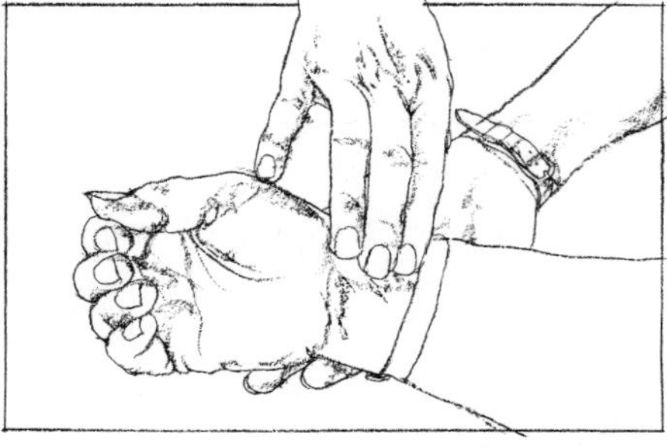

3. Using the second hand on your watch, count the number of beats for 1 minute.

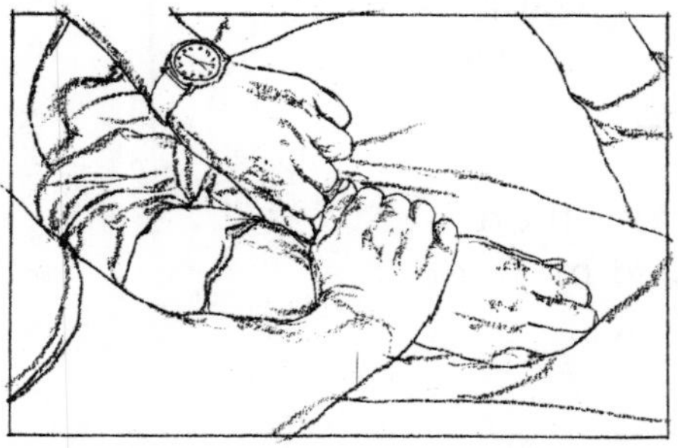

---

4. While you count the pulse rate, note the rhythm and force.

Rationale: A change in rhythm or force may indicate a problem.

---

5. Write down the pulse rate.

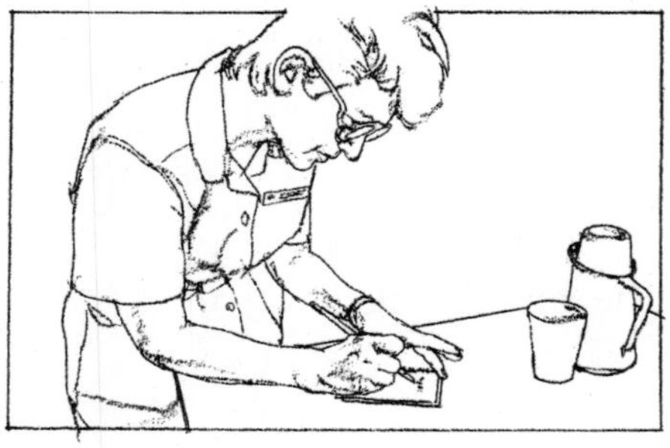

Rationale: The nurse assistant may become distracted and forget the rate.

Skill 22: Counting Respiration

Name: ______________________________ Date:

Procedure

Competency check

1. Count respiration by watching the rise and fall of the resident's chest. ☐

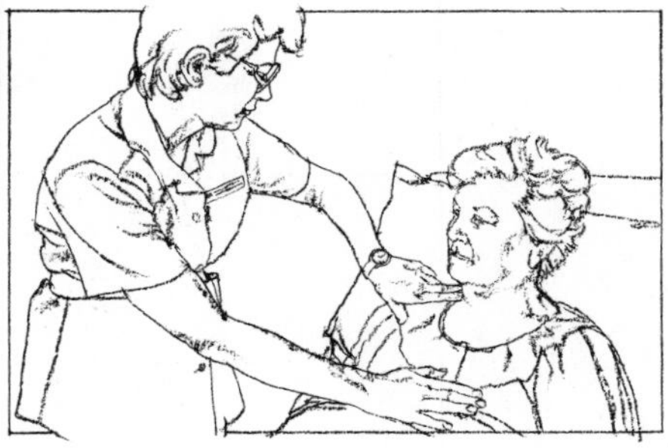

Rationale: This is one complete respiration.

2. Using the second hand on your watch, count respiration for 1 minute. ☐

3. Write down the respiration rate. ☐

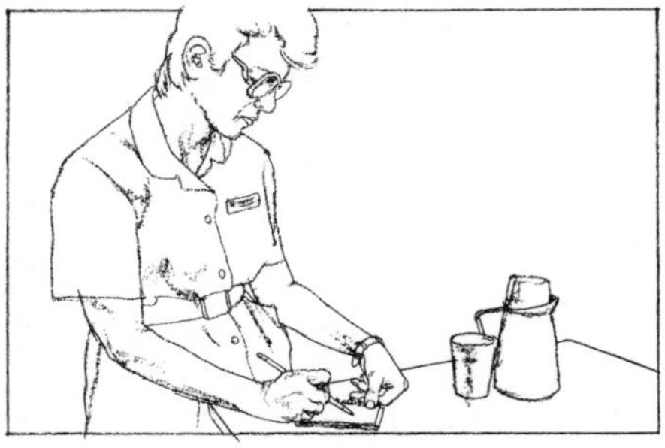

Rationale: The nurse assistant may become distracted and forget the rate.

Skill 23: Taking Blood Pressure

Name: ______________________ Date: ______________

Precautions

- Never put a cuff on an arm with a cast.
- Never put a cuff on an arm with an IV (intravenous infusion) in place.
- Never put a cuff on the arm on the side where resident has had a mastectomy (breast removal).
- Never put a cuff on an arm immediately following venipuncture (drawing blood for testing).
- Avoid putting a cuff on the weak arm if resident has had a stroke.

Procedure

Competency check

1. Before putting the cuff on the arm, open the valve (remember, left–loose) and squeeze all the air out of the cuff. ☐

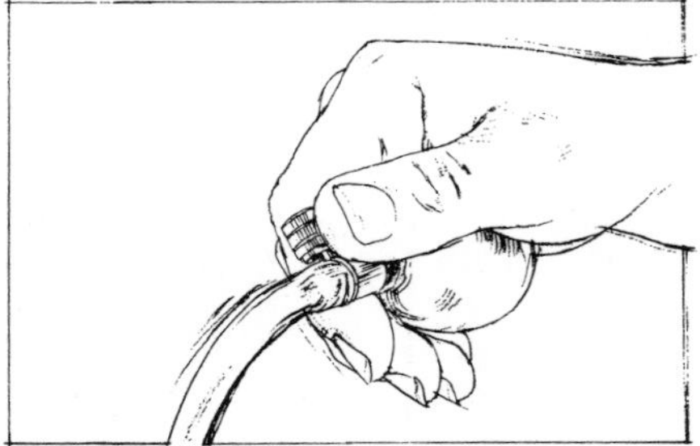

2. Put the center of the cuff's bladder 1 inch above the elbow on the inside of the arm, over the brachial artery.

Note: Move clothing on that arm out of the way.

Rationale: Proper positioning for accurate reading. Blood pressure should not be measured over clothing.

---

3. Wrap the cuff around the arm snugly and smoothly so that the bladder presses evenly against the arm.

Rationale: Cuff must be wrapped smoothly for an accurate measurement.

---

4. Clean the earpieces of the stethoscope with an alcohol wipe.

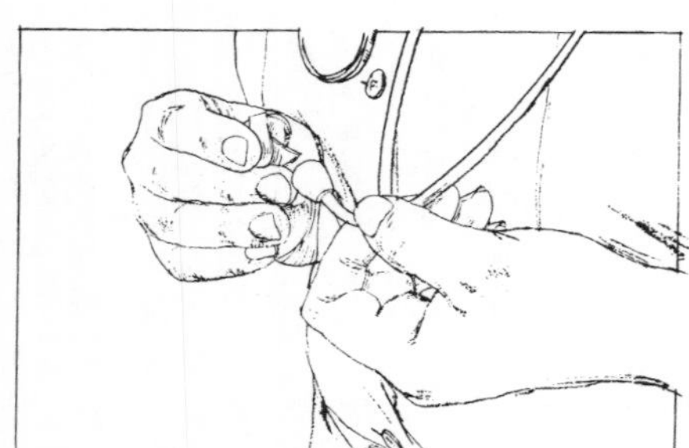

Rationale: Infection control measure

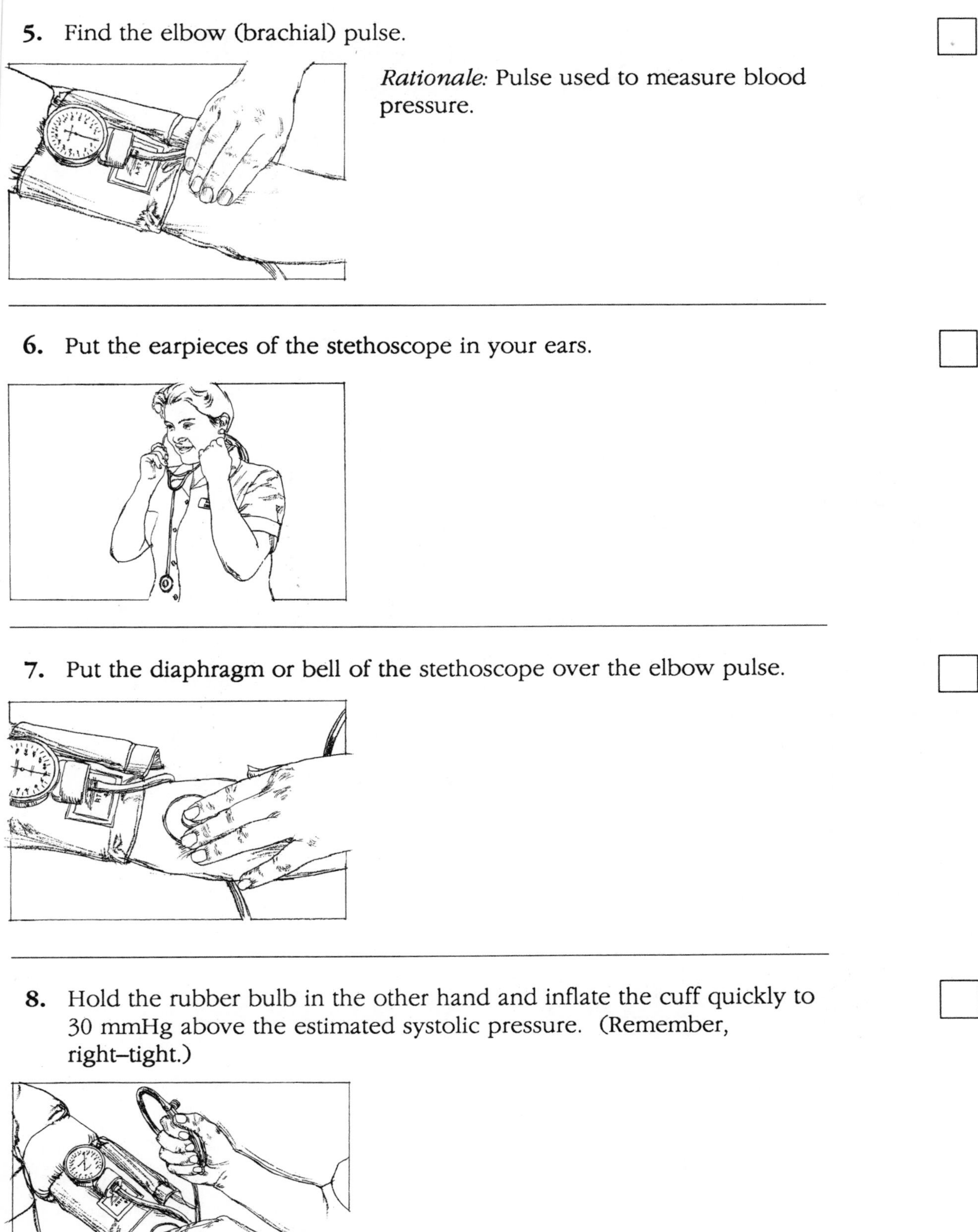

5. Find the elbow (brachial) pulse.

Rationale: Pulse used to measure blood pressure.

6. Put the earpieces of the stethoscope in your ears.

7. Put the diaphragm or bell of the stethoscope over the elbow pulse.

8. Hold the rubber bulb in the other hand and inflate the cuff quickly to 30 mmHg above the estimated systolic pressure. (Remember, right–tight.)

9. Let the air out of the cuff slowly. The reading when you first hear the pulse sound is the systolic pressure. Remember this number and go on.

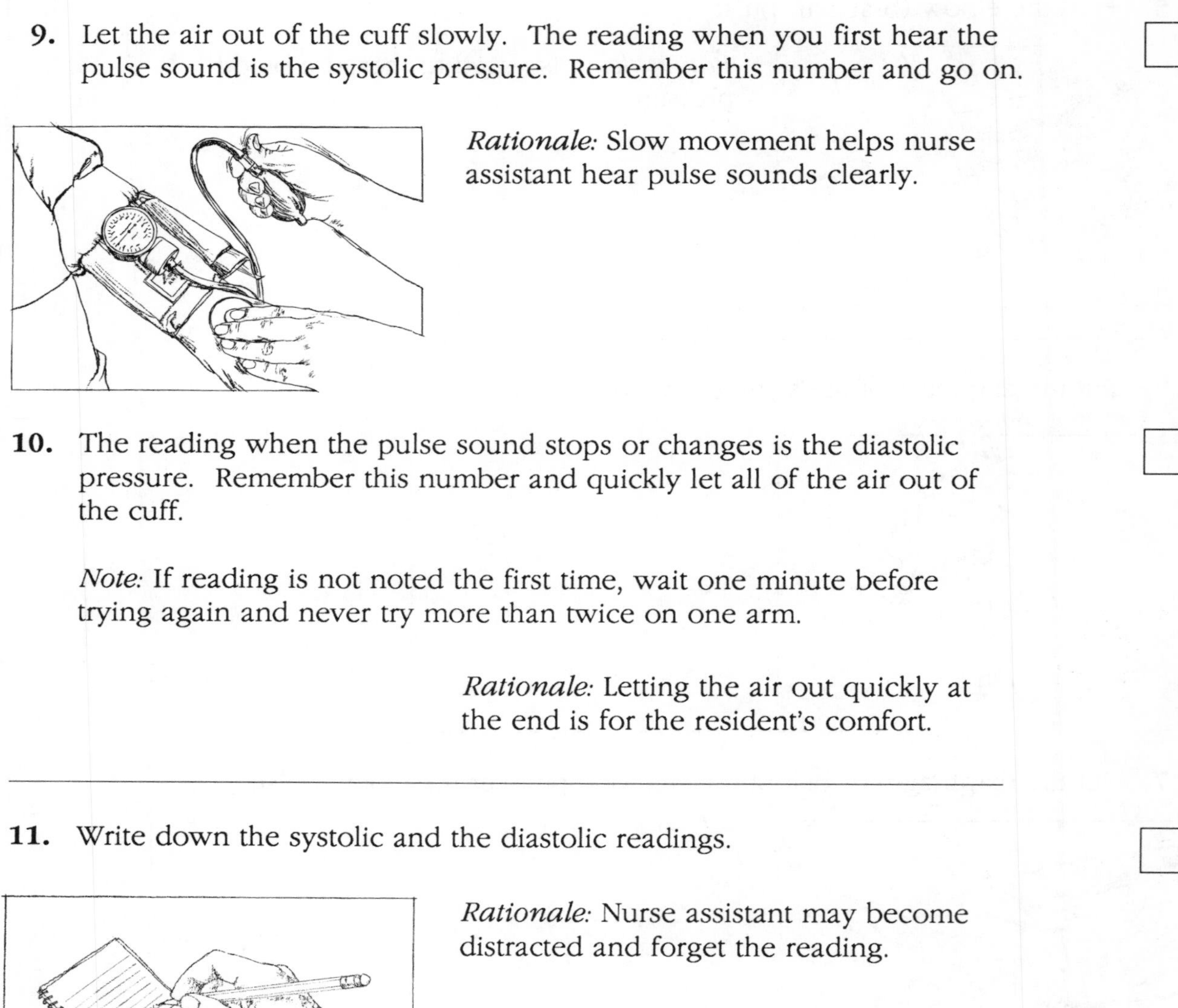

Rationale: Slow movement helps nurse assistant hear pulse sounds clearly.

10. The reading when the pulse sound stops or changes is the diastolic pressure. Remember this number and quickly let all of the air out of the cuff.

Note: If reading is not noted the first time, wait one minute before trying again and never try more than twice on one arm.

Rationale: Letting the air out quickly at the end is for the resident's comfort.

---

11. Write down the systolic and the diastolic readings.

Rationale: Nurse assistant may become distracted and forget the reading.

Glossaries

Glossary of Common Abbreviations
General Glossary

Glossary of Common Abbreviations

Abbreviations or shortened forms of words or phrases are frequently used in long-term care facilities to save time and space. Some common ones are listed here. Use may vary with facilities. Lists of acceptable abbreviations are usually available in a facility.

Abbreviation	Meaning
a.c.	Before meals
abd.	Abdomen
ad lib	As desired
ADL	Activities of daily living
Adm. (adm.)	Admitted or admission
AM (am)	Morning
amb.	Ambulatory
amt.	Amount
b.i.d.	Twice a day
BM (bm)	Bowel movement
BP	Blood pressure
c̄	With
c/o	Complains of
Ca.	Cancer
Cath.	Catheter
CBC	Complete blood count
cc	Cubic centimeter
CPR	Cardiopulmonary resuscitation
CVA	Cerebrovascular accident; stroke
dc (d/c)	Discontinue/discharge
DOA	Dead on arrival
DON	Director of nursing
dsg. or drsg.	Dressing
Dx.	Diagnosis
EKG	Electrocardiogram
ER	Emergency room
FBS	Fasting blood sugar
FF	Force fluids

fld.	Fluid
ft.	Foot or feet
h.s.	Hour of sleep
H_2O	Water
ht.	Height
I&O	Intake and output
in.	Inch
IV	Intravenous
Lab.	Laboratory
lb.	Pound
liq.	Liquid
LPN	Licensed practical nurse
LVN	Licensed vocational nurse
ml.	Milliliter
N.P.O.	Nothing by mouth
NA	Nurse assistant
neg.	negative
NKA	No known allergies
no., #	Number
noc	Night
O.T.	Occupational therapy
O_2	Oxygen
OJ	Orange juice
OOB	Out of bed
oz.	Ounce
p.c.	After meals
p.o. (per os)	By mouth
per	By, through
PM (pm)	Afternoon
prn	As necessary
P.T.	Physical therapy
q	Every
q.d.	Daily
q.h.s.	Every night at bedtime
q.i.d.	Four times a day

q.o.d.	Every other day
qh	Every hour
q2h, q3h, etc.	Every 2 hours, every 3 hours, etc.
R	Rectal temperature
RN	Registered nurse
ROM	Range of motion
$\bar{s}$	Without
S.O.B.	Short of breath
Spec. (spec.)	Specimen
SSE	Soap suds enema
Stat	Immediately
t.i.d.	Three times a day
T.P.R.	Temperature, pulse, respiration
tbsp.	Tablespoon
TLC	Tender loving care
tsp.	Teaspoon
U/a (U/A, u/a)	Urinalysis
VS (vs)	Vital signs
W/C	Wheelchair
wt. or wgt.	Weight

General Glossary

abduction: moving a body part away from the body

active range of motion: exercising your body joints by moving them without help

adaptive feeding equipment: feeding equipment designed to help residents feed themselves

adduction: moving a body part toward the body

AIDS (acquired immune deficiency syndrome): a condition which makes the body unable to fight off infection.

amputation: removal of a limb by surgery or accident

anal: area around the anus where the bowel movement comes out

antimicrobial: agent that destroys germs or slows down their growth

anus: opening of the body where the bowel movements come out

aspiration: breathing food or fluid into the lungs

assess: to gather information about a situation, and then make decision about the situation

auscultate: to hear

axillary: in the armpit or underarm

bacteria: one-celled organisms that can be seen only through a microscope. There are many kinds, only some cause disease.

balance: standing evenly on both feet without falling; having equal weight on both sides

base of support: the weight-bearing part of the body. When standing, the feet are the base of support

bladder: a pouchlike structure, sometimes shaped like a flat balloon, that may be filled with air or fluid. In the urinary system, the bladder is the sac where urine collects before it is passed outside the body. In a blood pressure machine, the bladder inside the cuff is inflated with air when taking a person's blood pressure.

blood pressure: force that blood exerts against the arteries as it travels through the body

body alignment: proper positioning of parts in relation to each other

body fluids: any liquid substance in the body, like blood, or that comes out of the body, like tears or saliva

body mechanics: the way your entire body adjusts to keep its balance as you move

body temperature: amount of heat in the body

bowel movement (BM): defecation, or elimination of semi-solid waste from the body

bowel training: process of helping the resident regain control of defecation

care plan: a written list of a resident's needs and goals for treatment and a plan to coordinate care so the goals can be achieved.

catheters: tubes that are inserted in the bladder so that it drains constantly

cc or ml: cubic centimeter or milliliter units of measurement. 1,000 cc or ml equal about one quart

clean: free from dirt, unsoiled but not sterile

clinical: the applied or "hands on" part of a nurse assistant's job

congenital: existing at birth

congenital deformity: a deformity that existed at birth

constipation: difficult, incomplete, or infrequent emptying of the bowels

contagious disease: disease that is easily spread from one person to another

contaminate: to touch something clean with something dirty

contaminated: unclean

contracture: abnormal stretching of muscle resulting in deformities

convulsions: muscle contractions; a sudden attack in which muscles tighten and relax

coordination: the ability to move muscles smoothly and easily when doing a task

cuff: part of a blood pressure machine, or sphygmomanometer, the cuff is a long piece of fabric that is wrapped around the arm to take a person's blood pressure

cyanosis: blue or gray color seen on lips, skin, and nail beds caused by lack of oxygen

decubitus ulcer: an open area of skin that results from poor circulation, continued pressure, friction (rubbing), or moisture from sweat, urine, and feces

defecate: to eliminate semi-solid waste from the rectum To have a bowel movement (bm)

dehydration: excessive loss of water from the body tissues

dental floss: a flat thread used to clean between the teeth

dentures: a set of false teeth

diarrhea: frequent liquid or watery feces

diastolic pressure: The pressure in the artery when the heart is at rest. When taking a person's blood pressure, this is the point at which the sound stops

disinfect: to kill most of the germs with a chemical solution in order to slow down the germs' growth and activity

dyspnea: difficulty with breathing

empathetic person: a person who can understand how someone is feeling and why they feel that way

EMS (emergency medical services system): a community-based system that delivers emergency care at the scene of an accident or disaster, and during transportation to a treatment facility or shelter

enema: putting fluid into the rectum and colon to stimulate a bowel movement

enteric: intestinal; having to do with the intestines

epilepsy: a disorder of the nervous system in which the major symptom is a seizure

evacuation: assisting persons away from an endangered area, or leaving an endangered area

extension: straightening, or unbending a body part

extremity: a hand or a foot

feces: semi-solid waste products of the bowel; stool

fever: abnormally high temperature

flexion: bending a body part

flossing: the use of dental floss to clean between the teeth

force fluids: encouraging a person to drink more

foreskin: a loose fold of skin that covers the end of the penis

Fowler's position: position of the resident when the head of bed is elevated.

friction: rubbing one object against another, e.g., rubbing skin against the sheets

gastrostomy tube: a feeding tube put into the stomach through a small surgical opening

genital: having to do with the reproductive organs

geriatric: having to do with older people

germs: tiny living things that cause disease and can be seen only with a microscope

graduated measure: pitcher with measurements marked on the side

hepatitis: inflammation of the liver

HIV (human immunodeficiency virus): the virus that causes AIDS

HIV transmitters: substances that carry HIV from an infected person to another.

hyperextension: stretching or straightening a body part beyond normal limits

immune system: the body's natural defense against disease

impaction: a hard stool that is wedged in the rectum

incontinent: unable to control passage of urine or feces

infection: condition that results when germs grow and multiply in the body

insulin: a hormone released by the pancreas that helps the body to use sugar.

isolation procedures: practices that prevent the spread of germs

labia: the folds of skin around the opening of the vagina

limb: an arm or a leg

manometer: a gauge on a blood pressure machine that measures systolic and diastolic pressure and shows them in millimeters of mercury (mm hg)

micro-organisms: bacteria viruses, yeasts, molds, and other tiny living things, which may or may not be harmful

millimeters of mercury (mm hg): measurement used for reading blood pressure shows how far up the air pressure has pushed the column of mercury on the mercury gauge of a blood pressure machine. Although a dial gauge does not use mercury, its measurements are also given in millimeters of mercury (mm hg) so that the two types of readings can be compared.

mitered corner: a particular fold of a sheet corner

mucous membranes: moist tissues inside of mouth, vagina, nasal cavities, and rectum

nasogastric tube: a feeding tube put into the stomach through the nose

observation: using your senses to gather information

oral: in the mouth

palpate: to feel

pancreas: a body organ near the stomach which releases insulin and digestive enzymes

passive range of motion: exercising of body joints by someone else

penis: part of the male reproductive and urinary systems

perineal care: cleansing of the genital and anal areas of the body

prompt: say something to remind someone what to do next

post-mortem care: care given after a physician says the resident is dead

prone: lying flat on stomach

prosthetic: a device that replaces a missing part of the body

pulse rate: the number of times the heart beats per minute

pulse: the beat of the heart

range of motion (ROM): the amount of movement present in a joint

rectal: in the rectum, the part of the intestine that is just inside the anus

rectum: section of large intestine leading to the anus

regular diet: food plan that provides the daily nutrients needed by the average person

rehabilitation: helping a resident to regain physical, mental, or social functions that may have been lost because of injury or disease

respiration: the act of breathing in and breathing out; inhaling and exhaling

restorative nursing: nursing care that helps residents increase their independence and abilities as well as restore lost functions

rigor mortis: stiffness of muscles that occurs after death

rotation: turning the joint

safety or transfer belt: a canvas or cloth strap that fits around the resident's waist and is used to help a person move or walk

safety vest or poncho: a canvas vest worn by the resident for safety

scrotum: the pouch of skin that holds the testicles

seizure: a sudden attack of which the resident may be unaware and/or during which the resident may show certain symptoms, such as convulsions; usually related to brain malfunction that can be the result of disease or injured brain tissue

shroud: bag-like garment used to hold the dead body

social reinforcement: using a combination of positive words and caring touch to communicate

sphygmomanometer: the instrument used to measure blood pressure, usually called the blood pressure machine

stethoscope: instrument that is used to hear pulse sounds when taking blood pressure

stool: feces; semi-solid waste that comes out of the rectum after a bowel movement

stump sock: special sock designed to prevent a stump from swelling

stump: end of a limb when the rest of the limb has been removed or missing since birth

supine: lying flat on back

systolic pressure: pressure in the artery when the heart is pumping. When taking a person's blood pressure, this is the point at which the first sound is heard after the air is let out of the bladder in the cuff

therapeutic diets: food plans prepared to help treat diseases or disabilities (also called special diets, modified diets, and restricted diets)

thrush: a fungus infection of the mouth

transmission: spreading or moving from one place to another

ulnar and radial deviation: bending the wrist from side to side

unconscious: the condition of a person who is not mentally alert but may be able to hear and feel

universal precautions: methods of making sure that every person who has direct contact with body fluids will be protected, in case the fluids are infectious, or carrying a disease

urinate: to void or pass urine

vagina: part of a woman's reproductive system; the birth canal

valve: on a blood pressure machine, the part of the bulb that opens and closes